THE GENETIC CO

A Guide to Health Problems in Purebred Dogs

DEDICATION

To my wonderful wife Susan
and my three phenomenal children—
Nadia, Rebecca, and David

THE GENETIC CONNECTION:

A Guide to Health Problems in Purebred Dogs

Lowell Ackerman, DVM, PhD, Dipl. ACVD

AAHA®
AMERICAN ANIMAL HOSPITAL ASSOCIATION

Many thanks to the AAHA Press Editorial Advisory Board:
Dr. Laurel Collins, ABVP
Dr. Richard Goebel
Dr. Charles Hickey
Dr. Clayton McKinnon
Dr. Richard Nelson, ABVP
Dr. Hal Taylor

Design and Typography
Sheryl Tongue

Cover Design and Illustration
Timothy Nyman

AAHA Press
12575 W. Bayaud Avenue
Lakewood, Colorado 80228

The Author and AAHA do not assume responsibility for and make no representation about the suitability or accuracy of the information contained in this work for any purpose, and make no warranties, either express or implied, including the warranties of merchantability and fitness for a particular purpose. Neither AAHA nor the Authors shall be held liable for adverse reactions to or damage resulting from the applicaton of this information. Rapid advances in veterinary medicine may cause information contained herein to become outdated, invalid, or subject to debate by various veterinary professionals. AAHA and the Author are not held responsible for any inaccuracies, omissions or editorial errors, nor for any consequence resulting therefrom. AAHA and the Author shall be held harmless from any and all claims that may arise as a result of any reliance on the information provided.

ISBN 0-94151-93-3

Contents

Foreword

The standards of physical and behavioral uniformity that define most modern breeds of dog can be met only through deliberate inbreeding. This leads, of necessity, to the production of animals displaying a comparatively high level of genetic homogeneity. One byproduct of homogeneity in outward traits in the absence of strong selection against it, however, is the expression of hidden, inherited disease traits. Until recently, even the most informed breeder or veterinarian could do little to accurately predict the likelihood that any given dog, or the offspring, would carry the genes that predisposed it to a particular disease. Fortunately, rapid progress in the development of a canine genetic map, coupled with improved clinical diagnostic testing, has led to a revolution in canine health care.

Although the following chapters focus largely on the descriptive features of canine diseases, the summaries should be put in the context of expected advances in the field of canine molecular genetics. In the coming years, diagnostic genetic tests will be developed for many common canine diseases. Breeders will have the option, and in some cases the responsibility, to test key dogs in their breeding programs to determine their carrier status for a variety of disorders. Judicious use of these tests can be expected to rapidly reduce the rate of specific diseases for some breeds and to eradicate them from others.

Not all decisions informed by the results of genetic testing will be simple. In some circumstances, a truly extraordinary dog, exemplifying the breed standard, will be found to be a carrier for a highly undesirable trait. In these situations, owners and breeders will be forced to make difficult choices about the ways in which their breeding programs should best be modified. Breeders will likely turn to veterinarians and their colleagues for advice on how to proceed. Clients will expect accurate risk assessment for their dogs and will want guidance on how best to proceed with their breeding programs. This may involve extensive restructuring of ongoing breeding programs. The most informed veterinarians will be in the best position to advise their clients accurately.

The following chapters represent a significant step forward in providing canine health practitioners with much of the necessary information in an accessible and easily referenced form. The author clearly and accurately presents data on the features of many inherited canine diseases, together with easy-to-follow explanations on the underlying genetics. Particularly useful is the author's effort to update the reader on recent advances in canine molecular biology and its associated terminology. In addition, where diagnostic genetic tests are already available, the author provides much descriptive information that readers will find valuable.

Thus, contained within the following pages is much of the data necessary to help readers incorporate modern molecular genetics into their daily practice. With the application of these new methods, we have every expectation that the next generation of purebred dogs will be healthier and longer lived than their predecessors, giving the next generations of owners even more satisfaction with their pets than they have enjoyed in the past.

Elaine Ostrander, PhD
Associate Member
Head, Program in Genetics
Fred Hutchinson Cancer Research Center

Preface

The roots of education are bitter, but the fruit is sweet.—Aristotle

Authoring a book on the genetics of medical conditions in purebred dogs did not seem to be such a daunting task in the beginning. After all, genetics has been around since the time of Gregor Mendel, and dogs have been around even longer. By all accounts, veterinary medicine is advancing in step with human medicine and the sky seems to be the limit in diagnostic and therapeutic possibilities. New breakthroughs in genetics make the matter even easier, with virtual certainty in diagnostic testing and the promise of genetic therapies tailored to our specific needs. Matching breeds with medical conditions should be a snap, right? So what's the problem?

Even though the above statements are true, we have good reason to suspect that man's best friend may not be benefiting fully from all of the medical marvels available today.

Although one dog with roundworms is much like another, many other medical problems are far more breed-specific than disease-specific. For example, progressive retinal atrophy (PRA) in the Irish setter (rod-cone degeneration type I) bears little resemblance (clinically or genetically) to PRA in the miniature poodle (progressive rod-cone degeneration). We have DNA tests to detect PRA in both of these breeds, but the tests are breed-specific; the Irish setter test won't work in the poodle, and vice versa.

As another example, von Willebrand disease is seen in the Doberman pinscher, Airedale, and dozens of other breeds. In the Doberman the condition typically results in a coagulation problem, whereas affected Airedales are almost always asymptomatic. And hereditary nephritis is sex-lined in the Samoyed but autosomal dominant in bull terriers and autosomal recessive in the English cocker spaniel.

Soon we realize that we don't have canine medicine any more. We have Labrador retriever medicine, German shepherd dog medicine, Bouvier des Flandres medicine, and on and on. We cannot assume that epilepsy in the keeshond is the same as epilepsy in the Belgian Tervuren, and research is bearing this out.

Accordingly, this book is the first to try to compile the current information available on medical conditions with a genetic basis and make it available in a form useful to the private veterinary practitioner, and potentially the conscientious breeder. The goal is to enable veterinarians to incorporate basic genetic counseling into their practices without having to consult dozens of other texts to find breed-relevant information.

The book is formatted to be of use primarily to busy veterinary practitioners and veterinary students. This is not a textbook on genetics, nor is it a tome on canine medicine. It is a collection of what is known about medical problems that are inherited, how they are genetically transmitted in different breeds, how they are best identified, and strategies to help prevent them from occurring in future generations.

This book should augment, not replace, the information provided in medical textbooks. And, because the book consists of information from a wide range of peer-reviewed sources, we cannot completely avoid the bias found in many published reports. This final critical analysis of the facts is a necessary exercise for us all, and something that makes veterinary medicine as much an art as a science. Note that due to the extensive reference list at the end of the book, references are cited by number (in parentheses).

This book is the most comprehensive collection of breed-specific medical information ever assembled. I hope that it will serve as a springboard for even more ambitious projects in the field. My sincere thanks to all the researchers, veterinary practitioners, and breeders who help projects such as this one to become a reality.

Lowell Ackerman, DVM

GENETICS 101

The Basics of Inheritance

Although this is not a book about genetics per se, at least a basic understanding of genetics is necessary to appreciate how dogs become susceptible to inherited problems and how they might best be diagnosed and treated. *Genes* are sequences of genetic material (DNA) that reside on *chromosomes* and provide directions for the body to produce specific structural proteins, enzymes, or polypeptides. At the very heart of the matter is an animal's *genotype*, the unique assortment of genes inherited from both parents. Even though we can't see the genotype with our eyes, we can see the outward product of this genotype, combined with environmental influences, the sum of which is known as the *phenotype*.

For example, we have before us an Irish setter that has developed the devastating eye disease progressive retinal atrophy (PRA). There is no doubt that the animal is affected, but the breeder is at a loss to explain it, as both parents appear completely normal and PRA has not appeared in the family before. Perhaps this is just a new mutation and not really a problem in the family lines?

IDENTIFYING GENOTYPE

Today, as at no time in the past, we can test the hypothesis. We have a test that will prove, in all likelihood, that both parents are carriers by identifying their genotype (their genetic makeup for the trait) as such, even though their phenotype (what we can see) is normal for the trait (they don't have evidence of clinical PRA). So, even though we can see the phenotype for traits (hemophilia, PRA, hip dysplasia, and so forth), in most cases we have to infer the genotype from observing how traits seem to run in families. Only in the past several years has it become possible to determine the actual genotype for several different conditions.

As our knowledge of genetics expands, judging genotype becomes less of a guessing game and more of a science. A new DNA test has allowed that to happen for progressive retinal atrophy in the Irish setter and for several other diseases as well. In addition, genetic information can be used for nonmedical advances. For example, a genetic testing company, VetGen, offers a coat-color prediction service for Labrador retrievers, known as ChromaGene®. This company has determined nine different coat-color combinations in the breed, the product of two different color genes, and pairing known gene types takes all the guesswork out of determining colors of the pups.

If you were to breed a black Lab (Type IV) with a yellow Lab (Type VII), the color distribution in the pups would be about 25% black, 50% yellow, and 25% chocolate. You could also breed a black Lab (Type I) with a yellow Lab (Type V) and get all black pups. Or you could breed a black Lab (Type III) to a yellow Lab (Type VII) and get 50% black pups, 50% chocolate pups, and no yellow pups. Now that's diversity! Because the new test lets you determine the genotype for coat color, you now can predict accurately the coat color (phenotype) of pups and use this information to select appropriate breeding pairs based on the coat color desired (see Table 1). A ChromaGene® test is also available for color genotype in the Doberman pinscher, American cocker spaniel, flat-coated retriever, poodle, and Scottish terrier.

Although the study of genetics has been with us ever since Gregor Mendel started planting peas, without knowing genotype, genetics has been a perpetual enigma for most people. To explain what we see (the phenotype), we often make up rules to help us infer which actual genes are involved (the genotype). This works fairly well for some problems (such as hemophilia) and not so well for others (hip dysplasia, for example). Just like the coat-color dilemma in Labrador retrievers, most disorders don't fit neatly into categories based on phenotype alone. In truth, neither did the pea plants, but that didn't stop Mendel from pioneering a new discipline.

Table 1 Coat Color Inheritance Chart

Coat Color	Test	Genotypes	Types
Black	EB	BBEE, BBEe, BbEE, BbEe	I, II, III, IV
Yellow with black nose	B	BBee, Bbee	V, VI
Yellow with liver nose	None needed	bbee	VII
Chocolate	E	bbEE, bbEe	VIII, IX

Source: VetGen

UNDERSTANDING GENETICS

To understand genetics, we try to make it as simple as possible. We like to believe that traits have to be dominant or recessive and appear either on the sex chromosomes or the autosomes. We enjoy nice, clean statistics such as "approximately 25% of offspring will be affected." In reality, the deeper we delve into genetics and statistics, the more we realize that, for most conditions, hard statistics don't apply unless we have a direct test for the genotype. Though we want black or white, without being able to actually determine genotype, genetics is more like shades of gray.

Some things are immutable. When an animal is born, it receives half of its genetic blueprint from the sire and half from the dam. This combination of genes is what accounts for the animal being a truly unique individual, not a clone of the parents. For any one genetic character, then, each parent contributes one version of the gene for that character, which we call an *allele*. The location of a gene on a chromosome is its *locus*.

X-Linked Recessive

- All offspring of two affected parents are affected.
- Affected females mated to normal males produce male offspring that are all affected, but female offspring that are phenotypically unaffected.
- The disorder can skip generations.

In the Irish setter example, the PRA disease allele is called *rcd1* for the specific form of rod-cone dysplasia seen in that breed. When an animal inherits the same version of an allele from both parents, we say it is *homozygous* for that trait. When the alleles differ in a gene pair, we say the animal is *heterozygous* for that trait. For an X-linked trait, affected males are *hemizygous* for the trait because they possess only one X chromosome, which they get from their mother. Whatever the combination, the pairing of actual genes is what constitutes the genotype.

Based on this pairing of genes, we have rules to determine the impact of genetic combinations on progeny. This is most applicable when a single gene pair determines how the trait will be expressed. This is known as *monogenic* inheritance, of which PRA in Irish setters is an example. Other traits, such as hip dysplasia, are caused by the product of multiple gene effects. This is known as *polygenic* inheritance. In a monogenic trait involving one pair of genes, four genotypic outcomes are possible, but only three phenotypic expressions, as alleles from mother and father combine in offspring. When two gene pairs are involved, 16 genotypic combinations are possible, and, assuming all genotypes are expressed equally, nine possible phenotypes (for example, coat color in the Labrador retriever). For every n gene pairs involved in a trait, there are 4^n possible genotypic outcomes and 3^n possible phenotypic expressions.

When you realize that most traits are controlled by many gene pairs, you start to appreciate just how complicated predicting genetic outcome can be. In addition, modifiers, incomplete penetrance, or variable expressivity may have a significant effect on phenotypic outcome.

Because accurately predicting genotypes with polygenic traits is difficult, and because environment can have profound influences, the genetic involvement in a trait is typically expressed as *heritability* (h^2), which is a mathematical representation of the variance in breeding values divided by phenotypic variance (772). The heritability of a trait can vary from 0 (no heritable component) to 1 (complete inheritance).

Dogs have 78 chromosomes (39 pairs), two of which are sex chromosomes. Females are XX, and males are XY. The rest of the chromosomes, which have nothing to do with sex determination, are called autosomes. Some traits, such as hemophilia, are transmitted on the X chromosome, but to date no disease traits seem to be transmitted on the Y chromosome. Accordingly, a trait can be *sex-linked* (actually *X-linked*, as no Y-linked traits have been documented) if it resides on the X chromosomes or

Table 2 Possible Outcomes for Hemophilia Gene

Female \ Male	X^HY (normal)	X^hY (hemophiliac)
X^HX^H (normal)	all normal	females carriers, males normal
X^HX^h (carrier)	½ females normal, ½ carriers; ½ males normal, ½ hemophiliacs	½ females carriers, ½ hemophiliacs; ½ males normal, ½ hemophiliacs
X^hX^h (hemophiliac)	all females carriers; all males hemophiliacs	all hemophiliacs

autosomal if it resides on one of the other chromosomes. Sex-linked traits and *sex-limited* traits have to be differentiated. An example of a sex-limited trait is cryptorchidism, the presence of undescended testicles, in that it can be seen only in males. This does not imply that a female cannot carry the gene for cryptorchidism or that it is sex-linked and carried on the Y chromosome, which we know is not the case.

Table 2 gives possible outcomes related to the hemophilia gene. Note that males are hemizygous for the trait and contribute their hemophilia allele only to their daughters.

Recessive and Dominant Traits

When two copies of a disease-causing gene (one from each parent) are required to cause a specific problem, we say that trait is *recessive*. Thus, PRA in Irish setters is recessive because, to manifest the disease, an animal must inherit a defective gene from both parents. If the parents of an Irish setter with PRA appear phenotypically normal, they both must be *carriers* (heterozygous for a recessive character) of the trait, because each contributes a disease-causing gene to their offspring. And, because the trait is recessive, both carrier parents appear normal.

When only one copy of a gene is necessary for a trait to be expressed, we say that trait is *dominant*. In our PRA example, the gene for normal retinal development is dominant. That's why carriers look outwardly normal even though they carry an abnormal allele as well as a normal one.

In the simplest terms, if one gene pair controls a trait, the conventional use is to capitalize the dominant form and use lower-case for the recessive form. For example, let's imagine that the coat color in a fictitious breed, the American car-chasing terrier (ACCT), is controlled by a single gene pair. The dominant presentation is black (B), and the recessive presentation is brown (b). Because black is dominant

X-Linked Dominant Traits

- Affected offspring must have at least one affected parent (unless the mutation is new).
- The disorder does not skip generations.
- Affected males mated to normal females transmit the disorder to all of their daughters and none of their sons.
- Normal offspring from an affected parent produce only normal offspring.

Autosomal Recessive Traits

- All offspring of two affected parents are affected.
- Approximately equal numbers of males and females are affected.
- The disorder may skip generations.
- Mating an affected animal and an unrelated normal animal produces all normal-appearing offspring.

Autosomal Dominant Traits

- Affected offspring must have at least one affected parent (unless mutation is new).
- The disorder does not skip generations.
- Approximately equal numbers of males and females are affected.
- Normal offspring from an affected parent produce only normal offspring.

Table 3 Possible Combinations in Pups with Different Parental Genotypes

	BB (black)	Bb (black)	bb (brown)
BB (black)	all black	all black	all black
Bb (black)	all black	¾ black ¼ brown	½ black ½ brown
bb (brown)	all black	½ black ½ brown	all brown

over brown, individuals with a heterozygous genotype (Bb) will appear black. Homozygotes will be either black (BB) or brown (bb).

If we don't have a genetic test to identify coat-color genotype, we would have to determine it the old-fashioned way, by progeny testing. If you were to breed a black dog (we know that at least one allele is B) to a brown dog (bb) and any of the puppies were brown (bb), the black dog would have to be a heterozygote (Bb). If all the pups were black (BB or Bb), the black parent is most likely a homozygote (BB). Similarly, if we were to breed two black dogs and got any brown dogs, we'd know that both parents had to be heterozygotes for the black color gene (Bb). This concept is illustrated in Table 3.

If things only were this simple! Although we indeed could give many examples of traits that are inherited in a simple fashion, many more aren't nearly as easy to determine. Or the phenotype is the expression of more than one gene pair. Consider the genotype example presented earlier for Labrador retrievers, in which nine different coat colors actually were possible (but 16 possible gene combinations). Also, some genes can affect more than one function, such as the genes affecting coat color that also can be associated with deafness or ocular anomalies, or both. When one gene affects two or more traits in the same individual, this is termed *pleiotropy*.

THE GENETICS OF DISEASE

The situation doesn't get easier when looking at the genetics of disease, because genes aren't the whole answer. Genes don't cause diseases. They code for proteins that may have developmental or maintenance roles. A golden retriever with X-linked muscular dystrophy, similar to Duchenne's muscular dystrophy in humans, inherits a gene that codes for a defective or absent form of dystrophin protein, which, in turn, is an important component of muscle. This animal has poorly functional dystrophin warranting a diagnosis of muscular dystrophy. If a magic therapy would provide dystrophin to the animal, that animal would appear phenotypically normal. Genotypically, however, it still would carry the gene mutation for muscular dystrophy.

A few more examples of genes, mutations, diseases, and mode of inheritance are in order. Fucosidosis is a devastating disease of English springer spaniels, transmitted as an autosomal recessive trait. Although the abnormal gene doesn't kill the dog, it codes for an absent or nonfunctional enzyme, α-L-fucosidase. If the enzyme isn't capable of breaking down its substrate, the substrate collects within cells and eventually kills them. When the organ is compromised severely, it will eventually lead to the dog's demise. Carriers appear outwardly normal. Their levels of fucosidase enzymes, however, are lower than normal, but not low enough to cause expression of the disease. The same is true for many of the bleeding disorders that have a defective gene that does not produce a protein or an enzyme important to clotting. Although carriers appear normal, their level of clotting factor is typically lower than normal, just not low enough to cause spontaneous bleeding problems.

Whether a trait is truly recessive depends on how hard we look at the phenotype. A dog with fucosidosis typically shows neurological signs early in life and has an abbreviated life span. This affected dog carries two copies of the abnormal gene. If a carrier, with one abnormal gene, has no outward problems as a pup but suffers from dementia and is euthanized at 7 years of age, can this truly be considered a recessive trait without influence? If the bitch that is the carrier of one hemophilia gene has no spontaneous bleeding episodes but has complications with bleeding during surgery, is she truly phenotypically "normal"?

Young Labrador retrievers with late-onset rod-cone degeneration have been demonstrated to have measurably reduced retinal function (541). In this is

Table 4 The Genetics of Coat Color (772, 884, 1134)

Locus	Allele	Effect	Locus	Allele	Effect
Agouti	A	Solid color	Extension	E^m	Black mask
	A^y	Yellow		E	Normal extension
	A^w	Gray		e^{br}	Brindle
	a^s	Saddle		e	Nonextension (yellow)
	a^t	Bicolor (tan)	Greying	G	Born black, turns blue
	a	Recessive black		g	Born black, stays black
Black	B	Black	Intensity	INT	Lightest tan
	b	Liver		int^m	Intermediate tan
Color	C	Color factor		int	Darkest tan
	c^{ch}	Chinchilla	Merle	M	Merle
	c^d	White with dark eyes		m	Non-merle
	c^b	Blue eyes	Spotting	S	Solid color
	c	Albinism		s^i	Irish spotting
Dilution	D	No dilution		s^p	Piebald
	d	Dilution (e.g., blue Doberman)		s^w	Extreme white piebald
			Ticking	T	Ticking
				t	Non-ticking

cutaneous asthenia, gene mutations that produce abnormal collagen are considered dominant because heterozygotes produce 50% abnormal collagen, whereas procollagen-processing mutations are considered recessive because heterozygotes usually have enough enzyme activity to convert procollagen to collagen. Thus, as we learn more about genetic conditions and our testing improves, suppositions about dominant and recessive traits will have less impact on our genetic counseling skills.

Dominance

Now let's take a look at dominance. A trait that is completely dominant is easy to spot because the parent is affected and so are offspring. In the case of a dog that is homozygous for a dominant trait, all pups will be affected. With a dog that is heterozygous for a dominant trait, that dog and 50% of its offspring will be affected. What happens in many instances is incomplete dominance or expression of a dominant trait with variable expressivity. That basically means the trait has dominant features with a spectrum of possibilities in the offspring. If penetrance of a dominant gene is complete, all progeny receiving the allele will express the trait. If penetrance is 50%, only half will express the trait. With variable expressivity, some genes may produce different degrees of expression of a phenotype, ranging from severe expression to absence of the trait.

For example, dermatomyositis in collies was originally believed to be an autosomal dominant trait, but now it is believed that, although the trait has dominant features, environmental components (likely viral infection) are required for full manifestation of the disorder. Other traits may be codominant, each contributing to the phenotype.

An example of a dominant trait is merling of coat color. The normal, recessive genotype is the homozygote, *mm*. The heterozygote, *Mm*, has the characteristic merle coat coloring. In the homozygous dominant animal, *MM*, the animal is nearly all white, has blue eyes, and is usually deaf. Although merle is a desirable feature in some dog breeds, the deafness and white coat color are completely undesirable. Breeders wishing to perpetuate merle in their lines will breed normal (*mm*) to merle (*Mm*) to achieve half typically colored offspring and half merle.

Epistasis

Until now, we've kept things quite simple, but that is not necessarily the case in the real world. Whereas we have portrayed the possibility of only one dominant and one recessive allele in gene pairs, this is not necessarily nature's reality. Some loci have a variety of different alleles that could participate in a gene pair. Nowhere is this more apparent that in coat coloration (see Table 4). When the action of one gene depends upon the action of another gene, referred to as epistasis. This is wonderfully illustrated with coat colors possible with different combinations of alleles from different loci. All breeds have all the loci mentioned, but they don't necessarily have all the possible alleles mentioned. Even though coat color genetics is one of the most difficult concepts in genetics, it is the facet that breeders tend to understand best. They'll know that an Isabella Doberman pinscher must be atatbbdd and that a blue and tan merle collie must be atatddllMmsi-. Can you determine the color in our hypothetical breed with the following genotype?

$a^{s}atBbc^{ch}c^{b}ddEe^{br}GGintintmms^{i}s^{i}Tt$

Here's a hint: Even recessives can act as dominants to those lower in the list. Don't strain yourself. Remember, the breed does not really exist!

In general, recessive disorders are often attributable to enzyme deficiencies, as heterozygotes with only 50% as much enzyme likely still have enough to perform needed functions. In contrast, dominant traits may be caused by defects in structural or substrate proteins, such that heterozygotes will be expected to be affected because these polypeptides are required in relatively large quantities (772). As more and more research accumulates, however, these suppositions seem to consist of more generalization than fact and each trait is best considered individually.

Cytoplasmic Inheritance

Most DNA is found within the nucleus, but mitochondria in the cytoplasm contain their own DNA, derived entirely from the mother's ovum. Sperm contain few mitochondria, and none survive fertilization. Therefore, defects in mitochondrial DNA can be passed only from the mother but are transferred to both male and female offspring.

We've learned a lot since Mendel began playing with peas, and new genetic tests that actually identify genotype deserve much of the credit. Some of the old rules just don't apply, though. For example, mitochondrial myopathy in Clumber and Sussex spaniels is believed to be a sex-linked but not an X-linked trait. The trait is believed to be passed from the mitochondrial DNA of the maternal line to both sexes. Therefore, hemophilia A is X-linked and is transmitted principally from mother to son, whereas mitochondrial myopathy is believed to be passed from mother to both sons and daughters.

Predicting Outcomes

Most traits that we recognize in veterinary practice, and that cause the most problems, don't seem to fit neatly into Mendelian patterns of inheritance (825). When we consider traits such as hip dysplasia, cardiomyopathy, seborrhea, allergies, epilepsy, diabetes mellitus, glaucoma, and colitis, no easy answers are forthcoming. If we presume that the problem is likely to be caused by more than one gene, we'll label it *polygenic*, but most of the time, this is impossible to prove without genotype testing. If we see a condition such as epilepsy, which might affect more than one member of a breed line, we might describe it as *familial*, without knowing precisely how the trait is passed within that family. When a disorder appears to be more common in some breeds than others, we call this a *breed predisposition*. Once again, in most instances we don't know the exact mode of inheritance.

This lack of specificity is difficult to reconcile with a desire to predict outcomes. Nearly everyone believes that German shepherd dogs are prone to hip dysplasia. We might say that the German shepherd dog has a breed predisposition or predilection for hip dysplasia. Yet, German shepherds are not one of the breeds most commonly afflicted with the disorder, especially when taking their popularity into account. If we cite statistics by the Orthopedic Foundation for Animals, German shepherds aren't even in the "top 20" list of breeds at risk for developing hip dysplasia.

Whenever possible, risk should include a correction for the prevalence of a breed within the population sampled. For example, if we were to run a hip dysplasia screening clinic and find that we had eight German shepherds and four St. Bernards with hip dysplasia, we might conclude that German shepherds have a higher incidence of the problem. When we compare these numbers with the prevalence of each breed in our clinic population, however, the incidence of hip dysplasia in St. Bernards might turn out to be more than twice that in German shepherds. Because our hospital has many more German shepherd dogs, they naturally would account for a larger number of affected individuals. For many conditions, the incidence might be high in mixed-breed dogs (mutts) just because they represent the largest segment of a hospital population.

As a fictitious example, let's say we have a clinic population of 10,000 dogs and, when we review our medical records, we see that we've diagnosed 43 cases of follicular dysplasia over the past 5 years. Of these, 27 cases were seen in mutts, 11 in Chinese shar peis, and five in Irish water spaniels. In this hypothetical situation, which has the highest incidence of follicular dysplasia? We cannot know until we see how the hospital population breaks down by

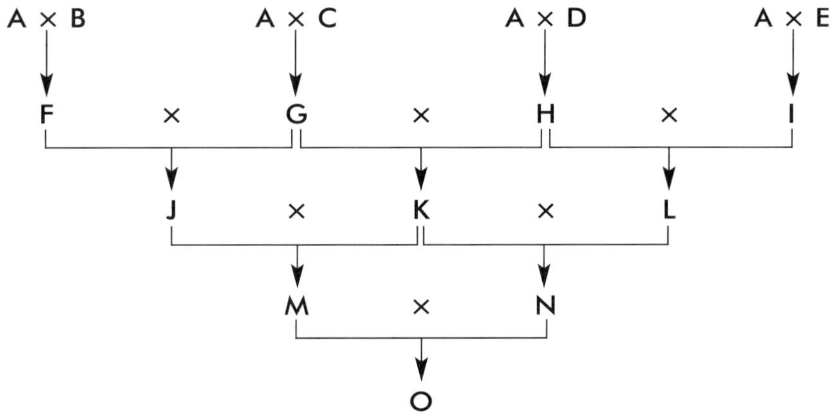

Figure 1 Example of linebreeding to concentrate the genes of a "superior" dog (A)

breed. It seems that 3,723 dogs in the practice are mutts, 89 are Chinese shar peis, and 12 are Irish water spaniels. According to our study, then, the condition is really seen in less than 1% of mutts, over 12% of Chinese shar peis, and more than 40% of Irish water spaniels. The lesson is that, without accounting for breed numbers in a population, we could easily draw inaccurate conclusions.

Calculating *relative risk*, accounting for the prevalence of a breed, is sometimes expressed as an *odds-ratio*, wherein numbers greater than 1 represent increased risk and numbers lower than 1 represent decreased risk. Thus, a breed with an odds ratio of 4 has four times the risk of the general canine population of developing a specific condition. Even with odds ratios, breed predisposition is only a rough guide to prevalence of disease. As long as individual breeders decide which qualities they wish to emphasize in their matings, overall breed statistics don't tell us much.

Linebreeding

Most breeders practice *linebreeding*, in which they find an animal with desirable traits and try to concentrate those traits in descendants of their foundation pair. This practice is what has created the breeds we see today (1054). It isn't the same as inbreeding *per se*, as most conscientious breeders don't breed brother to sister or sister to father, and so on, but they do create more concentrated gene pools in their family lines.

Even though all forms of linebreeding involve inbreeding, not all forms of inbreeding involve linebreeding. For example, a breeder might want to base a line on a show-winning dog and, therefore, breeds him with four unrelated but promising bitches. All pups have the same sire. The breeder then mates offspring from different litters together but does not breed full siblings from the same litter. All pups have the same grand-sire. This is repeated for another generation. All resulting pups have the same greatgrand-sire (Figure 1). With typical breeding, pups share 50% of their genes with their parents, 25% with their grandparents, and 12.5% with their great-grandparents. In this case on intense linebreeding, pups share about 47% of their genes with their greatgrand-sire, almost as much as their relationship to their parents (322).

Of course, while using linebreeding to concentrate desirable genes, this also can increase undesirable traits the foundation dog had but that weren't evident (recessive or incompletely dominant). The extent of inbreeding can be calculated as an inbreeding or consanguinity coefficient.

Outbreeding

Outbreeding is a technique to dilute rather than concentrate the genes of a family line. Sometimes it is used to undo the effects of linebreeding, and other times it is used to increase the fitness in the breed—so-called *hybrid vigor*.

Selection

Purebred dog populations have been subjected to strong selection, which has resulted in extreme differences between breeds and decreased heterogeneity within breeds (1054, 1055). Even so, a Portuguese water dog from a breeder's line in California may have little in common with that of a breeder from Maine, except for the ancestral genes they share.

Back to our discussion on hip dysplasia—this also explains why some lines of German shepherds have no incidence of hip dysplasia whatsoever and other lines are severely plagued by the condition.

> **Inbreeding**
>
> Inbreeding is not necessarily the cause of genetic problems in animals. Many colonies of laboratory animals with limited heterogeneity that are used for research do not become genetic invalids. Dog breeders, however, do not breed for uniformity but, instead, to produce different, and hopefully exceptional, animals. In fact, some traits that breeding associations prefer are associated with conditions that are detrimental to the animal's health (672). Most populations of animals not already subjected to rigorous artificial selection carry a number of recessive genes that, when homozygous in an individual, produce disease (821).

That's why quoting breed predispositions is so difficult. Problems run in family lines more than the breed in general. Having said this, a great deal of this book cites studies that allude to breed predispositions. At this point, it is a necessary evil until more tests allow genotype evaluation for specific traits. Odds-ratios, too, reflect only the population being sampled.

Despite Darwin's contentions to the contrary, survival of the fittest isn't an apt description for the role that genetics play in dog breeding. An animal with excellent conformation who is sterile contributes none of his or her genes to the breed. On the other hand, a mutt can impregnate every purebred bitch in a neighborhood if given the opportunity, and half of his genetic structure will be conserved in the offspring.

Veterinary medicine has also contributed to propagation of genetic disease in purebred dog lines. Without effective treatments for conditions such as demodicosis, malocclusion, allergies, entropion, and others, many animals might not have an appearance that would make breeders rush to breed them. Medical intervention that alters phenotype positively is more likely to propagate genotype. By the same token, as veterinary medical science has reduced the frequency of infectious, parasitic, and nutritional diseases in the dog, problems of a genetic nature become more significant.

Genetic Versus Congenital Anomalies

Finally, we should differentiate genetic and congenital abnormalities. The term *congenital* merely implies that a trait was present at birth. It does not mean that the disorder is heritable. Throughout this book, when discussing congenital problems, nongenetic forms are not explored further.

DNA—THE FABRIC OF LIFE

DNA is a fabulous device for conserving everything that makes us who we are. Whether you believe in evolution or divine intervention, DNA contains a lot more than just the genes that code for all our features. This residual DNA isn't entirely without function, though. It can come in handy when you're trying to create a genetic linkage map. That's because large chunks of this DNA consist of repetitive sequences of nucleotides that stand out from the rest. These serve as markers on a genetic map and are known as *microsatellites* (666).

Microsatellites have more to offer than just their role as signposts. They have considerable variability (which molecular geneticists call polymorphism), making them unique identifiers of individuals and their offspring. This is one way to identify an individual dog, as well as progeny, and has become a voluntary part of the DNA identification for the different purebred registries. If a sire has six repetitive sequences relative to a specific marker and the dam has eight, the offspring will have one copy from each parent. By comparing findings at multiple markers, the accuracy of predicting parentage becomes a virtual certainty (57).

Linkage

Taking this property of polymorphism one step further, imagine that we're not so much interested in parentage as in genetic diseases that individual dogs within a pedigree may be carrying. Perhaps we find that in a family of standard poodles, when an individual has two copies of eight repetitive sequences at a given microsatellite (homozygous), it develops sebaceous adenitis. In that instance, we have a genetic-linkage test for sebaceous adenitis (in this family at least) because we believe the trait to be *linked* to the pattern of repetitive sequence at a specific microsatellite. Not only that. If a dog has one copy with eight repetitive sequences and one with six, we can identify it as a likely carrier and use this information for genetic counseling.

In other families, other alleles of the same microsatellite may be associated with the disease gene. Preliminary studies in this example suggest that the linkage distance between the gene and the marker is about 3 centiMorgans. This means there is a 3% chance that the marker and gene could be separated during meiosis and lead to an incorrect result, or that genotype can be predicted with 97% accuracy. This is illustrated in Figure 2.

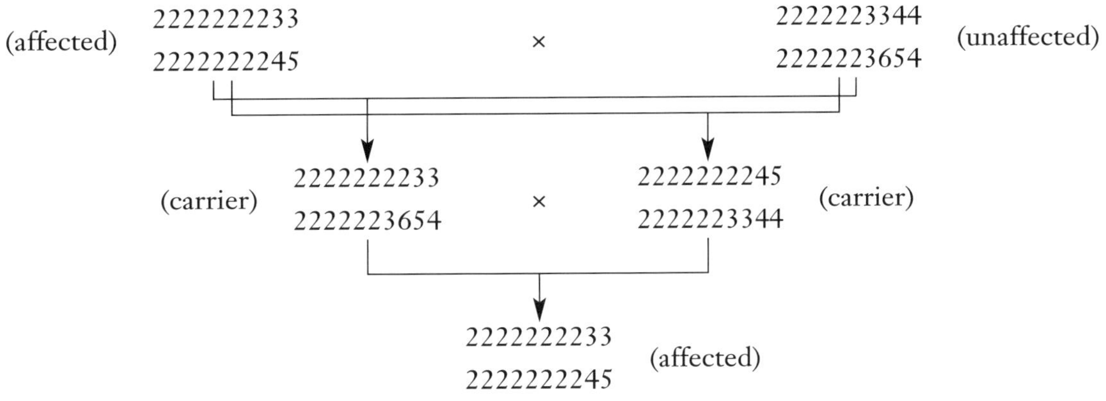

Figure 2 Example of linkage testing

Referring to the figure, for a given microsatellite, animals homozygous for eight repetitive two's seem to develop sebaceous adenitis. In this example, the F1 generation includes heterozygotes that are identifiable by examining the repetitive units. The offspring produced in the next generation is homozygous for the trait and will likely be affected.

Genetic Mapping

A project is under way to map all the genes in all the chromosomes in the domestic dog, creating a reference text of the canine genome. Scientists have been rigorous at their task, developing the markers to serve as cornerposts on the map and orienting the markers on the individual chromosomes. A preliminary canine map already has been constructed from more than 600 highly informative canine-specific markers, known as microsatellite markers (764, 907). Radiation hybrid mapping provides a different yet complementary view of the genome (851, 1081).The next job is to determine the order and spacing of genes and traits of interest on the chromosomes of the canine genome.

Genetic Disorders for Which DNA Testing is Already Available

- Linkage test for copper toxicosis in Bedlington terriers
- Pyruvate kinase deficiency in basenjis
- Progressive retinal atrophy (PRA) in Irish setters and Cardigan Welsh corgis
- Linkage test for PRA in poodles, Portuguese water dogs, English cocker spaniels, and Chesapeake Bay retrievers
- von Willebrand's disease in Doberman pinschers, Shetland sheepdogs, poodles, Scottish terriers, Pembroke Welsh corgis, and Manchester terriers
- Fucosidosis in English springer spaniels
- Glycogen storage disease type Ia in Maltese
- Globoid cell leukodystrophy in the West Highland white terriers and Cairn terriers
- Phosphofructokinase deficiency in springer and cocker spaniels
- Muscular dystrophy in golden retrievers
- Cerebellar ataxia in pointers
- Mucopolysaccharidosis I in Plotthounds
- X-linked severe combined immunodeficiency in Cardigan Welsh corgis and Basset hounds
- Congenital stationary night blindness in Briards
- Cystinuria in Newfoundlands
- Renal dysplasia in Shih tzu, Lhaso apso, and soft-coated wheaten terriers

Approximately 250 individual genes have been identified so far in the canine genome. By locating the actual defective genes or by identifying genetic markers, researchers are able to design DNA tests that tell whether a dog is affected, clear, or a carrier of the disorder. Experts predict that as many as 350 inherited disorders may eventually be deciphered using DNA analysis.

Of course, there are likely many more genetic disorders than this to differentiate, but when we lump different forms of PRA together as one entity, or as elbow dysplasia or cutaneous asthenia, the number approximates 350. As might be expected, answers will come faster for single-gene defects than for polygenic problems. The American Kennel Club (AKC), the United Kennel Club (UKC), and others are also using a DNA program for their registries. Not only will this information be used for identification and parentage verification, but it also will provide a stockpile of material to advance genetic and health research issues.

Instructions for DNA Brush Sample Collection

- Wash hands before collecting sample.
- If dog has been eating or drinking, wait 10 to 15 minutes before taking samples.
- Open cheek swab collection package.
- Remove collection brush without touching the bristles.
- Place brush between lip and gum of dog to be tested.
- Gently brush inside surface of cheek for 15 seconds.
- Place brush in mailing package provided. Do not place in zip-lock bag.
- Follow instructions regarding other brushes to be used.
- Prepare paperwork and mail sample to laboratory.

Considering that the research is being done internationally, it is remarkable that the work is being organized so thoroughly that it is avoiding duplication of efforts. This is largely to the credit of the Dog Genome Project (http://mendel.berkeley.edu/dog.html), a collaborative effort of the Fred Hutchinson Cancer Research Center in Seattle, the University of California, and the University of Oregon. The genetic map created so far has been a joint project of the Fred Hutchinson Cancer Research Center and the James A. Baker Institute for Animal Health at Cornell University.

In addition, DogMap (http://ubeclu.unibe.ch/itz/dogmap.html) is an international collaboration of 46 laboratories from 20 countries, under the auspices of the International Society for Animal Genetics (ISAG), dedicated to constructing a low-resolution canine genetic marker map. Further descriptions of these organizations are provided in the appendix.

Although baffling at the outset, the basics of molecular genetics are important in appreciating how precise the testing has become and the possibilities, as well as limitations, for genetic counseling. Recalling your days in introductory genetics (or its mention earlier in the chapter), you should remember that dogs have 39 pairs of chromosomes (a total of 78, with 76 autosomes and 2 sex chromosomes), composed almost entirely of proteins and nucleic acids. Despite decades of research and international cooperation, the canine genome has not yet been completely karyotyped such that chromosomes can be identified unequivocally (98, 1021), but that should become a reality in the near future. Chromosomes 1–21 have been fairly well defined but there are some major gaps in the latter autosomes.

The nucleic acids are deoxyribonucleic acid (DNA) and ribonucleic acid (RNA). The DNA consists of nucleotides containing four bases (adenine, thymine, cytosine, guanine), and the DNA in each chromosome is about 150 million nucleotide pairs long, about 3 billion nucleotides long in the entire canine genome. Given an alphabet with only four letters, it may seem improbable that this could account for all the genetic diversity in the world. Given also that these nucleotide triplets code for only 20 amino acids, it seems difficult to forge a plausible argument. Because those four nucleotides can occupy any position along the DNA sequence, however, even a 10-nucleotide stretch can form 4^{10} (more than 1 million) different combinations.

Imagine this as a combination lock: Instead of a 3-number sequence, you have an amino acid sequence of nucleotide triplets (e.g., CAT-TAG-GAC-ATT) that can code for an almost endless list of proteins. Instead of 10 nucleotides, consider 150 million, and you start to get a feeling of the potential for diversity.

If you recall the age-old model of the DNA double helix as a twisted ladder, those nucleotide base pairs form the rungs that connect the individual strands of DNA via sugar molecules. The rungs aren't haphazard; they're complementary. A binds only to T, and G binds only to C. Therefore, when the strands separate, each half can serve as a template for the other. If one strand starts with the sequence ATC, the other must be TAG. It's complementary!

Given 4 bases that can be arranged in groups of three (*codon triplets*), 64 (4^3) combinations are possible, but only 20 amino acid products. This

Table 5 Amino Acids and their DNA Triplet Codon

Amino Acid	Abbreviation	DNA Triplet Codon
Alanine	Ala	GCT, GCC, GCA, GCG
Arginine	Arg	AGA, AGG, CGT, CGC, CGA, CGG
Asparagine	Asn	AAT, AAC
Aspartic acid	Asp	GAT, GAC
Cysteine	Cys	TGT, TGC
Glutamic acid	Glu	GAA, GAG
Glutamine	Gln	CAA, CAG
Glycine	Gly	GGT, GGC, GGA, GGG
Histidine	His	CAT, CAC
Isoleucine	Ile	ATT, ATC, ATA
Leucine	Leu	TTA, TTG, CTT, CTC; CTA, CTG
Lysine	Lys	AAA, AAG
Methionine	Met	ATG
Phenylalanine	Phe	TTT, TTC
Proline	Pro	CCT, CCC, CCA, CCG
Serine	Ser	AGT, AGC, TCT, TCC, TCA, TCG
Threonine	Thr	ACT, ACC, ACA, ACG
Tryptophan	Trp	TGG
Tyrosine	Tyr	TAT, TAC
Valine	Val	GTT, GTC, GTA, GTG
Start	Beg	ATG
Stop	End	TAA, TAG, TGA

provides much opportunity for redundancy in the system. The average protein the DNA codes for is about 1000 amino acids long, which also means that it is 3000 codons in length (3 codons to 1 amino acid). Combined with codons that initiate reading and complete reading, the arrangement of codons is called an *open reading frame* (ORF).

Genetic diseases usually cause problems because the mutation creates a poorly functioning facsimile of the normal gene product. This often happens from innocent-appearing mishaps that result in an altered product. A *point mutation* occurs when there is a base substitution, insertion, or deletion in a DNA sequence.

Table 5 lists amino acids and their DNA triplet codon.

Mutations

Even though DNA replication is remarkably efficient, mistakes occasionally do happen. A base substitution that results in a stop codon halting the process prematurely is called a *nonsense mutation*; the resulting polypeptide will be shorter than usual, and probably not functional. PRA in the Irish setter, for example, is the result of a nonsense mutation in the cGMP-PDE-beta gene. A *missense mutation* occurs when a base is substituted for another, which potentially results in a different amino acid occurring in the chain.

In some cases, the resultant polypeptide probably won't be functional. In other cases, however, because of redundancy built into the system, a base substitution won't change the amino acid product (e.g., CAT and CAC both code for histidine). This is referred to as a *silent mutation*. Hemophilia B is characterized by a substitution of A for G at nucleotide 1477 in the gene for canine factor IX, resulting in the substitution of glutamic acid for glycine at position 379 in the factor IX molecule (772).

In contrast to missense mutations, in which only one amino acid in a sequence is affected, if a base is inserted or deleted in the DNA strand, it has the potential to alter the reading of the entire coded sequence downstream because the triplet codons are now out of their original sequence. This is known as a *frameshift mutation*. An example is X-linked nephritis (772). In simple terms, take the phrase "how are you" and insert the letter "b"

Story of a Mutation

We know that the genetic code is actually written with triplet codons, such that 3 nucleotide bases together code for a single amino acid. Thus, using the 4 bases, adenine (A), thymine (T), guanine (G), and cytosine (C), we can construct a chain of bases that code for amino acids that will form an enzyme, a protein, or a polypeptide. DNA is read three bases at a time, and these three bases correspond to specific amino acids. Accordingly, TATAGACAACAT would be read as tyrosine (TAT)-arginine (AGA)-glutamine (CAA)-histidine (CAT).

Redundancy is built into the system. For example, both TAC and TAT code for tyrosine, so if the T in position 3 happens to be replaced by the base C, the final product is not affected (a silent mutation). Now, given our sequence above, imagine that a point mutation occurs that deletes the third base in the sequence (T). With the bases after that point shifting one to the left, the first codon becomes TAA, which is a stop codon and arrests the process. If the deletion were to occur to the fourth base (A), the resulting peptide would be changed to tyrosine (TAT)-aspartic acid (GAC)-asparagine (AAC), which is completely different from the peptide normally produced.

after the letter "h" in "how." What do you end up with? The shift results in, "hbo ware eyo u." You can imagine what would happen to a genetic sequence.

Considering that a point mutation happens by chance, that it can affect any bases in a DNA sequence for a peptide, and then it passes to future generations, it shouldn't be surprising that similar disorders in different breeds can result from very different gene mutations. That's why the DNA test for PRA in Irish setters won't work in miniature poodles. Although the final clinical result is similar, the underlying genetic disorder couldn't be more different. When you combine the incidence of mutations with the fact that 70% of all mutations are recessive, it isn't difficult to see how they can be propagated.

If you have a dog that has other superior attributes but carries a recessive trait that isn't evident even to the trained eye, it shouldn't be surprising that the dog will be bred intensively. If that recessive trait isn't present in the other breeding stock, all of the offspring (F_1 generation) will be phenotypically normal but some of the offspring will carry the trait. If that generation is bred to unrelated stock, all of the next generation (F_2) will also be phenotypically normal, with even a smaller percentage being carriers. If bred to related stock that also carry the mutation, however, the recessive trait will start to be manifested.

Dogs have 78 chromosomes, which contain about 50,000 to 100,000 different genes. A gene is that portion of DNA that codes for a specific sequence of amino acids, which in turn make proteins, enzymes, or polypeptides. As you might expect, DNA segments are not packed like a passenger train with genes end to end. There are leaders and trailers before and after genes and within the gene, and there are some noncoded regions called *introns* that separate coded regions of "expressed sequences" called *exons*.

When DNA is being replicated, DNA polymerase can add nucleotides only at the 3' end of a growing strand. Some like to refer to the 5' end as being upstream from the 3' end and the 3' end as downstream relative to the 5' end. If you envision the DNA double helix as two snakes intertwined, with the 5' end being the head and the 3' end being the tail, the snakes are actually facing in different directions from one another. As the helix unwinds and acts as a template, a new strand is continually formed from the 3' end.

Because replication cannot occur from the 5' end of the other strand, however, small segments (Okazaki fragments) are created and then joined together with an enzyme, DNA ligase. Transcription then occurs via messenger RNA and translation by ribosomal DNA. Messenger RNA also includes sequences before (leader) and after (trailer) the gene that are necessary for ribosomal attachment and mRNA processing.

Microsatellites

In a simple world, you might consider the genome as a passenger train, with the genes as cars coupled to one another. In reality, it's not that orderly. This unsophisticated look is what actually gives us an opportunity to learn a lot from the canine genome. If the genome were arranged like a train, researchers would have to isolate each gene (car) to learn anything. But, lucky for us, nature has provided spacers, known as microsatellites, that can act as markers for traits. You might consider them as dining cars spaced between collections of passenger cars.

Right now, we have a few hundred useful microsatellites, but once we identify about 1,000 markers or so, we'll be well on our way to having a higher-resolution map of which markers are inherited along with which specific genes (586, 603, 665). Then, by measuring these markers, we can tell with some accuracy the genetic makeup of an individual for that specific trait, without having to measure the actual gene.

To use our train example once more, when train cars are unhitched and transferred to other trains, which passenger cars always seem to go along with the same dining car? Identify a specific dining car, and you know which passenger cars you'll find there, too. Obviously, the closer the gene (car) is to the marker (dining car), the greater is the probability that the two will be transferred together. A gene that is farther away from the marker may not be transferred 100% of the time, and this would affect the specificity of the test.

PCR

PCR, polymerase chain reaction, is a method of taking small bits of DNA or RNA that is specified by a probe and amplifying it by making millions of copies so a sufficient amount is available to be detectable by more routine laboratory tests. The important thing is to make sure we have identified a DNA sequence that is specific for the disease of interest. Otherwise, we might find that our test isn't measuring what we think it is.

Segregation Ratio

For any given trait, we often assume that separation of alleles during meiosis is an independent event, known as *segregation*. The ratio of different types of genotypes that will result is known as a segregation ratio. In most cases, segregations at multiple loci are considered to be independent of one another, so that the chance of obtaining a gamete with a particular allele at the first locus and a particular allele at the second locus is simply the product of the probabilities associated with each allele independently.

For some genes, however, given the fact that there are thousands of genes and only 78 chromosomes, some genes can be expected to be closely situated on a chromosome and may move together during meiosis. If we calculate the recombination fraction, the proportion of gametes from one parent that can have resulted only from crossing-over during meiosis in that parent, the map distance between the two can be calculated by multiplying by 100. So, if the recombination fraction for two loci is 50% (0.5), the map distance between the two loci is 50 (0.5 × 100) centimorgans (cM). The entire canine genome is about 26 Morgans.

Linkage and Lod Scores

When two loci are very close on a chromosome, their recombination fraction is low and the loci are said to be linked. This is the principle between linkage groups and the creation of linkage maps. Linkage is often expressed in terms of a *Lod score*, which is the log of the odds supporting linkage between two markers or between a marker and a disease gene. A Lod score of three or greater is considered sufficient evidence that linkage exists.

Once enough markers have been discovered, separation of genes and markers becomes less of an issue. Researchers look for single mutations that are co-inherited with the disease gene in all affected individuals and absent in all unaffected individuals. Thus, copper toxicosis in Bedlington terriers is tested using a genetic linkage test. The test, however, does have limitations: A known affected dog in the pedigree must be available to test related dogs, the marker must have genetic variation, and occasionally the gene and marker can become separated. At this point in time, with current technology and identified markers, there is about an 85% possibility of a disease gene being close enough to a marker to detect linkage.

To be the most specific, a test might actually look at the gene sequence. This involves cloning the gene, which is an involved and expensive process, but it is an extremely accurate assessment. The PRA test in Irish setters is an assay that tests the actual gene. Accordingly, the specificity is near 100%.

Candidate Genes

Identifying specific genes in the dog gets simpler when the basic research has already been done in another species (773). We call these *candidate genes* because we're searching for genes in the dog similar to genes that have been described already in other species. If a gene has been identified for a specific disease in both mice and humans, there's a very good chance that the same gene causes the problem in dogs. As dogs and humans share about

> **Genetic Databases**
>
> The Internet is a great source of information on genetic databases for humans and animals, although addresses (Universal Resource Locators or URLs) do change from time to time. Try accessing Online Mendelian Inheritance in Man (OMIM) at
>
> http://www3.ncbi.nlm.nih.gov/omim/
>
> and Online Mendelian Inheritance in Animals (OMIA) at
>
> http://www.angis.org.au/Databases/BIRX/omia/

80% of the same genes, this isn't a far stretch. Thus, when breakthroughs in human genetics identify a deafness gene (Cx26) or a diabetes mellitus gene (IDDM10) or a glaucoma gene (TIGR), dogs will likely benefit from those efforts.

Predicting Genotype

For now, the goal is to create a map of the canine genome and identify microsatellites (markers) useful in predicting genotype. Initially, we'll have a low-resolution map, and we'll improve on resolution as we identify more markers and more genes. In the not-too-distant future, we should have a map with a resolution down to about 5 to 7 centiMorgans. Absolute genetic identification of disorders is a little farther down the road for most other disorders. This is actually very much like the tests we use to diagnose systemic infectious agents. The first immunologic tests available for detecting heartworm were antibody tests. Although the tests were sensitive, there was always the worry of making a wrong diagnosis because of cross-reactivity. Antigen tests removed most of those doubts. If actual antigens from an infectious agent could be detected, the diagnosis could not be in much doubt. The same holds true for genetic testing. Linkage tests are a starting point, but eventually will be replaced by direct tests. It just takes time.

The possibilities are limitless. Progressive retinal atrophy (PRA) in the Irish setter is inherited as an autosomal recessive trait. This means that an affected individual inherits a defective gene (*rcd1*) from each parent. The good news for veterinarians, even without a DNA test, is that an electroretinogram can identify this affected individual by 6 weeks of age. That way it won't contribute its PRA genes to future generations. The bad news for veterinarians and breeders is that carriers of the trait cannot be identified clinically, even through sophisticated procedures such as electroretinography. Therefore, genetic counseling is a hit-or-miss enterprise until the animal produces affected offspring. With direct DNA testing, though, you can absolutely identify the animals that are affected, clear, or carriers.

That's got to be good news for Labrador retriever breeders, because labs are also prone to PRA but a clinical diagnosis can't be made until the dogs are 4 years of age, and not even by electroretinography until they are 18 months of age. Unfortunately, the specificity of DNA testing is also one of its limitations. The gene that causes PRA in Labrador retrievers (*prcd*) is different from the one in Irish setters (*rcd1*), so the same DNA test can't be used.

Miniature schnauzers have yet another form of PRA (*pd*), and so do Siberian huskies (*XLPRA*), collies (*rcd2*), and others. In Norwegian elkhounds, two different forms of PRA (*erd*, *rd*) have been identified. Accordingly, although the DNA test for PRA in Irish setters is a breakthrough, it will take time before genetic disorders are fully identified on an individual breed basis, and tests subsequently developed. For the most part, the research is being driven by individual breed clubs that are providing funds for researchers to work on specific problems in their breeds.

Is epilepsy in the Belgian Tervuren transmitted by the same gene as in the German shepherd dog? Is hip dysplasia in the bloodhound transmitted by the same genetic mechanism as in the rottweiler? Expect breakthroughs on single-gene defects in the near future for most popular breeds. Miracles related to unlocking the secrets of polygenic traits will take a little longer.

GENETIC COUNSELING

With new methods of identifying genetic diseases, veterinarians may think they will have an easy time advising breeders. With the new technologies, though, come new responsibilities. This is especially true when a trait is highly entrenched in a breed. For example, approximately 75% of Bedlington terriers either are affected with copper toxicosis or are carriers of the trait. Because a DNA linkage test is now available for copper toxicosis, should we advise breeders to breed only animals that are "clear" for the trait? Unfortunately, things aren't that simple.

Linkage-Based Testing

The DNA linkage-based test is not the same as a direct DNA test and isn't nearly as infallible. Linkage-based tests measure the presence of microsatellites that may be located close on a chromosome to the gene for a genetic disorder such as copper toxicosis, rather than detecting the gene itself. The tests are valid only if the family line includes animals affected with the condition, and sufficient polymorphism is present in the microsatellite to reveal trends.

Even under perfect circumstances, the linkage-based test for copper toxicosis could be wrong 1% to 5% of the time. Still, it is a handy tool until a direct DNA test is developed. A dog that tests as marker type 1/1 is 90% likely to be completely clear of the trait. About 95% of dogs that are 1/2 are carriers of the trait. Those that are 2/2 are mostly affected (about 72%), but some are carriers (about 24%). The results of the test can be formally registered with the Orthopedic Foundation for Animals.

Direct DNA Tests

Even with direct DNA tests that detect animals that are clear, affected, or carriers with almost absolute certainty, enforcing a "clear only" policy of breeding may not be possible. It may not even be desirable. For a trait such as copper toxicosis in Bedlington terriers, or von Willebrand disease in Doberman pinschers, or collie eye anomaly in collies, the incidence may be too high to advise breeding only animals that test "clear." In so doing, we may select a very small number of animals to become the foundation for a new breed line. Although this is laudable, this narrow gene base conceivably could concentrate other deleterious genes instead. Accordingly, if mating only clear-to-clear animals is not possible, breeding clear to carrier may be necessary until a large enough population of clear animals is created so the gene pool isn't quite so shallow and will preserve some genetic diversity.

Breeding Responsibilities

Actually, breeding carrier to clear (as long as we can identify carriers) with regard to recessive traits will achieve our goal of not producing any affected animals. To breed two carriers or any affected animals, however, is never desirable. Breeding two carriers is acceptable only if the trait is prevalent in the breed, or if it is of minimal medical significance. Under this policy, we will be able to establish breeding lines of only clear animals within a few generations. Affected individuals can always be eliminated, but selecting against heterozygotes (carriers) is desirable, as they are most responsible for disseminating the trait in family lines (1055).

In genetic counseling, it is important to assume genetic responsibility for individual animals and eugenic responsibility for the fate of the breed. Our breeding strategies, therefore, cannot be shortsighted. Breeding control can be achieved by mass selection or progeny testing, of which individual or mass selection is the most practical method for most veterinarians and breeders.

Mass Selection

- Select breeding animals based on superior physical characteristics and lack of genetic problems.
- In successive generations, breed only animals from the top 10% of those available.
- If genetic problems are seen in offspring, consider their parents to be unsuitable for breeding.
- Rate of disappearance of a defect depends on the mode of inheritance.

Mass or Individual Selection

With mass or individual selection, the breeder selects the animals to be bred based on their superior characteristics. Whereas many breeders select their breeding stock based on conformation or other physical characteristics that exemplify the breed standard, genetic counseling is intended to temper enthusiasm for physical traits with a more holistic picture of genotypic as well as phenotypic health. As veterinarians, we also should exert some self-discipline in not just focusing on one health aspect (e.g., von Willebrand status) but, rather, on the whole animal. Otherwise, in our zeal to rid a line of one disease, we may inadvertently foster another.

Selection works best at eliminating dominant traits from a population. After all, because all animals that carry the dominant allele develop the trait, it is theoretically possible to eliminate a dominant trait in one generation. This is complicated, however, by the fact that some dominant traits (e.g., dermatofibrosis) don't appear until later in

Table 6 Possible Selection Index

	Factor	Score	Out of
Health	CERF evaluation	15	20
	Family history of hypothyroidism	9	10
	Family history of immune disorders	3	10
	Dental evaluation	5	5
	PennHip	4.5	5
	Subtotal	**36.5**	**50**
Conformation	Coat characteristics	8	10
	Body conformation	6	10
	Stance/gait	7	10
	Subtotal	**21**	**30**
Behavior	Temperament	7	10
	Trainability	9	10
	Subtotal	**16**	**20**
	Total	**73.5**	**100**

life when animals already have been bred, or for traits with incomplete dominance or variable expressivity, in which an affected animal may not be detected, yet carry the trait.

With recessive traits, selection can quickly remove homozygous affected animals from breeding, but if heterozygotes cannot be detected, carriers will persist in the population. The final elimination of the trait from a breed requires identifying carriers and ensuring that no carriers are bred to one another. Even though this doesn't eliminate the deleterious allele from the population, it does ensure that no affected animals are produced.

Selection of Breeding Animals

There are many ways to select animals for breeding purposes. Some breeders select animals based on their conformation—their appearance. Perhaps they think the individual has an exceptional topline, or head shape. This, however, does not take genetic health into consideration, so this method is not the best to recommend during genetic counseling. Another method is to set "culling levels" for traits. For example, the breeder may eliminate all dogs that have less than perfect hip conformation, or test "positive" for carrier status of von Willebrand disease, or other diseases. Although this allows for many characteristics to be considered, it tends to be too rigid for a flexible breeding program. Perhaps the best option for the conscientious breeder and accommodating veterinarian is a selection index scheme.

The selection index is a numerical score assigned to an animal that provides a relatively objective measure of overall suitability for breeding. The index can be customized for each situation, but to be fair, it should be consistent among all dogs evaluated. In my own selection index for show breeders, I typically assign 50 points for health concerns, 30 points for conformation, and 20 points for behavior. For performance dogs, I might assign 50 points for health concerns, 30 points for performance factors, and 20 points for behavior. For pet owners who are not interested in show or performance, more weight can be given to health and behavioral concerns.

In creating a selection index, more significance could be attributed to certain traits and less to others while remaining constant within groups. For example, a collie breeder who is trying to eliminate collie eye anomaly from her lines but has a negligible incidence of hip dysplasia may assign more of the health points to CEA evaluation. The heritability of individual traits is also important when assigning significance. For example, chest width has a heritability of about 80%, whereas litter size has a heritability of only 10%–20%. The lower the heritability, the more generations will be required to see improvement. Table 6 gives an example of a possible selection index for our fictional collie breeder.

Table 7 Using Selective Index to Evaluate Individual Dogs

Factor	1	2	3	4	5	6
CERF	15	17.5	5	10	0	12.5
Thyroid	9	2	4	7	8	7
Immune	3	5	4	5	8	8
Dental	5	3	5	3	4	4
Hips	4.5	3	2	3.5	4	4
Coat	8	8	9	8	9	7
Conformation	6	7	10	8	7	7
Stance/gait	7	6	9	8	8	7
Temperament	7	5	10	7	7	8
Training	9	6	10	7	8	7
TOTAL	73.5	62.5	68	56.5	63	72.5

Although the evaluation is subjective in most cases, observer consistency is what makes the selection criteria relatively objective. In the example above, our collie has no evidence of collie eye anomaly but, because carrier status cannot be determined and there is some family history, genotype cannot yet be confirmed as "clear." Although hypothyroidism has been a growing concern for collie breeders, this dog tested in normal range and is registered with the OFA thyroid registry.

A brother of this dog's grandfather developed hypothyroidism at 6 years of age but so far is the only family member to be so diagnosed. This dog was not as lucky in immune-mediated disorders. The maternal grandmother had been diagnosed with systemic lupus erythematosus and there have been scattered cases of cutaneous lupus erythematosus, pemphigus foliaceus, and dermatomyositis. This dog and its siblings, however, have not shown any evidence of problems.

A dental evaluation showed perfect dentition, although the breeder did not consider this an important factor (but the veterinarian did, given the results of previous dental evaluation he had done on collies). This dog scored in the top 10% for the breed on the PennHip evaluation, earning a score of 4.5 of a possible 5. Based on her assessment of the dog's performance at dog shows and the judges' comments, the breeder provided the scores for conformation. The veterinarian and the breeder jointly evaluated temperament. Although the dog performed well in the show ring, he did seem somewhat tentative when being handled but didn't demonstrate any direct evidence of aggression.

In the comparison of the six dogs for breeding selection (Table 7), the selection index allows us to weigh our options more objectively. We also can change the relative weightings if the breeder suddenly discovers that a trait is more important than was realized originally. In this example, the dog that would have scored best in the show ring (Dog 3) would not be a top choice because of features that a judge would not see.

Progeny Testing

Progeny testing evaluates prospective breeding stock by estimating genotype. It is cumbersome because large numbers of animals and their progeny must be followed. Males are scrutinized most

Progeny Testing

- Males should be selected for foundation duty based on truly exemplary physical characteristics and scrutiny for genetic anomalies in all body systems. Health information on parents and siblings also should be evaluated.
- Males should be bred to unrelated, phenotypically similar females.
- Thirty to forty progeny should be obtained for each male, recording all animals, even stillborn pups.
- Progeny must be kept long enough for the trait to be expressed.
- Once proven, the male should continue to be used until a better replacement animal is determined. Affected animals should be culled.

intensely because one male can yield 15 litters in the time one female produces a single litter (672). Mass selection is preferred until the incidence of a disease in a breed line has been significantly diminished. To rid a line completely of a trait, however, requires progeny testing. Of course, once DNA tests are available for most traits, these exercises in selection will not be needed.

Because recessive disorders represent the majority of genetic problems and because they are so insidious, most genetic counseling is involved with determining heterozygotes, which carry the trait but appear normal themselves. Once heterozygotes are identified, they don't have to be culled. They are quite suitable for house pets. If they are of extraordinary value for other qualities, however, they may even be bred. Two carriers should not be bred unless circumstances dictate this as a necessity, and a carrier should never be bred to an affected individual.

Hardy-Weinberg Law

Sometimes the magnitude of the problem is not immediately obvious. We can bring it more sharply into focus with something called the Hardy-Weinberg law. This law helps us predict genotype frequencies with a simple algebraic formula, where p^2 is the frequency of the homozygous dominant gene pairing, 2pq the heterozygotes, and q^2 the frequency of the homozygous recessive gene pairing, with the individual gene frequencies, p + q, equaling one. The Hardy-Weinberg law applies as long as there is no mutation (allelic changes), migration ("new blood"), or active selection for a trait. While the Hardy-Weinberg law is very useful in canine genetics, it must be remembered that dog breeding invalidates some of the basic tenets of the law, since matings don't occur randomly or without selection, the way they might in nature. Also, the population is rarely in equilibrium since breeders often bring in breeding animals from outside the local population. As such, gene frequencies predicted by the Hardy-Weinberg law may not be completely accurate. Still, much useful information is provided.

Let's examine this with our American car-chasing terrier (ACCT) and the incidence of an autosomal recessive trait, von Willebrand disease (vWD), in this breed. Because vWD in the ACCT is autosomal recessive, we have difficulty distinguishing between the homozygous dominant and the heterozygote; von Willebrand factor testing does not convincingly differentiate the two in this breed. The only phenotype we can conclusively demonstrate is the homozygous recessive, those affected with von Willebrand disease.

We did a survey with the local ACCT club and found that, of 1,000 dogs, 53 had von Willebrand disease. The ACCT club seemed happy that the incidence of the disorder in the breed was of the order of only 5%. Using the figures from the survey, the genotype frequency for homozygous recessive (q^2) is 0.053 and the gene frequency (q) is the square root of 0.053, or 0.23. We know the sum of p and q equals 1, and q=.23, so p must equal 0.77, and p^2, the proportion with the homozygous dominant genotype, equals 0.59. Based on these numbers, we would predict that 2pq, or 0.35 (35%), is the likely proportion of heterozygous carriers in the population.

What does this exercise in algebra tell us? Well, it tells us that, although only 5.3% of American car-chasing terriers actually have von Willebrand disease, an incredible 35% of the ACCT population are carriers of the trait, and not detectable by conventional means. This breed club has a potentially serious problem and would be best advised to invest money is a genetic test to detect heterozygotes. In the interim, however, our goal is to identify heterozygotes by other means so we are able to discern animals that are homozygous normal. We'll have to do the best we can with vWD testing and progeny testing to differentiate normal homozygotes from normal-appearing heterozygotes.

We have no problem identifying our dogs that are homozygous recessive. They are the ones with von Willebrand disease. We also know that the normal-appearing parents of these affected animals are heterozygotes, carriers of the trait. Nevertheless, most of the other heterozygotes, which we would like to avoid breeding, are clinically indistinguishable from the homozygous normal animals that we would like to use in our breeding program. For example, because we know that the parents of affected animals are carriers, it follows that at least one of each of the parents (grandparents of the affected animal) must also be a carrier. Inferring genotype from a family tree is known as *pedigree analysis*.

Test Mating

To establish a foundation stud to rid a line of a recessive disorder, such as von Willebrand disease in the American car-chasing terrier, it is helpful to confirm that the animal is not a normal-appearing carrier of the trait. This can be done with a *test mating*. We know that affected animals are homozygous recessive, so breeding our potential foundation stud to an affected animal should answer this question with near certainty. If he is a carrier of the trait, we would suspect that half of the offspring

Table 8 Probability of Animal of Unknown Genotype Being Homozygous Dominant or a Carrier for a Recessive Trait Based on Pups Produced by Breeding to an Affected Individual

# Normal Offspring	Chances of Being Homozygous Dominant (%)	Chances of Being a Heterozygous Carrier (%)
1	50.0000	50.0000
2	75.0000	25.0000
3	87.5000	12.5000
4	93.7500	6.2500
5	96.8750	3.1250
6	98.4375	1.5625
7	99.2187	0.7813
8	99.6094	0.3906
9	99.8047	0.1953
10	99.9023	0.0977

Table 9 Probability of an Animal Being Homozygous Dominant for a Recessive Trait, Based on Pups Produced by Breeding to a Heterozygous (Carrier) Individual

# Normal Offspring	Chances of Being Homozygous Dominant (%)	Chances of Being a Heterozygous Carrier (%)
1	25.0000	75.0000
2	43.7500	56.2500
3	57.8125	42.1875
4	68.3594	31.6406
5	76.2695	23.7305
6	82.2022	17.7978
7	86.6516	13.3484
8	89.9887	10.0113
9	92.4915	7.5085
10	94.3687	5.6313
11	95.7765	4.2235
12	96.8324	3.1676
13	97.6243	2.3757
14	98.2182	1.7818
15	98.6637	1.3363
16	98.9978	1.0022
17	99.2483	0.7517

will be affected. If he is homozygous normal, none of the offspring should be affected.

The number of offspring needed for evaluation is simply a function of how sure we want to be. A carrier crossed with an affected animal produces offspring with a 50% chance of being affected. In a litter of *n* normal pups, the chance of a carrier remaining undetected is 0.5^n and the chance that the animal is a non-carrier is $100–0.5^n$% Accordingly, there is only a 3% chance that the stud is a carrier if there are five pups, all normal, and less than a 1% chance that he's a carrier if there are seven or more pups, all normal. If any affected pups are produced, the dog must be a carrier, heterozygous for the von Willebrand disease trait. This can be easily expressed as a table (see Table 8).

For some recessive genetic conditions, breeding affected individuals in a test mating is not possible.

For example, in some of the lysosomal storage diseases, affected animals may not survive until maturity. In these cases, a test mating can be done with our prospective stud and a known carrier, such as a dam that previously has produced an affected individual. In this case, in a litter of *n* normal pups, the chance of the prospective stud being a carrier and remaining undetected is 0.75^n. In this situation, 11 pups, all normal, would be required to be 95% sure, and 16 pups to be at least 99% sure, that the prospective stud was not a carrier. If any affected pups are produced, the prospect must be a carrier, heterozygous for the von Willebrand disease trait. Table 9 gives these probabilities.

Although establishing harsh criteria to rid breeds of genetic disorders by completely eliminating affected animals and carriers may seem reasonable, this is neither practical nor realistic. Because each animal carries between 50,000 and 100,000 different genes, ridding lines of all deleterious alleles is not possible. If carriers can be determined, however, breeding phenotypically normal dogs is a real possibility by never breeding two carriers together. If we are aware of heterozygotes, we can safely breed carriers with known normal individuals and we will never see cases of the disorders we are trying to avoid. Isn't that what genetic counseling is all about?

Trying to overcome polygenic traits takes longer and is more troublesome. Obviously, the higher the heritability of a trait, and the more ruthless we are at selecting superior individuals for breeding, the more successful our selection process will be. This response to selection (R) also can be described as an algebraic function, $R = h^2S$, where R is the response to our breeding strategy, h^2 is the heritability of the condition, and S is the selection differential, the phenotypic superiority of the parents we selected versus the general population from which they came. The result is that the mean improves; it doesn't mean that the pups will be superior to their parents.

Hip dysplasia provides a good example of how selection pressure improves the standard, albeit slowly. Let's say we create a scoring system for hips in which 0 represents severe dysplasia and 100 represents perfect hips. In our American car-chasing terrier, the mean hip score for the population is 55 and the heritability of the trait is believed to be 0.25. To try to improve hip joint morphology in the breed, we mate a stud with a hip score of 88 with a bitch scoring 92. The average score of the parents is 90, which is 35 points higher than the mean. Should that produce terriers with great hips? The response to selection (R) is 0.25×35, or 8.75. Thus, in the litter produced, the mean hip score for the pups is predicted to be 63.75 (55 + 8.75). We've managed to shift the whole bell-shaped curve of hip scores to the right, but not by the magnitude you may have expected. Now you see why creating real improvement with polygenic traits takes so long, even when using superior breeding animals.

Regardless of the mode of inheritance of a trait, genetic counseling is always more effective when veterinarians and breeders work as a team. This includes keeping records of affected animals, as well as those that are clear for a disorder. Registries are wonderful tools for genetic selection, if they are nonjudgmental so as to encourage free exchange of information. Closed registries release only information of animals certified as having desirable phenotype. Open registries provide information on specific animals and those to which they are related, including both desirable and undesirable phenotypes.

As we attempt to scrutinize genetic reports in the literature, we must note that study bias is rampant in clinical research, even studies published in peer-reviewed journals (901). *Nonselection* is defined as failure to include a subject or subjects from the population of interest in the experiment or study group; *nonresponse* is the failure to include a subject or subjects from the study population in the results and analyses of the study (901). Thus, for a disorder as common as hip dysplasia, incidence data by breed are often contentious. Because submission of radiographs to most registries is voluntary, owners with dogs that are most likely to have hip dysplasia may see no reason to pay to have the radiographs submitted to the registry. This leads to substantial nonresponse bias and underestimation of the actual prevalence of hip dysplasia in these breeds.

This isn't a far-fetched argument. Owners with dogs that have clinical evidence of hip dysplasia aren't likely to ask to have radiographs taken, as they know their animal won't be certified. Other owners, who have radiographs done thinking their animal is "clear" and learning that it has hip dysplasia, may elect not to have those radiographs sent to the registry.

Nonselection bias also plagues hip dysplasia statistics. Even if the registry decides to petition a national breed club, such as the American Car-Chasing Terrier Club of America, and asks all registrants to participate in a cost-free hip evaluation plan to gather breed statistics on hip morphology, bias still potentially exists. If the breed club has a strong policy of encouraging the breeding of only disease-free dogs, might there be dog owners who don't agree with those policies and, therefore, don't belong to the club? Or might there just be a sizeable population of owners of the breed who don't belong to the breed club because they are pet owners, not breeders. In any case, results cannot be extrapolated to the entire breed, just the frame selected for study.

Much of the research on which breed statistics for genetic disorders have been based is subject to nonresponse and nonselection bias. When bias is not addressed, readers are left to make their own assumptions based on the results reported. Sadly, this book also depicts bias, because it includes published reports from peer-reviewed journals that are not free of their own bias.

For example, if a teaching hospital reports in the literature that it has had 12 cases of tetralogy of Fallot over a 5-year period and the breed most often affected was the American car-chasing terrier (ACCT), can we safely assume that a breed predilection for tetralogy of Fallot is present in the ACCT? Perhaps, on careful scrutiny of the cases, all reported cases of tetralogy of Fallot were reported to have come from one line and one specific family. A survey of other ACCT owners and breeders from around the country failed to reveal another case of the disorder in this breed. Still, veterinarians for decades to come will quote the largest study of congenital cardiac diseases done to reveal that the ACCT had the highest incidence of tetralogy of Fallot. And that fact also will be propagated in books like this one, until a better-designed study comes along that will refute the original.

APPLICATION FOR VETERINARIANS

Why do veterinary practitioners need knowledge of genetic diseases and selection pressures? Despite the fact that genetics is a critical component of veterinary medicine in general, the discipline holds very real implications for effective medical practice. Issues of legal liability and medical competence also have to be addressed.

Although some veterinarians believe that breeders represent too small a segment of their practice to warrant gaining proficiency in genetics and genetic counseling, this is a poorly conceived argument. In most circumstances, when someone purchases a dog, whether from a pet store or a breeder, the dog must be evaluated by a veterinarian within a fixed time period (usually 2–5 business days) and found to be fit. During that visit, most astute practitioners will discern the most common anomalies, such as luxating patellae, umbilical hernias, congenital cataracts, heart murmurs, and the like. If the veterinarian finds the animal to be unfit, the purchaser often has the option of returning the animal, either for a refund or an exchange, depending on the seller's policies.

Let's investigate what happens when a veterinarian determines the pup to be fit. The purchaser, now the owner of the dog, starts to notice strange behavior in the dog at 4 months of age. The dog is an English springer spaniel, and, unsure of the diagnosis, you refer it to a neurologist. The final diagnosis is fucosidosis, with a grave prognosis. The dog will be dead before a year of age, but not before getting progressively more impaired than it is now. The owner asks the specialist how this could have been avoided and is informed of a simple blood test that should have been performed on the parents of the affected dog, which would have identified them as carriers.

The owner now has a dog that was accepted as a family member, which will die shortly, will incur a huge veterinary bill, and has little hope for satisfactorily resolving the problem. Should the owner have expected more from the veterinarian selected to do the post-purchase examination? Should the veterinarian have informed the owner that he or she was examining the animal only for obvious problems the dog had at that point in time, and not for problems that may be prevalent in the breed but not yet evident?

The problem was driven home to the American public in an exposé that appeared in *Time* magazine on December 12, 1994. The correspondent concluded that up to 25% of the 20 million purebred dogs in the country—1 in 4—were afflicted with a serious genetic problem, with costs of about $1 billion annually in veterinary bills and lost revenues from stillborn pups that couldn't be sold (583).

At least 13 states now have pet lemon laws that give purchasers of dogs (or cats) some recourse against people who sell dogs (or cats) that develop genetic problems of which the purchasers were not advised. Typically, the liability is limited to the cost of the animal. Once veterinarians become involved, however, the total costs of diagnosis and treatment are often many times the cost of the animal itself. Whether veterinarians share any culpability when they perform post-purchase examinations without advising owners of breed-related problems is something that should be discussed and settled within the profession, and hopefully not in the courts.

Currently, most veterinarians are not involved in the pet selection process until after the fact. This puts them and their clients at a distinct disadvantage. If a client asks, "Where can I get a good cocker

Miniature Schnauzer Adoption Questionnaire (©Pet Health Initiative, 1999)

Information to be Provided by Seller

Name of Business ____________________ Telephone ____________________

Address ____________________

Name of Dog ____________________

Date of Birth __________ Weight __________ Color __________

Identification: Microchip implant __________ Tattoo __________ Collar/Tag__________

Registration (e.g., AKC, CKC)____________________

Purpose: Show Quality______ Pet Quality ______ Breeding ______ Non-breeding ______

Question	Yes	No	Don't Know	Documents provided
Any evidence of problem behaviors in this animal?	______	______	______	______
Is there a history of problem behaviors in the family?	______	______	______	______
Any evidence of allergies in this animal?	______	______	______	______
Is there a history of allergies in the family?	______	______	______	______
Any evidence of urolithiasis in this animal?	______	______	______	______
Is there a history of urolithiasis in the family?	______	______	______	______
Any evidence of hypothyroidism in this animal?	______	______	______	______
Is there a history of hypothyroidism in the family?	______	______	______	______
Any evidence of comedo syndrome in this animal?	______	______	______	______
Is there a history of comedo syndrome in the family?	______	______	______	______
Any evidence of hyperlipidemia in this animal?	______	______	______	______
Is there a history of hyperlipidemia in the family?	______	______	______	______
Any evidence of pancreatitis in this animal?	______	______	______	______
Is there a history of pancreatitis in the family?	______	______	______	______
Is this animal free of orthopedic diseases (OFA, GDC, PennHip)?	______	______	______	______
Are parents registered with OFA or GDC?	______	______	______	______
Is this animal free of congenital heart disease?	______	______	______	______
Are both parents free of heart disease (OFA)?	______	______	______	______
Is this animal free of heritable eye diseases (CERF)?	______	______	______	______
Are both parents registered with CERF?	______	______	______	______
Is this animal free of von Willebrand disease?	______	______	______	______
Are both parents free of von Willebrand disease?	______	______	______	______
Has this animal received regular veterinary evaluations?	______	______	______	______
Any irregularities determined by veterinary evaluation?	______	______	______	______
Are all vaccinations current?	______	______	______	______
Did the veterinarian perform fecal evaluation for parasites?	______	______	______	______
Is this animal now free of parasites?	______	______	______	______
Was the heartworm test negative and is this animal on preventative therapy?	______	______	______	______
Medical/behavioral money-back guarantee provided?	______	______	______	______

Signature ____________________ Date __________

Table 10 Risk of Being a Carrier if Related to an Affected Dog (AR Trait)

Category	Relationship	Degree of Relationship	Minimum Carrier Risk
1	Parent, Progeny	1	100%
2	Full sibling	1	66.6%
3	Grandparents, aunts, uncles, half-siblings, grandchildren	2	50%
4	Niece, nephew	2	33.3%
5	Great grandparent, first cousin, half aunts & uncles, great-grandchildren	3	25%
6	Great-great grandparent, first cousin once removed, second cousins	—	12.5%
7	Great-great-great-grandparent, first cousin twice removed, third cousins	—	6.25%

spaniel?" few veterinarians take this opportunity to offer preemptive genetic counseling. On their own, few prospective dog owners know where to look for a dog or what questions to ask. All too often, they purchase a dog with "papers," mistakenly believing that this is some certificate of genetic superiority, a "Good Housekeeping Seal of Approval." Most people would be genuinely surprised to learn that this dog could be blind, have epilepsy, be dying of a lysosomal storage disease, and bear little resemblance to the breed it is supposed to represent, and would still qualify to get "papers." They are expecting assurances from "papers" while the registries are only doing what they are mandated to do—to register purebred dogs produced as offspring of registered purebred dogs.

Veterinarians often are at a loss when clients inquire as to where they might buy a problem-free purebred dog. Though the standard answer is often "a good breeder," we must appreciate that prospective dog owners have no way of differentiating a good breeder from a bad one. Because the goal is to match owners with healthy, well-adjusted dogs, veterinarians probably should spend more time on objective criteria by which clients can select dogs, rather than the source of dogs that owners select. If clients are educated to buy dogs only from sources that focus strongly on health and behavioral issues, these same clients become better and more informed consumers, regardless of where they shop.

At present, we have a great need for veterinarians to take a firm stand in favor of routine genetic counseling, and to learn everything there is to learn about new methods of testing and treatment. Blaming breeders or registries is not the answer, especially as they are now funding most of the current research, providing DNA samples for breed-related databases, and encouraging education in this area. In actuality, if veterinarians aren't careful, they'll be busy playing catch-up to client breeders who have a better knowledge of genetic developments in their particular breeds!

Risk Calculations

During the course of genetic counseling, veterinarians often are asked to comment on the risks of certain matings. For example, a breeder may want to know the risk of progressive retinal atrophy in her pups from the mating of a specific stud and bitch. If the mode of inheritance is known for the breed, and carrier status can be determined by family history or diagnostic testing, the assessment is simple. If the condition is inherited as an autosomal recessive trait in the breed and both potential parents are known to be carriers, it is simple to advise that each pup has a 25% chance of being affected.

If we don't know the carrier status of each potential parent, we often can use statistics to give an approximation of the risk. For example, with an autosomal recessive trait, when an affected animal results, both parents must be obligate carriers of the trait. If a full sibling is affected but our animal of interest is not, there is a two-thirds chance that it is a carrier and a one-third chance that it is not. A table (see Table 10) can be used to determine carrier risk depending on the relationship to dogs that are known to be affected.

The probability of producing a homozygous recessive (affected) puppy also can be calculated from looking at known carriers and affected animals

Table 11 Generational Factors in Producing Affected Pups

Generation	Factor (Affected)	Carrier (Factor)
1	1	0.5
2	0.5	.25
3	0.25	.125
4	0.125	0.0625
5	0.0625	0.03125

Generation	1	2	3	4

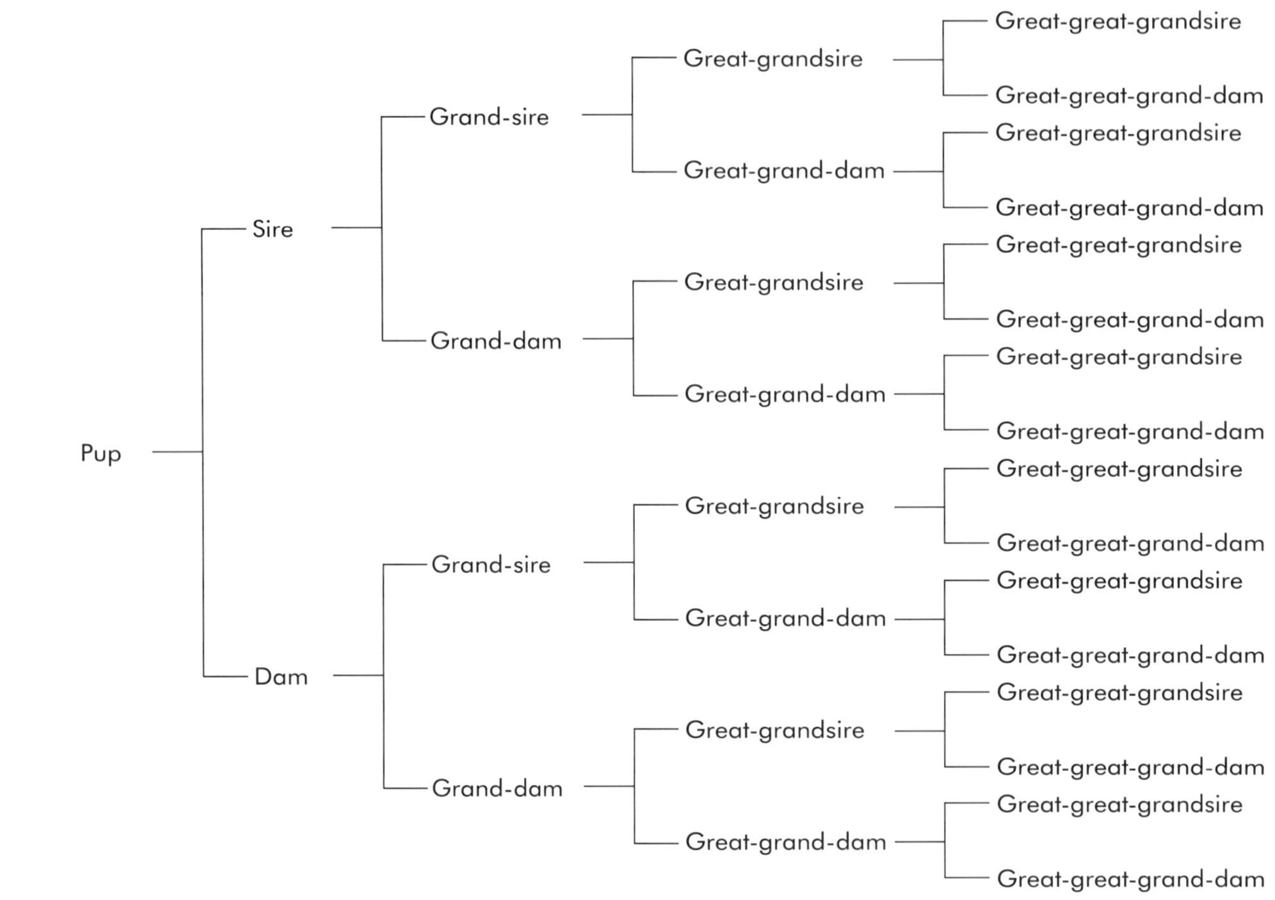

in the pedigree. Depending on how far back in the pedigree you need to look to find affected and carrier animals, you can produce a rough measure of the likelihood of producing an affected pup. One factor is assigned if an individual of the pedigree is affected, depending on generation, and half that amount is assigned if the individual of the pedigree is a carrier (see Table 11).

For example, if a pup has an affected uncle on its father's side but his grandfather appeared clinically normal, that grandfather (generation 2) must have been a carrier (0.25). On the pup's mother's side, her maternal great-grandfather (generation 4) was affected (factor 0.125). The risk of the pup being affected is $0.25 \times 0.125 = 0.03125$, or just over 3%.

Sometimes the situation is more complicated and simple statistics cannot be used to accurately predict risk. In these cases, risk still can be approximated using Bayesian risk calculations. This calculation has four steps. (1) Specify the prior risk of the potential breeding animal being a carrier, given a normal appearance. For autosomal recessive traits, this would be two-thirds chance of being a carrier and one-third chance that it is not a carrier. For autosomal dominant traits, there would be a 50% possibility of carrier status and 50% chance of not being a carrier. (2) Determine conditional probabil-

Table 12 Bayesian Risk Calculation

	Carrier	Not Carrier
Prior	1/2 (dominant) or 2/3 (recessive) (a)	1/2 or 1/3 (b)
Conditional	Disease-specific (c)	Disease-specific (d)
Joint	a × c (e)	b × d (f)
Posterior	e/e+f	f/e+f

Table 13 Probabilities of Being a Carrier Using Bayesian Risk Calculation

	Carrier	Not Carrier
Prior	0.5	0.5
Conditional	1–0.80 = 0.20	1–0.14 = 0.986
Joint	0.5 × .20=.10	.5 × .986= .493
Posterior	.10/.593=.17	.493/.593=0.83

ities based on known data such as disease prevalence, test results, and age of onset. Given this information and family history, it is important to determine all possible genetic configurations for individuals in the pedigree. (3) Multiply all probabilities together for each configuration to yield the joint probability for that configuration. (4) Calculate posterior probabilities from these joint probabilities. Each posterior probability has a denominator, which is the same for all posterior probabilities (the sum of all joint probabilities); the numerator is the sum of the joint probabilities for each specific genetic configuration. Table 12 summarizes the results.

For example, a breeder brings to the hospital two 3-month-old pups from a bitch with cutaneous asthenia. One of the pups is obviously affected and, as the sire is normal, you conclude that this pup is a carrier. You don't have positive confirmation of the mode of inheritance, but most cases are believed to be autosomal dominant, and electron microscopy and biochemical testing of dermal collagen are beyond the financial means of this breeder. A literature search suggests that about 80% of carrier pups show evidence of the disease by 12 weeks of age. The chances of a spontaneous mutation causing cutaneous asthenia is approximately 1 in 20,000 (q^2). This translates to a population carrier frequency of 0.014. The breeder wants to know the likelihood that the normal-appearing pup will eventually manifest cutaneous asthenia.

The first caution to give the breeder is that the assessment is only as good as the assumptions used in the calculations. Accordingly, given that the pup looks normal but has an affected sibling, you reason that the pup could either be a carrier that is late in manifesting the condition or is homozygous for the normal allele. The prior risk, thus, is 0.5 for each possibility. We do know, however, that 80% of carrier pups would have shown evidence by now, so that means there is still a 20% conditional probability that the pup is a carrier.

In calculating the conditional probability that it is not a carrier, we also must consider the likelihood of a spontaneous mutation—which is approximately 1 in 20,000. From this number the carrier frequency can be calculated. According to the Hardy-Weinberg law, this is 2pq. If the chances of a spontaneous mutation are 1/20,000 (q^2), then

$$q = 0.007,$$

$$p = 1 - q\ (0.993) \text{ and}$$

$$2pq = (2)(0.993)(0.007) = 0.014.$$

This is the odds of the pup being a carrier, so 1 – 0.014 or 0.986 is the conditional probability of not being a carrier. The joint probability for each option then is calculated by multiplying the prior and conditional probabilities for those options. Finally, the posterior probability, which is most likely to be accurate given all the possibilities, is the joint probability for each option divided by all the joint probabilities for all options. In this case, given the assumptions and probabilities, the normal-appearing pup has a 17% chance of being a carrier and an 83% chance of not being a carrier (i.e., homozygous normal). This is illustrated in Table 13.

Practice Makes Perfect

Case 1: A cocker spaniel breeder takes your advice and performs DNA testing for phosphofructokinase deficiency on a prospective breeding pair. The potential sire is clear, but the bitch is determined to be a carrier. What are the odds that this mating will result in affected pups?

Because the sire is clear, he must be homozygous for the normal allele (PP). The bitch, as a carrier, has the heterozygous genotype Pp. A mating of these two would produce roughly 50% homozygotes (PP) and 50% carriers (Pp), but *no* affected individuals (pp). Given the new technology, which allows genotypic determination for this trait in cocker spaniels, the occurrence of affected individuals can be completely eliminated even when it may be difficult to completely eliminate the recessive allele itself from a population.

Case 2: A Westie breeder is hoping to raise pups without craniomandibular osteopathy (CMO), an autosomal recessive trait. She considers herself fortunate in that the sire she selected has no direct history of the trait. Only a brother of the grandfather of that dog has developed CMO. On the bitch's side, an aunt was affected. What are the chances of this union creating a pup with CMO?

In this case, on the father's side there is an obligate carrier three generations back. On the mother's side there is an obligate carrier two generations back. Using the multiplication factors provided, the probability is 0.25 × 0.125 or 3.125%.

Case 3: A Norwegian elkhound was a grandson of a bitch that produced *erd* in some of her pups, an autosomal recessive form of progressive retinal atrophy (PRA) in the breed. The breeder would like to use this dog as her foundation stud but wants to be sure he isn't a carrier of the trait. She breeds him to a known affected bitch, which produces four pups, all pronounced "normal" at 1 year of age by a veterinary ophthalmologist. The breeder wants to know the likelihood that he is not a carrier of PRA, given this breeding data.

Because the dog is obviously not affected, he could be either homozygous dominant or a carrier. In this test mating, in a litter of *n* pups, there is 0.5^n chance of a carrier remaining undetected. From the chart presented earlier, we can see that after producing four normal pups, there is a 93.8% chance that he is a homozygote, and a 6.2% chance that he is a carrier. If necessary, one more litter can be used to remove almost all doubt.

Case 4: An American car-chasing terrier (ACCT) breeder requests a consultation on preventing the rare autosomal recessive disease Quasimoto's parathyroiditis, which often results in the dog's death by 9 months of age,. The potential sire's full brother died of this disease at 6 months of age (confirmed at necropsy) but shows no evidence of the disease himself (now 2 years of age). The bitch selected for the breeding has no family history of the disorder. The condition has a population frequency of 1:40,000. A carrier detection test is available, with a false positive rate of 10% and a false negative rate of 6%. The potential sire tests negative, and the bitch tests positive. What are the risks for an individual pup to develop Quasimoto's parathyroiditis?

In this case, we assume that the potential sire is not affected but both parents must be carriers (Qq) if the dog's brother was affected (qq). When two carriers are bred, the typical ratios expected are ¼ affected, ½ carriers, and ¼ clear. His prior risk, based on this alone and assuming he is not affected, is two-thirds (0.66) that he's a carrier (Qq) and one-third (0.33) that he's not a carrier (QQ). The prior risk for the bitch with no family history is determined based on disease frequency, not family history. With a disease frequency (q^2) of 1:40,000 (0.000025), q must equal the square root of 0.000025, which is 0.005. Since p + q = 1, p = 0.995 and the population carrier frequency is 2pq or 2 (.005) (0.995) ≈ 0.01. Therefore, her prior risk is only 0.01 that she's a carrier and 0.99 that she is not a carrier.

We have more information to consider, however, because we have to evaluate this prior risk in light of our diagnostic testing. For this, we calculate conditional risk based on the chances of false test results. There is still a 6% chance that the sire is a carrier (false negative rate) even with a negative test result but a 90% chance that he is not a carrier (given a false positive rate of 10%). There is a 94% chance that the bitch is a carrier (given a false negative rate of 6%) and a 10% chance that she is not a carrier (false positive rate).

Sire

	Carrier	Not Carrier
Prior	2/3	1/3
Conditional	.06	.90
Joint	0.04	0.30
Posterior	0.118	

Dam

	Carrier	Not Carrier
Prior	0.01	0.99
Conditional	0.94	0.10
Joint	0.0094	0.099
Posterior	0.087	

Bayesian Risk Calculation (*Source:* Hodge, 1998)

The joint probabilities then are calculated by multiplying each prior risk by its respective conditional risk. In this case, the sire has a joint risk of 0.04 ($2/3 \times 0.06$) that he's a carrier and 0.30 ($1/3 \times 0.9$) that he's not a carrier. The bitch has a joint risk of 0.0094 (0.01×0.94) that she's a carrier and 0.099 (0.99×0.1) that she's not a carrier. The posterior risk for each animal then is calculated by dividing the joint risk of being a carrier by the joint risks of being either a carrier or a noncarrier. In this case, the sire has a posterior risk of 0.118, calculated as 0.04/(0.04 + 0.30) and the bitch has a posterior risk of 0.087, calculated as 0.0094/(.0094 + 0.0990).

So what are the chances that this mating would produce a pup with Quasimoto's parathyroiditis? Because the mating of two carriers would be expected to produce an affected pup about 25% of the time, the risk of a pup's having the disease from that mating would be calculated by multiplying the posterior risk that the sire is a carrier (0.118) by the posterior risk that the bitch is a carrier (0.087) $\times$ ¼ = 0.0026.

THE FUTURE

With the advancement of the dog genome project, disease genes are being detected regularly. Over the next several years, many diseases will be detectable with virtual certainty, thanks to molecular genetics. Veterinarians will have to embrace genetics as a "new" discipline within their practices, just to keep up with advances. In time, the costs associated with DNA testing will come down, these tests will be used more routinely, and prevention of genetic diseases that have plagued dogdom will become a realistic goal. The next step will be to use this technology to treat the animals in which disease could not be prevented.

Gene therapy involves the transfer of normal genes into the cells of individuals with genetic disease. This will most likely involve somatic cells rather than germ cell lines. Cloned genes will most likely be transferred via viral (probably retroviral) vectors. The normal structural gene will be cloned into the viral genome and introduced to somatic cells, then introduced into the body. The first diseases to be treated will most likely be recessively inherited inborn errors of metabolism and localized conditions, such as progressive retinal atrophy. Even though gene therapy has had some limited applications in humans and dogs, major technological hurdles remain before they become mainstream medicine. In any case, the next decade will be an exciting time to be practicing veterinary medicine!

CHAPTER 1

Cardiovascular System Disorders

Genetic diseases of the cardiopulmonary system are some of the best studied in veterinary medicine. Although congenital heart disease accounts for less than 10% of the clinically significant cardiovascular diseases diagnosed in small animal patients, it is the most common cause of cardiovascular disease in animals less than 1 year of age (691). Most diagnoses are based on auscultation and echocardiography.

AORTIC STENOSIS

Subaortic stenosis (SAS) is a congenital heart disease involving a narrowing or stricture just below the aortic valve. The stricture is usually an abnormal fibrous ring of tissue that results in a reduction of blood flow pumped from the heart. This condition causes the cardiac muscle to overwork, and thereby increases the oxygen needs of the heart itself (523). The result can be arrhythmias and, potentially, sudden death. Congenital SAS is observed most often as an inherited trait in larger breeds including the Newfoundland (106) and is strongly suspected to be inherited in Bouvier des Flandres, boxers, bull terriers, English bulldogs, German shepherd dogs, German shorthaired pointers, golden retrievers, Great Danes, rottweilers, and Samoyeds (126, 575, 645, 691, 789, 1020). The pattern of transmission is most compatible with an autosomal dominant trait with variable expressivity (576), at least in the Newfoundland (789).

Most puppies with SAS do not develop signs of illness until approximately 6 to 18 months of age. While many cases are asymptomatic, clinical signs observed may include coughing, fainting (syncope), exercise intolerance, irregular heart rate, and lethargy. Chronic turbulence and high-velocity blood flow past the aortic valve can predispose a dog to infective endocarditis (377). A pronounced cardiac murmur will typically be heard during auscultation. The systolic murmur is loudest over the left fourth intercostal space near the costochondral junction and radiating into the ascending aorta and forward over the carotid arteries (106). The murmur may also be prominent over the right cranial thorax. Murmur intensity and duration are significantly correlated with aortic flow velocity (560).

The diagnosis of congenital SAS is based upon physical examination (i.e., heart murmur), radiography, electrocardiography, and echocardiography (Figure 1-1). Echocardiography may reveal abnormal subvalvular or aortic valves, and there may be sudden acceleration of blood flow in the left ventricular outflow tract with turbulent, high-velocity systolic flow across the aortic valve and, often, concurrent aortic regurgitation. Cardiac catheterization with blood pressure measurements and angiography can also help determine the severity of the defect.

Treatment of SAS is difficult and often discouraging because many of these dogs either die suddenly or develop heart failure. Acute death, often without previous clinical signs, commonly occurs at 1 to 3 years of age. Surgical correction of the problem is seldom attempted because a heart/lung bypass procedure is recommended (717). The use of balloon valvuloplasty catheters has been suggested to relieve the problem, thus alleviating the need for the expensive and risky surgery (247). The results of this procedure are not as good in dogs as in humans, and the practice has been largely discontinued. The reason is that many stenotic lesions in dogs have substantial obstruction below the level of the valve. They open with surgery but tend to reobstruct within 3 months in most cases. Prevention is the best approach and can best be accomplished with genetic counseling. Animals with a family history of SAS should not be used in

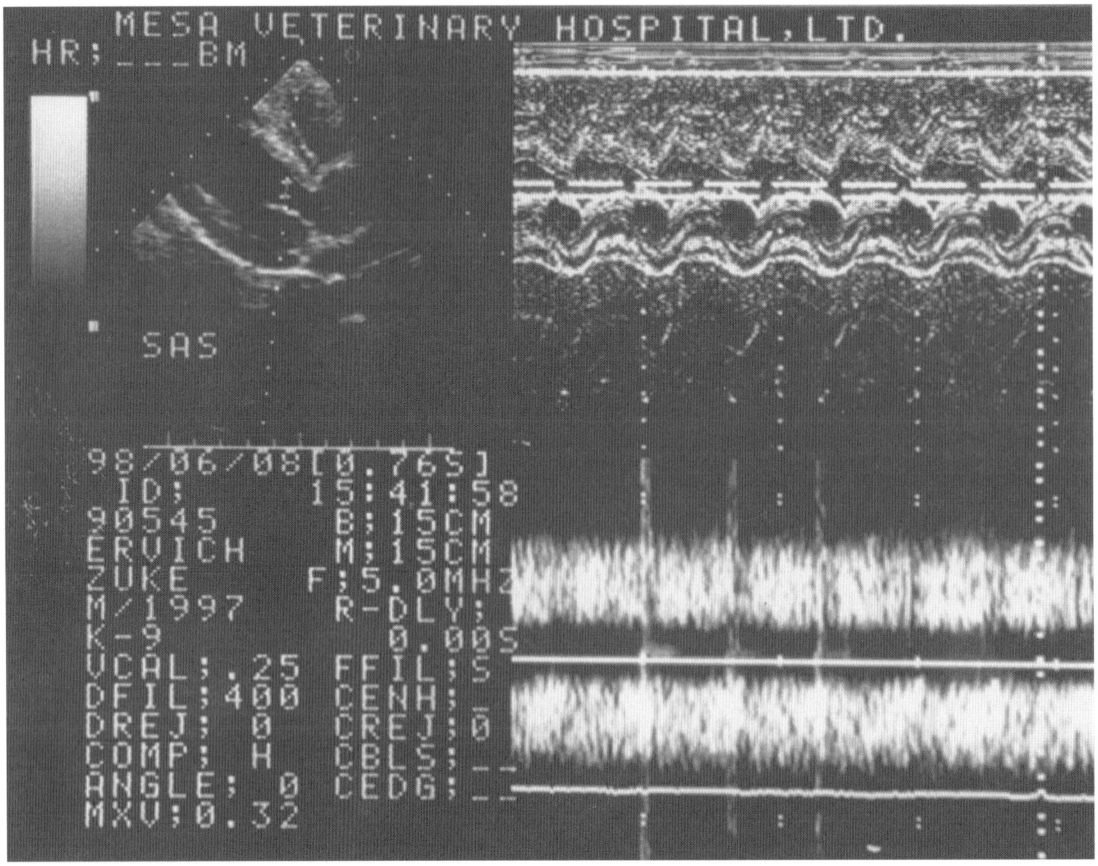

Figure 1-1 **Echocardiogram demonstrating subaortic stenosis**
Courtesy of Dr. Kenneth Jeffery, Mesa Veterinary Hospital, Mesa, Arizona

breeding programs, especially in breeds with a high incidence of the condition.

ATRIAL SEPTAL DEFECT

Atrial septal defect is a congenital cardiac anomaly resulting in communication through the interatrial septum. It is most commonly reported in the boxer, Doberman pinscher, Old English sheepdog, and Samoyed (375). Currently, a genetic basis for the disorder has not been documented. Clinical signs may be absent with small defects, or may include exercise intolerance, dyspnea, and syncope. The diagnosis is suspected when auscultation reveals a systolic murmur over the pulmonic and tricuspid valves and is confirmed by echocardiography. Severely affected animals develop and are treated for congestive heart failure.

CARDIOMYOPATHY

Dilated cardiomyopathy (DCM) refers to a defect of the heart muscle in which the heart muscle becomes thin and stretched, much like a balloon. In this condition, the heart is not an effective pump, and eventually affected dogs succumb to heart failure. The condition is seen most commonly in the Airedale (1036), American cocker spaniel (674, 690), boxer (126, 690, 1036), Dalmatian (333), Doberman pinscher (139, 985, 1036), English cocker spaniel (236, 1000, 1036), golden retriever (126), Great Dane (674, 690), Irish wolfhound (674), Newfoundland (674, 1035, 1036), Old English sheepdog (126), St. Bernard (1036), Scottish deerhound (690, 965), and standard poodle (1036). In all, dilated cardiomyopathy has been reported in at least 38 breeds (1036, 1037). Doberman pinschers are affected more than all other breeds combined, and the majority of dogs with DCM are males (138). It is also apparent that many Dobermans with the condition are linebred, and involvement of related dogs is common (139). A familial trend has been documented in the boxer (374). Therefore, there are at least two dog breeds (boxer, Doberman pinscher) in which the condition is believed to be familial (676). Dilated cardiomyopathy is also recognized as a distinct entity in young Portuguese water dogs (226), and

OFA Registry

The Orthopedic Foundation for Animals (OFA) maintains a heart disease registry, and certification can be issued to an animal of at least 12 months of age. Provisional certification for dogs under 12 months of age is possible, but full certification requires subsequent examination at 12 months of age or older. The breed registry number indicates the age at evaluation and the qualifications of the examiner (e.g., cardiologist, specialist, practitioner). Careful clinical examination with critical cardiac auscultation is used for screening purposes, and echocardiography with Doppler is the preferred method for establishing a definitive diagnosis. The OFA provides details regarding examination, identification, and classification of congenital heart diseases. For more details on the OFA, see Appendix.

research is currently underway to study the molecular and genetic basis of the disorder in this breed.

Deficiencies of myocardial troponin-T and creatinine kinase MB isoenzyme may play a role in the energy deficiency characteristic of myocardial failure in dogs with dilated cardiomyopathy (780). A respiratory chain defect of myocardial mitochondria may be involved (652). Some evidence also suggests that autoimmunity plays a role in the development of cardiomyopathy. Approximately 30% of English cocker spaniels with cardiomyopathy had circulating mitochondrial antibody, and there is a strong association between the disorder and a particular complement C_4 phenotype (236). Hypothyroidism does not appear to be a contributing factor to the development of cardiomyopathy, at least not in Doberman pinschers (178).

Although a genetic tendency is suspected, long-term studies are not yet available. In human medicine, it has been reported that about 25% of patients with cardiomyopathy have a genetic cause. In some breeds, especially the Doberman pinscher and American cocker spaniel, a nutritional mechanism has also been implicated. Boxers seem to have an autosomal genetic association, likely dominant in nature, with incomplete penetrance. Genetic analysis is under way, with the hope that a gene marker may someday allow for screening of breeding pairs.

The specific cardiomyopathy found in boxers is characterized by severe ventricular arrhythmias, and affected dogs may die suddenly; others develop more progressive congestive heart failure. Three different clinical types are often reported: Type I, which is typically asymptomatic but with cardiac arrhythmia; Type II, characterized by syncope or episodic weakness with or without ventricular arrhythmia, and; Type III, characterized by the clinical signs of heart failure (676). Continuous ambulatory electrocardiography (Holter monitoring) is sometimes necessary to confirm the diagnosis.

In Doberman pinschers, cardiomyopathy is characterized by cardiac rhythm disturbances, ventricular dilatation, systolic dysfunction, and myocardial failure (676). Doberman pinschers with cardiomyopathy often have episodes of ventricular tachycardia. If these last more than 30 seconds, the dog is at risk of dying suddenly (140). In cocker spaniels, a systolic murmur or a gallop rhythm may be auscultated.

On echocardiography, left ventricular and left atrial dilation are common, as is decreased systolic function (674). Larger left ventricular volumes are detected in Dalmatians, compared to the other breeds (333).

Some boxers and Doberman pinschers with dilated cardiomyopathy have a defect in L-Carnitine (an amino acid) levels in the heart muscle (513, 514). These dogs occasionally respond to carnitine supplementation. Although the underlying cause of dilated cardiomyopathy in these dogs remains unknown, an inherited defect resulting in carnitine deficiency of the heart muscle may be important, especially in boxers. Whether this is true in other breeds has yet to be determined.

Studies in the American cocker spaniel seem to suggest that taurine (another amino acid) may be implicated, as it is in the feline form of the disease (343). Supplementation of both taurine and carnitine is recommended in this breed, and though myocardial function may not return to normal, it may improve enough to allow discontinuation of

Cardiomyopathy

Cardiomyopathy is common in the dog and the vast majority of cases reported are dilated cardiomyopathy. Hypertrophic cardiomyopathy is quite rare in dogs, but a hereditary form has been reported in pointer dogs (126).

Most American cocker spaniels with cardiomyopathy have plasma taurine concentrations below 50 nmol/mL. Supplementation of both taurine and L-Carnitine are often recommended in this breed.

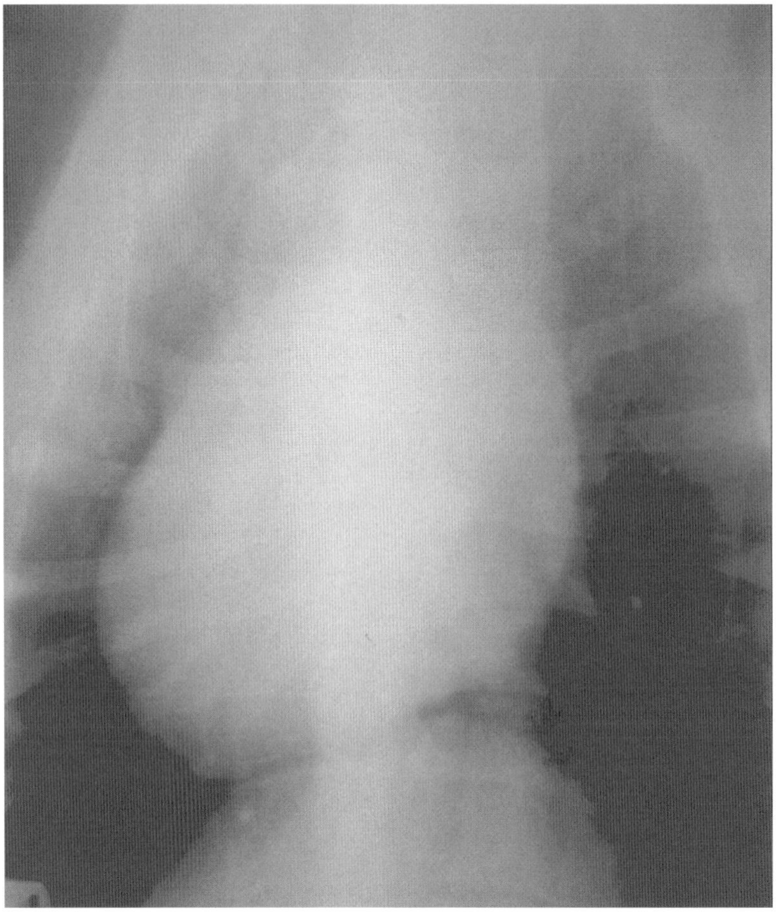

Figure 1-2 Chest radiograph of a dog with cardiomyopathy
Courtesy of Dr. Kenneth Jeffery, Mesa Veterinary Hospital, Mesa, Arizona

cardiovascular drug therapy and allow a reasonable quality of life in most dogs (529, 837). As if this isn't confusing enough, some researchers suspect that viruses might also be involved, because some research on humans indicates that this might be the case in people.

Early in the course of the disease, affected animals appear clinically normal. About 25% to 30% of Doberman pinschers with echocardiographic evidence of cardiomyopathy are completely asymptomatic (138). Only when the dogs show signs of heart failure do most owners seek veterinary attention. Early signs might include depression, coughing, exercise intolerance, weakness, respiratory distress, decreased appetite, and even fainting. In some breeds, especially the Doberman pinscher, sudden death may be the first clue that something was wrong (143). Thus, routine, thorough veterinary examinations are important, especially in the young and middle-aged adult. In some cases, the heart rate is increased, but radiographs, electrocardiograms (EKGs), and echocardiograms are required for definitive diagnosis (Figure 1-2).

Studies have also shown that most dogs (especially Doberman pinschers) with early cardiomyopathy have ventricular premature contractions (VPCs), evident on electrocardiograms, which are indicators of increased risk to developing actual cardiomyopathy. These VPCs may not be evident all the time when electrocardiograms are taken, so 24-hour studies with a Holter monitor are sometimes necessary, just as they are in people.

In addition, signal-averaged electrocardiography (SAECG) can be used to try to identify ventricular late potentials, which are seen in some patients with damaged myocardium (141). Although not foolproof, this is one method of identifying Dobermans at increased risk of dying suddenly but without overt evidence of congestive heart failure. For postmortem evaluation, the presence of attenuated wavy myocardial fibers is the best presumptive evidence that the dog suffered from cardiomyopathy (1034).

Digoxin is often used to treat the condition, and sometimes so are beta-1 blockers, calcium channel blockers, and vasodilators. L-Carnitine is helpful in some cases, especially in the boxer,

American cocker spaniel, and Doberman pinscher breeds. Taurine and carnitine supplementation is helpful in some American cocker spaniels. Coenzyme Q10 seems to be a valuable nutritional adjunct to many cases of dilated cardiomyopathy. Antiarrhythmic therapy with drugs such as sotalol and procainamide is important in the boxer (675).

Affected animals should be excluded from breeding programs, even though they may not be diagnosed until after they have already been mated several times. Family history is important when selecting which animals should be used for breeding. Until more is learned about the heritability of the condition, to make breeding recommendations regarding parents and siblings of affected animals is premature.

CHRONIC MITRAL VALVULAR DISEASE (ENDOCARDIOSIS)

Chronic mitral valvular disease is the most common acquired cardiac abnormality of dogs. It is a degenerative process, most typically involving the atrioventricular valves and resulting in mitral regurgitation, rupture of the chordae tendineae, and potentially, left-sided heart failure. There is some similarity to mitral valve prolapse in humans. An underlying connective tissue defect is postulated. There is thought to be a genetic tendency to experience degeneration of the collagen in the heart valves. The insufficiency increases in frequency and severity with advancing age, and chronic mitral valve insufficiency is estimated to be present in more than half of dogs 9 years of age and older.

The canine condition is most commonly reported in the Afghan hound, American cocker spaniel, beagle, Boston terrier, bull terrier, Chihuahua, dachshund, fox terrier, German shepherd dog, Great Dane, Japanese chin, Maltese, miniature poodle, miniature schnauzer, and Yorkshire terrier (126, 228, 376, 627). In the Cavalier King Charles spaniel, 30% to 50% may be affected by 5 years of age, and development is believed to be a polygenic threshold trait with gender influencing threshold levels (228, 1019). Males are affected more often and more severely than females.

Mild forms of valvular insufficiency likely result in few, if any, clinical signs early in the course of the condition. In most cases, the clinical presentation is prolonged over years until valvular degeneration eventually results in mitral regurgitation and left-sided heart failure. The onset, however, can be rapid and severe if the chordae tendineae rupture.

Many older pets have mild heart murmurs that develop as a consequence of aging. Early valvular insufficiency is usually a clinical diagnosis based on detecting a heart murmur. In the early stages, few, if any, changes are noticed on radiographs, electrocardiograms (ECGs), or echocardiograms. As impairment increases, echocardiography will eventually detect thickened heart valves and dilated heart chambers.

Because valve replacement surgeries are not routinely performed in dogs, most treatment options involve a variety of medications. In the earliest stages, the dogs are not treated—not even with very-low-salt diets, although moderate sodium restriction is probably desirable. Eventually, many different drugs are needed to combat the effects of heart enlargement and impending heart failure.

Making breeding recommendations for dogs with chronic valvular disease is difficult, as it is an acquired disease that typically isn't manifested until later in life, when an animal has likely finished its breeding career already. Most Cavalier King Charles spaniels that develop the condition do so by 5 years of age, and breeding stock preferably can be screened at this age before being used for breeding. Otherwise, it is best to select breeding animals based on a family history of no chronic valvular disease for several generations.

Endocardiosis

Chronic mitral valvular disease appears to be polygenic in nature and some breeds have an extremely high incidence of the condition. For instance, in the Cavalier King Charles spaniel, 30%–50% of dogs may be affected by five years of age. Family history can be critical to successful genetic counseling, as can waiting until animals are older before breeding them.

FEMORAL ARTERY OCCLUSION

Common human conditions, such as arteriosclerosis, atherosclerosis, and thrombosis, are actually rare in dogs. Nevertheless, thrombosis of the femoral arteries in the Cavalier King Charles spaniel is considered a primary form of vascular disease rather than just an extension of thromboembolism (128). Because this breed is also prone to mitral valve disease, an underlying connective tissue disorder may be present that renders the Cavalier King Charles spaniel susceptible to cardiovascular disease. Fortunately, the condition rarely results in any clinical signs, as dogs have extensive collateral circulation in their hind limbs via lateral circumflex femoral and distal caudal femoral arteries. The diagnosis is suspected when clinicians detect a weak or absent femoral pulse in one or both hind legs. The condition seems to be familial but with no clear mode of inheritance determined to date. Affected dogs should not be bred, but there is insufficient information to make breeding recommendations for other family members.

HYPERTENSION

High blood pressure, or hypertension, has been reported in dogs. Although the primary form, essential hypertension, accounts for more than 90% of human cases, secondary hypertension is much more common in dogs (121, 987). Still, essential hypertension in the dog is believed to have a polygenic mode of inheritance (970), and has been reported in the Labrador retriever and Siberian husky (79, 802).

Essential hypertension may not be apparent in the dog, or it may result in ocular, cardiac, or central nervous system abnormalities (987). The diagnosis is confirmed by determining elevated systolic or diastolic pressures by direct or indirect methods (262). Antihypertensive drugs used with humans have been used successfully in dogs. Affected animals should not be used for breeding, but there is insufficient information to make breeding recommendations for other family members.

PATENT DUCTUS ARTERIOSUS (PDA)

Patent ductus arteriosus (PDA) is the most common congenital heart defect in dogs. It is inherited as a polygenic threshold trait with a high rate of heritability in some breeds (106, 576). This means that the trait is controlled by a number of different genes and has a threshold, although the degree of patency can vary from a large patent ductus to a blind-ended diverticulum.

This defect occurs when normal fetal communication between the nonfunctional lungs and the aorta fails to close after birth. This results in blood being shunted into the pulmonary artery and overperfusing the lungs. At the same time, the rest of the body is not getting adequate circulation.

Breeds at increased risk include the bichon frisé, Chihuahua, collie, English springer spaniel, keeshond, Kerry blue terrier, Maltese, miniature poodle, Pomeranian, Shetland sheepdog, toy poodle, and Yorkshire terrier (126, 576). Females with this condition outnumber males by a three-to-one margin (126, 127). PDA appears to be transmitted as a genetic trait in Australian border collies (181).

Although most puppies with PDA show no clinical signs early in life, a heart murmur is detected upon first examination. The characteristic machinery murmur is loudest high in the left axillary region on the left side of the thorax over the craniodorsal cardiac base (106). Other puppies may develop acute heart failure and have difficulty in breathing, show exercise intolerance, or develop a cough. Even though most dogs with PDA are diagnosed early in life, some are not identified until they are adults. These dogs have changes similar to younger dogs but also are likely to have increased frequency of ventricular arrhythmias and reduced left ventricular shortening fraction (379).

The diagnosis of PDA is normally made by the characteristic murmur, electrocardiogram (EKG), chest radiographs, and ultrasound examination (Figure 1-3). With echocardiography, continuous retrograde flow is noted from the patent ductus arteriosus into the pulmonary artery. In most cases, PDA results in left-sided congestive heart failure. High pulmonary vascular resistance might result in high, right-to-left shunting, called "reversed PDA."

If there is evidence of cardiac failure, medical stabilization is necessary. Surgery is needed to correct the condition. The surgery should be done as soon as possible, ideally before 5 months of age, to minimize secondary damage to the heart and lungs. The success rate with surgery is over 90%, and, if completed early enough, the prognosis is excellent for a normal life expectancy. If uncorrected, the puppies usually do not live more than the first year or two, and 50% die within the first year of life (377).

An alternative to ligation is the use of intravascular embolization coils (307) or a vascular occlusion device (391), which can be introduced via percutaneous catheterization. A right-to-left shunting PDA (reversed PDA) should not be ligated, as the ductus acts as a relief valve, sparing the heart from right heart overload (199). Affected animals, and those with a prominent family history of PDA, should not be bred.

PULMONIC STENOSIS

Pulmonic stenosis (PS) refers to a stricture or incomplete opening through the pulmonic valve within the heart. In most cases, the underlying defect is pulmonic valve dysplasia (377). The valve is located between the right ventricle and the pulmonary artery, which delivers blood from the heart to the lungs. Many dogs with pulmonic stenosis are asymptomatic but do have a heart murmur. As they get older or if the condition is severe, they show evidence of exercise intolerance, fainting (syncope), coughing (rarely), or fluid accumulation within the body.

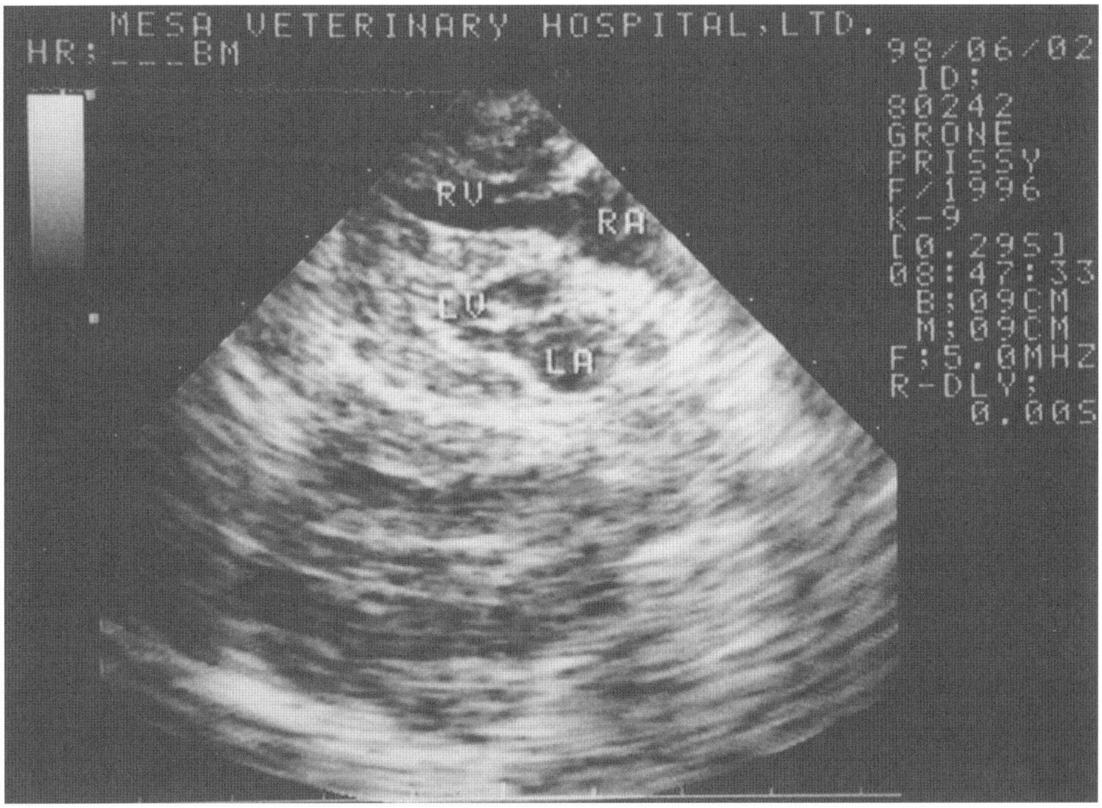

Figure 1-3 Echocardiogram demonstrating patent ductus arteriosus
Courtesy of Dr. Kenneth Jeffery, Mesa Veterinary Hospital, Mesa, Arizona

This condition is most prevalent in the American cocker spaniel (1029), beagle (106, 691), Chihuahua (106, 691), English bulldog (691, 1029), fox terrier (106, 316, 691), mastiff (1029), miniature schnauzer (691, 1029), Samoyed (691, 1029), and West Highland white terrier (126). Boykin spaniels may also be at increased risk. The condition does not seem to have a sex predilection except in English bulldogs, in which 80% are males (126). A hereditary component, likely polygenic, has been established in the beagle (106, 127) and English bulldog (1029). In the English bulldog, PS is associated with, and probably caused by, a coronary artery anomaly (127).

An accurate diagnosis of pulmonic stenosis is made through physical examination, radiographs, electrocardiogram (EKG), and either echocardiogram or cardiac catheterization. The systolic murmur is loudest over the left side of the thorax at the heart base, over the pulmonic valve area and pulmonary artery (106). On echocardiography, sudden acceleration of blood flow may be noted in the right ventricular outlet, with turbulent, high-velocity systolic flow across the pulmonary valve and into the main pulmonary artery. Abnormal valvular and subvalvular anatomy may be detected. Quite often, it is necessary to inject a contrast agent to visualize the defect, via angiography, on a series of radiographs.

Many cases of pulmonic stenosis are mild and don't require therapy. More severe blockages will result in heart failure and, therefore, require corrective surgery. One such technique is balloon valvuloplasty (353), which is effective in more than 50% of cases. If this approach isn't possible, surgery (valvulotomy or patch grafting) may be necessary. Care must be taken in surgical approaches in the English bulldog and perhaps the boxer, because of the potential anomalous coronary artery. Affected animals should not be used in breeding programs.

SICK SINUS SYNDROME

Sick sinus syndrome is a clinical syndrome associated with irregular discharge of the sinoatrial node, causing severe bradycardia. An underlying genetic susceptibility is suspected but undocumented, and the condition is seen most commonly in the miniature schnauzer (1005). It is characterized by periods of sinus arrest, which may be clinically apparent or may result in dizziness or syncope. Animals recover soon after the attack. Sudden death is a rare sequel.

The diagnosis can be confirmed by electrocardiography in which sinus bradycardia is associated with absent P waves and periodic supraventricular tachycardia. The treatment of choice is pacemaker implantation. Medical therapy may be needed to manage supraventricular dysrhythmias. Affected animals should not be bred.

TETRALOGY OF FALLOT

Tetralogy of Fallot, the most common cause of cyanosis in the dog, has four components: ventricular septal defect; overriding of the interventricular septum by the aorta; pulmonic stenosis; and right ventricular hypertrophy. This affliction is uncommon but is reported most often in the English bulldog (576, 645, 691), golden retriever (126), keeshond (127, 576, 645, 691), Labrador retriever (126), Siberian husky (126), toy poodle (126), and wire fox terrier (126). The condition is rare enough, though, that relative risks cannot be reliably assigned for these breeds. A hereditary component has been established in the keeshond (127, 822) as a severe manifestation of conotruncal hypoplasia, which is transmitted as an autosomal recessive trait with variable expressivity (576).

Affected dogs have right-to-left shunting of blood and develop chronic hypoxia, cyanosis, and exercise intolerance (377). Although some animals have no audible murmur, most display the systolic ejection murmur of pulmonic stenosis or a holosystolic murmur of the septal defect (106).

Definitive correction requires bypass surgery, but most cases are managed with palliative surgery to increase pulmonary perfusion, and medications to effect β-adrenergic blockage (1099). Total surgical correction requires cardiac bypass, which is not practical in most veterinary facilities.

TRICUSPID VALVE DYSPLASIA

Tricuspid dysplasia is a congenital abnormality of the right atrioventricular valve, characterized by anomalies of the chordae tendineae, papillary muscles, and valvular tissue. It is seen most commonly in the borzoi (712), boxer (126), German shepherd dog (126, 691), Great Dane (691, 712), Great Pyrenees (712), Irish setter (712), Labrador retriever (in which it is presumed familial) (691, 712), Newfoundland (712), Old English sheepdog (712), shih tzu (712), and Weimaraner (691, 712). Clinically, a murmur (systolic regurgitant murmur over tricuspid valve area) is apparent, but an electrocardiogram might not show classic evidence of right-sided heart enlargement. In the Labrador retriever, atrial tachyarrhythmias are most commonly seen (712).

The diagnostic test of choice is an echocardiogram. High-velocity retrograde systolic flow across the tricuspid valve into the right atrium may be noted. Abnormal anatomy or stenosis of the valve may be detected. Affected dogs are eventually treated for cardiac insufficiency and arrhythmias. It is best not to breed affected animals, especially Labrador retrievers, in which evidence of inheritance is the most convincing.

VASCULAR RING ANOMALIES

Vascular ring anomalies include persistent right aortic arch (which accounts for 95% of cases), aberrant right subclavian artery, aberrant left subclavian artery, double aortic arch, persistent right ductus arteriosus with normal aortic arch, aberrant intercostal arteries, and persistent right dorsal aorta (1066). Persistent right aortic arch is a developmental anomaly in which the aorta is formed by the right fourth aortic arch instead of the left fourth aortic arch. In about 40% of cases, a retroesophageal left subclavian artery is also present. It is most commonly reported in the American cocker spaniel (126), Boston terrier (1066), German shepherd dog (106, 1066), Great Dane (106, 209), and Irish setter (576, 1066).

In this anomaly, the esophagus and trachea are encircled by a vascular ring consisting of the aorta on the right, the pulmonary trunk and base of the heart ventrally, and the ligamentum arteriosum on the left (384). It is actually more of a gastrointestinal disorder than a heart disease because it often results in regurgitation and aspiration pneumonia rather than cardiac dysfunction (Figure 1-4).

The diagnosis is typically made via contrast esophagraphy, or angiography. Mild cases require no treatment, and more pronounced debility requires ligation and division of the ligamentum arteriosum (744). Accordingly, although this is a congenital disease, it is not included in the OFA congenital heart disease registry. Affected animals should not be bred.

VENTRICULAR ECTOPY

Ventricular ectopy includes premature ventricular complexes, ventricular bigeminal or trigeminal rhythms, ventricular couplets, and ventricular tachycardia. An inherited ectopy of German shepherd dogs that results in sudden cardiac death has been reported, but the mode of inheritance has not

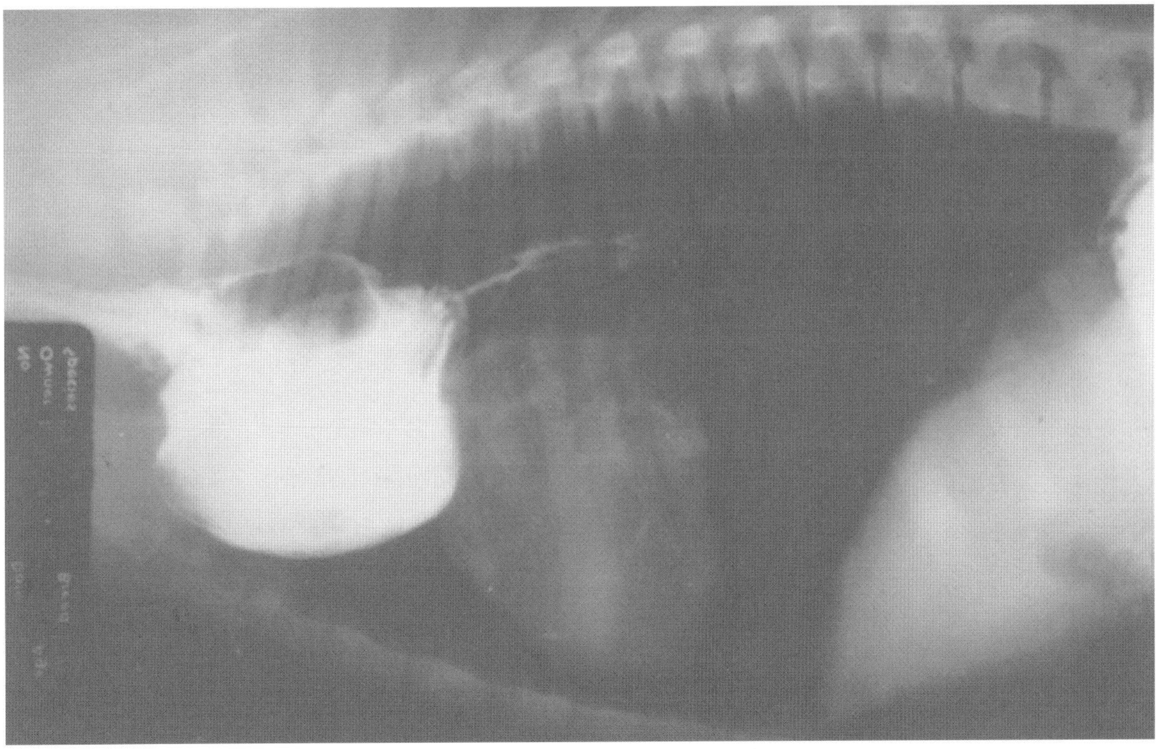

Figure 1-4 **Contrast study to demonstrate persistent right aortic arch (PRAA)**
Courtesy of Dr. Kenneth Jeffery, Mesa Veterinary Hospital, Mesa, Arizona

been identified (714). Breeding studies suggest that the disorder is not sex-linked and not a simple autosomal dominant trait (713).

Affected dogs develop arrhythmias by 12 months of age and typically die suddenly during this period (713). Dogs with ventricular tachycardia have the greatest risk of dying (714). Antiarrhythmic therapy is the cornerstone of treatment. Some dogs become less prone to arrhythmia as they get older. Regardless, no affected animals should be used in breeding programs.

VENTRICULAR SEPTAL DEFECT

Ventricular septal defect (VSD), a common cardiac abnormality, refers to an abnormal opening or hole in the wall between the left and right ventricles of the heart. This creates a communication between the two ventricles. English bulldogs are at least five times more likely than the general dog population to have ventricular septal defects (645). Other breeds at risk include the Brittany spaniel (126), chow chow (126), English springer spaniel (122), keeshond (122), Newfoundland (126), Samoyed (126), and Siberian husky (645).

In the English springer spaniel, VSD is believed to be inherited either as an autosomal dominant trait with incomplete penetrance or as a polygenic trait (122). In the keeshond, the condition is associated with malformation of the conotruncal septum, which is an autosomal recessive trait with variable expressivity (576). Affected animals have a pronounced heart murmur, but if the opening is small, the animal may be completely asymptomatic. If the hole is large, clinical signs usually develop by 1 year of age and include a cough, exercise intolerance, and poor growth.

The diagnosis is confirmed by the sound of the murmur and characteristic changes on radiographs, electrocardiograms, and echocardiography. In most affected animals, the holosystolic murmur is best heard along the right cranial thorax at the cardiac base (106). Less often, maximal intensity is detected over the pulmonic valve area and pulmonic artery. With echocardiography, the septal defect can often be imaged in multiple imaging planes and color flow doppler can discern the pressure gradient. Abnormal systolic flow across the septal defect is evident, and often of high velocity. Cardiac catheterization with angiography is sometimes done to determine accurate pressure changes and ascertain the exact size of the opening.

Dogs with very small defects often remain normal, and occasionally the defects close spontaneously. Definitive treatment requires cardiopulmonary bypass surgery to close the defect.

Alternative surgery includes restricting the overperfusion of blood into the lungs by suturing a band around the pulmonary artery, thereby better equalizing the pressures within the heart. If the band is placed too tight, a right-to-left shunt or right heart failure might result. This can be corrected by loosening or removing the band. Many of these patients still develop congestive heart failure or cardiac rhythm disturbances and require additional medical therapy. Affected animals should not be bred, and close relatives should be evaluated thoroughly before being included in a breeding program.

CHAPTER 2

Dental Disorders

Dental disorders are important not only for health reasons but also because abnormal dentition is important to breeders as an aesthetic issue. Dogs on the show circuit and those used for breeding are expected to have dental features representative of the breed. Formal registries have not yet been established for dental disorders, although veterinary dentists routinely perform "bite" evaluations for breeders. Unfortunately, most of the information on heritability of dental disorders has not been provided by controlled studies, and reports are sparse in the peer-reviewed literature.

BRACHYGNATHISM

Brachygnathia, also known as overshot jaw and mandibular distoclusion, is a condition in which the mandible is significantly shorter than the maxillae (240) (Figure 2-1). It is seen most commonly in the saluki but is reported in a great number of breeds (278). The condition is sometimes called "shark mouth" in the Pembroke Welsh corgi, and "pig jaw" in the cocker spaniel. Brachygnathism is an inherited defect, and affected individuals should not be used for breeding (460). Some of the breeds that present with brachygnathism are:*

Afghan hound	Akita	American cocker spaniel
Australian shepherd	basset hound	beagle
bearded collie	bichon frisé	bloodhound
Bouvier des Flandres	Brittany spaniel	Cavalier King Charles spaniel
Chesapeake Bay retriever	Chihuahua	Chinese shar pei
collie	Dachshund	Dalmatian
Dandie Dinmont terrier	Doberman pinscher	English cocker spaniel
English foxhound	English setter	Fox terrier (smooth and wire)
German shepherd dog	German shorthaired pointer	German wirehaired pointer
giant schnauzer	Great Dane	Great Pyrenees
greyhound	Ibizan hound	Irish setter
Italian greyhound	Jack Russell terrier	Maltese
miniature schnauzer	Norfolk terrier	Norwich terrier
Norwegian elkhound	Old English sheepdog	otter hound
Pembroke Welsh corgi	poodle (standard)	pug
rottweiler	Saluki	Scottish terrier
Sealyham terrier	Shetland sheepdog	silky terrier
soft-coated wheaten terrier	Tibetan spaniel	Tibetan terrier
whippet		

*List compiled by Gregg DuPont, DVM, Dipl. AVDC

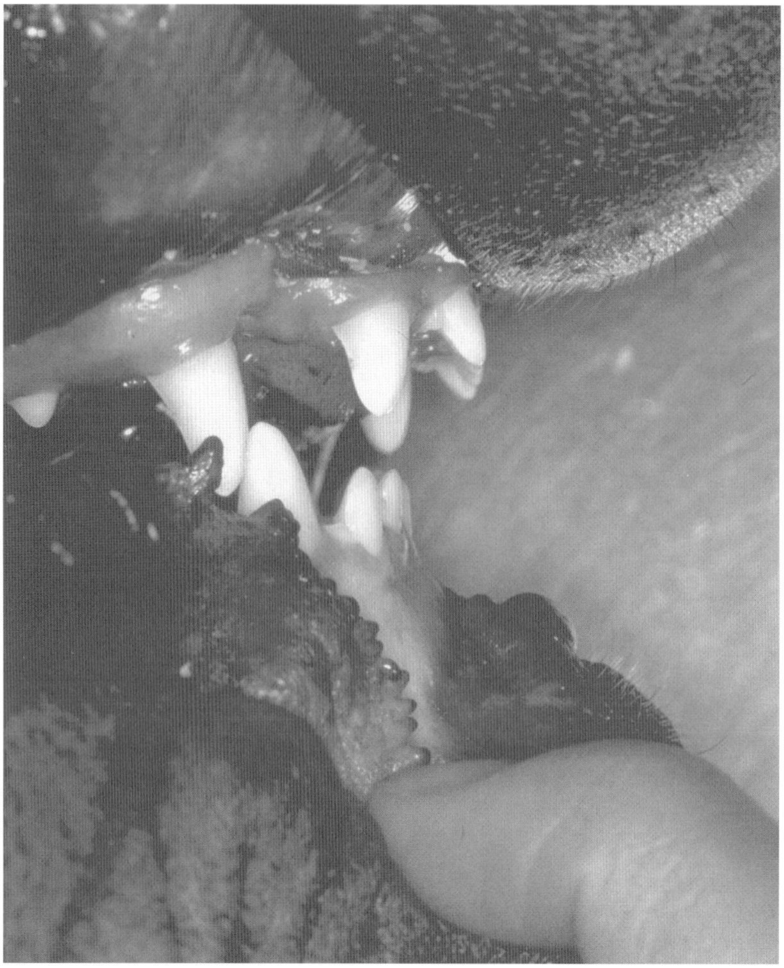

Figure 2-1 **Brachygnathia/base narrow**
Courtesy of Dr. Kenneth Lyon, Mesa Veterinary Hospital, Mesa, Arizona

MALOCCLUSION

Malocclusion denotes any abnormality in how the upper and lower teeth meet. Breeders refer to occlusion as "bite." Most malocclusions have mild clinical significance but, because they are presumed to be hereditary, are of primary concern to breeders (522).

In most breeds, the scissors bite—in which the teeth of the upper jaw are positioned just in front of those of the lower jaw—is preferred (621). To a certain extent, however, "normal" varies with the breed, in terms of preferred occlusion.

Malocclusion often results from achondroplasia, a defect in cartilage growth and development that is transmitted as an autosomal dominant trait with variable expressivity (621). The gene pattern responsible for this condition is prevalent in several breeds, including the dachshund, basset hound, miniature poodle, and Scottish terrier (621).

There are many different types of malocclusion and different methods of evaluation. An occlusal (bite) evaluation is an important part of the classifying process. Most breed standards include only information about the relationship of incisors and the number of teeth that should be present, but occlusal evaluation is much more involved (893). Systematic evaluation involves observing the symmetry and morphology of the head and teeth, making sure all teeth are present (and no extras), evaluating occlusion of the incisors, canine teeth and premolars, judging the relationship between the temporomandibular joint and the angle of the mandible, and observing the occlusal plane of the upper and lower arches (373, 456, 894). Standardized forms are available for veterinary dentists to use to evaluate "bite" and judge which animals are most suitable for breeding.

Level bite is a malocclusive disorder in which the front teeth meet end to end rather than the top incisors being just slightly in front of the bottom incisors. It is most commonly reported in the

Belgian Tervuren (620) and is considered a minor form of prognathism (621). It is acceptable in some breeds, such as the borzoi, Lhasa apso, Newfoundland, Old English sheepdog, schipperke, and Skye terrier (278).

Reverse scissors bite occurs when the upper incisors fall just behind the lower incisors. This is acceptable in many breeds, including the Afghan hound, Boston terrier, boxer, bulldog, bullmastiff, English toy spaniel, French bulldog, Pekingese, and shih tzu (621). If an actual gap is present between the upper and lower teeth, it is more correctly referred to as prognathism.

Open bite occurs when a gap of at least 5 mm is present between the top and bottom incisors when the mouth is closed. It can occur on its own, such as in the briard, or with other forms of malocclusion. Although it is suspected to be a recessive trait, this has yet to be proven (621).

Wry mouth is a version of either brachygnathia or prognathia that affects only one side of the head, the left or the right. Abnormal in all breeds, it has been reported in the Belgian Tervuren, Border terrier, Brittany, bull terrier, Cairn terrier, Cavalier King Charles spaniel, Chesapeake Bay retriever, Chihuahua, Clumber spaniel, Dalmatian, Doberman pinscher, English bulldog, English setter, German shepherd dog, Great Dane, Maltese, miniature schnauzer, Pekingese, poodle, rottweiler, Shiba Inu, standard poodle, and standard schnauzer (278, 620).

Anterior crossbite is a common bite abnormality, occurring when the maxillary incisors are lingual to the mandibular incisors in occlusion (240). If more than the incisors are involved, the condition is correctly referred to as prognathia. Anterior crossbite is reported most commonly in the Australian shepherd, Belgian Tervuren, Chesapeake Bay retriever, miniature schnauzer, poodle, soft-coated wheaten terrier, and standard schnauzer (620). Anterior crossbites have been attributed to jaw size discrepancies and to retained maxillary primary incisors, both of which are likely to be inherited (240). Typically, no treatment is required, although the condition can be corrected orthodontically.

Posterior crossbite occurs when the mandibular premolars or molars occlude buccal to their maxillary counterparts. This is presumed to be an inherited condition and is reported most commonly in dolichocephalic breeds (240) such as the borzoi, collie, and Shetland sheepdog. No treatment is required in most cases, but in severe cases, extraction is the treatment of choice.

Base-narrow canines are lingually displaced mandibular canines, believed to be genetic in nature (240). Although the exact cause has not been determined, it may result from retained deciduous mandibular canines or when the mandible is short in relation to the maxilla. It is seen most commonly in the Cairn terrier, German shepherd dog, miniature schnauzer, poodle, Shiba Inu, and standard schnauzer (620). Clinically the condition is manifested as permanent mandibular canine teeth erupting lingual to the deciduous teeth, resulting in retained deciduous teeth and lingually deviated permanent teeth. The treatment of choice is orthodontic correction.

Rostrally displaced maxillary canines, also known as lance canine, are seen most commonly in the Shetland sheepdog and Shiba Inu (620). This is considered to be a heritable condition (240). The treatment of choice is orthodontic correction.

All pups should have dental evaluations at 8 weeks of age and then again at 6 to 7 months of age to check for proper occlusion and possible retention of deciduous teeth. If the permanent teeth have been displaced, the condition can be corrected with orthodontic movement. This can be started at 6 to 10 months of age. Animals requiring orthodontic procedures should not be used for breeding.

MISSING TEETH

Anodontia is the complete absence of teeth, and oligodontia refers to several missing teeth, but not all. Puppies are expected to have 6 upper and 6 lower incisors, 2 upper and 2 lower canines, and 6 upper and 6 lower premolars. In the adult dog, the count for incisors and canines remains the same, except that adults have 8 upper and 8 lower premolars and 4 upper and 6 lower molars.

Dentition is sometimes expressed as a formula in which the numerators reflect the count on one side of the maxilla and the denominators are counts on one side of the mandible. The sum is doubled to express the total tooth count.

Although anodontia is rare, oligodontia and hypodontia (a few missing teeth) are common in

Canine Dental Formulas

Deciduous

$$2\left(\frac{i3}{3}\ \frac{c1}{1}\ \frac{p3}{3}\right) = 28$$

Permanent

$$2\left(\frac{I3}{3}\ \frac{C1}{1}\ \frac{P4}{4}\ \frac{M2}{3}\right) = 42$$

Dental formula for dogs in which i/I, c/C, p/P, and -/M stand for incisors, canines, premolars, and molars of deciduous and permanent dentition, respectively.

Table 2-1 Some Breeds with Oligodontia and the Teeth Most Commonly Missing*

Breed	Teeth most commonly missing	Breed	Teeth most commonly missing
Affenpinscher	ND	Jack Russell terrier	Premolars
Afghan hound	ND	Keeshond	ND
Bedlington terrier	Canine teeth	Komondor	Premolars
Belgian Tervuren	Premolars	Labrador retriever	Premolars
Border terrier	Upper lateral incisor	Lhasa apso	Incisors
Borzoi	Premolars	Maltese	Incisors
Chinese crested dog	ND	Manchester terrier	First premolars
Clumber spaniel	ND	Miniature poodle	ND
Dandie Dinmont terrier	Incisors, premolars, canines	Norwegian elkhound	ND
		Pomeranian	ND
Doberman pinscher	Premolars	Poodle (standard)	ND
Fox terrier (smooth and wire)	ND	Rottweiler	ND
		Shetland sheepdog	ND
German shepherd dog	First premolars acceptable	Shih tzu	ND
		Skye terrier	Premolars and molars
Great Dane	ND		
Havens, toy	ND	West Highland white terrier	ND

*NOTE. This list was compiled by Gregg DuPont, DVM, Dipl. AVDC, and Kenneth Lyon, DVM, Dipl. AVDC.
ND = Not determined

many breeds of dog (240). Oligodontia is inherited as an autosomal recessive trait in the fox terrier (673). Radiography should be used to confirm the diagnosis and differentiate the condition from delayed eruption, which is a familial trait in Tibetan terriers and soft-coated wheaten terriers (240). Table 2-1 lists some breeds with oligodontia, along with the teeth most commonly missing.

POLYDONTIA

Polydontia can be attributable to supernumerary or extra teeth, or to retained deciduous teeth. The condition is prevalent in some breeds (240). In the greyhound, it may be seen in one-third of dogs examined (268).

Breeds in which supernumerary teeth are reported most commonly include the boxer, bulldog, bullmastiff, Doberman pinscher, collie, golden retriever, and Labrador retriever (278, 620). These extra teeth should be extracted if they are causing the other teeth to be crowded.

The deciduous or puppy teeth are normally erupted completely by 8 weeks of age and then fall out and are replaced by the permanent teeth. The permanent teeth are usually completely in place by 6 to 7 months of age. The retention of deciduous teeth seems to have a strong genetic basis, but the actual mode of inheritance has not been characterized (621). Retained primary teeth are reported in the affenpinscher, border terrier, Brussels griffon, bull terrier, Chihuahua, English cocker spaniel, Irish setter, Italian greyhound, komondor, Maltese, Manchester terrier, papillon, West Highland white terrier, and Yorkshire terrier (278). A mode of inheritance has not been determined.

The diagnosis is made by visual inspection and comparison to a chart showing when the permanent teeth should have erupted. The treatment of choice is to remove the retained deciduous or supernumerary teeth, being careful not to disturb or disrupt the underlying tooth bud. Information on which to base breeding recommendations is insufficient.

PROGNATHISM

Prognathism, also known as undershot jaw and mandibular mesioclusion, occurs when the mandible is significantly longer than the maxilla. Brachycephalic dogs are sometimes described as having relative prognathism because their mandible is normal and the maxillae are shortened (240), and this constitutes a normal breed characteristic. This is to be expected in the affenpinscher, Boston terrier, boxer, Brussels griffon, Chinese pug, English bulldog, French bulldog, and Lhasa apso. In these breeds, the prognathic deformity results from the inherited defect in development of the bones in the base of the skull (460). Breeds in which this condition has been reported include the following:*

Afghan hound	Akita	American cocker spaniel
American Eskimo	American Staffordshire terrier	Australian shepherd
Beagle	Belgian sheepdog	Belgian Malinois
Belgian Tervuren	Bichon frisé	Border terrier
Bouvier des Flandres	Brittany spaniel	Bull terrier
Cavalier King Charles spaniel	Chesapeake Bay retriever	Chihuahua
Chinese shar pei	Clumber spaniel	Collie
Dalmatian	Dandie Dinmont terrier	Doberman pinscher
English cocker spaniel	English foxhound	English setter
Fox terrier (smooth and wire)	German shorthaired pointer	German wirehaired pointer
Giant schnauzer	Great Dane	Great Pyrenees
Ibizan hound	Irish setter	Italian greyhound
Jack Russell terrier	Komondor	Kuvasz
Lakeland terrier	Maltese	Mastiff
Miniature schnauzer	Newfoundland	Norfolk terrier
Norwich terrier	Norwegian elkhound	Old English sheepdog
Otter hound	Pekingese	Pembroke Welsh corgi
Pointer	Pomeranian	Poodle (standard)
Rottweiler	Saluki	Schipperke
Sealyham terrier	Shih tzu	Silky terrier
Soft-coated wheaten terrier	Staffordshire bull terrier	Standard schnauzer
Sussex spaniel	Tibetan spaniel	Tibetan terrier
Weimaraner	Welsh springer spaniel	West Highland white terrier
Whippet		

*List provided by Gregg DuPont, DVM, Dipl. AVDC

CHAPTER 3

Dermatologic Conditions

Even though skin problems are commonly encountered in veterinary practice, genetic information is sparse for some of the more common dermatologic entities. No DNA tests are available for any skin condition, and there is a registry for only one (sebaceous adenitis in standard poodles). Despite the advances made in histopathologic diagnosis, genetic counseling for dermatologic conditions is hampered by a lack of concrete genetic information on these entities.

ACANTHOSIS NIGRICANS

Acanthosis nigricans is a poorly understood condition in dogs in which the skin becomes blackened, specifically in the axillary and groin areas. It is presumed to be inherited because it is diagnosed almost exclusively in the dachshund. An autosomal recessive or a polygenic inheritance has been proposed (21). The condition differs significantly from its human counterpart in that acanthosis nigricans in humans is associated with insulin resistance (866).

The process typically starts in the armpits and groin, and the skin becomes thick, greasy, and heavily pigmented (948). Although inflammatory pigmentation is common in dogs, this specific condition is distinct. The role of allergies in this condition has not been fully explored. Secondary yeast infection is commonly encountered.

The diagnosis is verified by biopsies for histopathologic assessment. Treatment is sometimes successful with topical therapies, oral vitamin E, topical corticosteroids, and injectable melatonin (768, 936).

Affected animals probably should not be bred. Because a mode of inheritance has not been conclusively documented, though, and because the condition is more cosmetic than life-threatening, it is difficult to be dogmatic about recommending that parents and siblings not be used for future breeding.

ACQUIRED AUROTRICHIA

Also known as *gilding syndrome*, this is a condition of miniature schnauzers in which the color of the coat changes from normal to gold, especially along the topline (1114). The mode of inheritance is unknown. Most dogs are 2 to 3 years of age when the condition is first detected. Diagnosis can be confirmed by biopsies for histopathologic assessment.

No treatment is necessary, as the animal's health is not compromised. Approximately half regrow a normal coat within 2 years. Until more is known about the genetic nature of this disorder, affected animals should not be bred unless they are truly superior in other important aspects. No screening tests are currently available for carriers.

ACRAL LICK DERMATITIS

Also known as *lick granuloma*, this is a disorder in which dogs continue to lick at their limbs, abrading the skin and creating ulcers and raw, weeping areas (Figure 3-1). The cause is still a matter of debate. Once thought to be caused by boredom, more contemporary views suggest a disorder of sensory nerves (1070) or an obsessive-compulsive disorder (77).

Although no direct mode of inheritance has been established, there are clear breed predilections. Those most commonly reported with the disorder are the Doberman pinscher, German

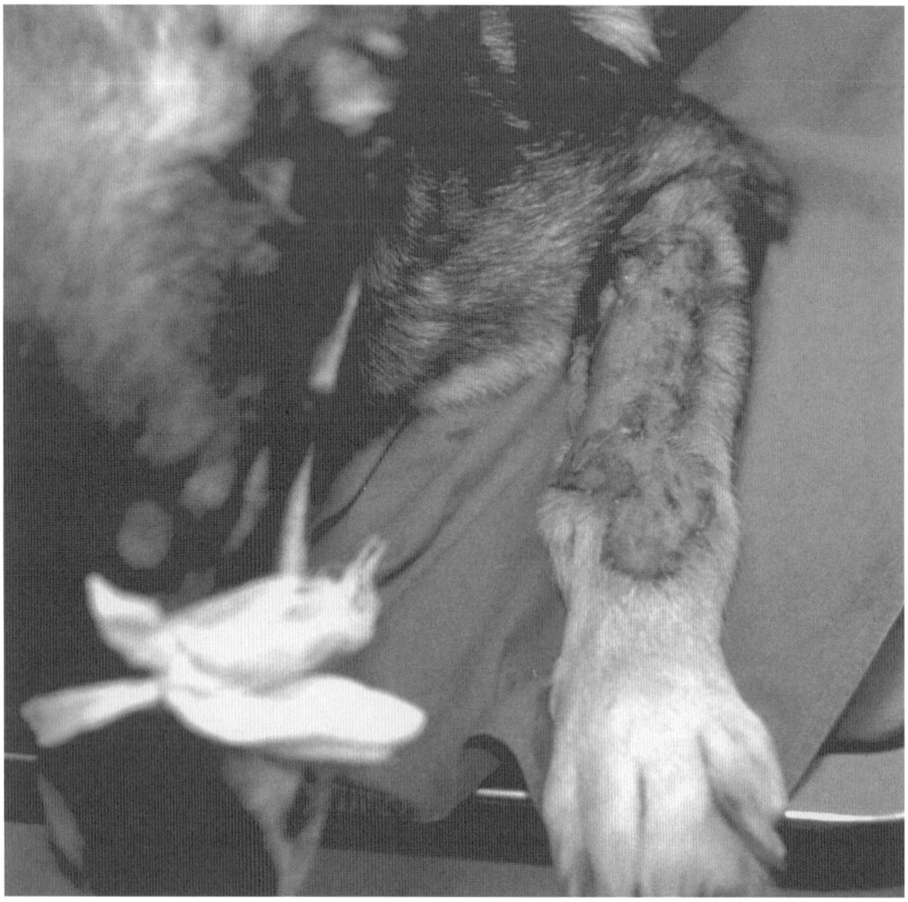

Figure 3-1 Acral lick dermatitis
Courtesy of Dr. Lowell Ackerman, Mesa Veterinary Hospital, Mesa, Arizona

shepherd dog, Great Dane, Irish setter, and Labrador retriever (89, 564, 768).

Biopsies should be done to confirm a diagnosis, as many other conditions can appear similarly. Treatment for acral lick dermatitis is frustrating. Even though bacterial infection is not the primary cause of the condition, treatment for deep pyoderma is an important component of therapy. Regarding the stereotypical licking at the affected area, some dogs respond to topical corticosteroids, some to antidepressant drugs, some to antiobsessional drugs, some to narcotics, and others to drugs that inhibit the effect of narcotics (267, 371, 671, 1110). Electrostimulation (shock collars) has also been used successfully to manage the condition (280), as has radiation therapy (877). Each case should be assessed individually.

Acral Lick Dermatitis

Acral lick dermatitis has been a confusing entity to deal with, as veterinarians have postulated genetic, behavioral, and neurologic etiologies. While certain breeds seem to be predisposed, a familial trend has not been convincingly demonstrated. In all likelihood, the condition represents a final clinical endpoint for numerous underlying problems.

The mode of inheritance is not known, so it is best not to breed affected animals, but insufficient information is available to prove that the condition is passed to future generations. No screening tests are available for carriers. Researchers are beginning to collect detailed behavioral and pedigree analyses of related dogs affected with acral lick dermatitis, with the hope of determining a mode of inheritance.

ACRAL MUTILATION SYNDROME

Acral mutilation syndrome is a bizarre sensory neuropathy in which animals lose pain sensation in their toes. This starts at about 3 to 5 months of age in affected animals. They initially just chew at their feet but will do extensive damage and even mutilation. The condition is presumed to be autosomal recessive and has been reported in

English pointers, German shorthaired pointers (768), and English springer spaniels (641). A similar condition has been reported in Czechoslovakian shorthaired pointers (83). A deficiency in growth or differentiation of primary sensory neurons may be involved (83).

Diagnosis requires electromyography, in which nerve potentials are measured and found to be abnormal. There is no effective treatment. Affected animals should not be bred, and the parents should be considered obligate carriers of the trait. Siblings are suspect carriers, and no screening tests are available to detect carriers.

ALBINISM

True albinism is rare in dogs and is inherited as an autosomal recessive trait (768). Albinos do have melanocytes but have a biochemical defect in that they lack the tyrosinase necessary to synthesize melanin. Despite the rarity of albinism, disorders associated with partial albinism are not uncommon. These conditions may be associated with neurological or ocular problems. These disorders are covered in other chapters. Congenital deafness has also been associated with merle color pattern in dogs (797).

Piebaldism, or partial albinism, is a congenital disorder characterized by discrete patches of leukoderma. In humans, it is inherited as an autosomal dominant trait (65) and is thought to represent either a defect in the migration of melanoblasts from the neural crest to the skin or a failure of melanoblasts to survive and differentiate into melanocytes once they reach the skin. The condition arises from mutation of the *c-kit* tyrosine kinase receptor gene or the gene coding for the *c-kit* ligand (794).

Waardenburg syndrome is associated with deafness, white coat, and blue or heterochromic irides and has been described in the bull terrier, collie, dalmation, Great Dane, and Sealyham terrier (12).

Even though most practitioners are familiar with deafness and its association with white coat color, and eye pigmentation and its association with deafness, it is important to recognize that a variety of ocular defects, such as microphthalmia, cataracts, and mesodermal dysgenesis, may also be involved (406). Affected animals should not be bred.

ANASARCA

Anasarca refers to a generalized edematous condition seen in newborn pups. It is most commonly reported in the English bulldog, where affected animals are referred to as walrus pups (181). While some researchers consider the trait to be recessive in nature (802), the mode of inheritance is currently unknown with certainty.

While the trait is lethal in many cases, other pups may be mildly affected with subcutaneous edema only, or accompanied by fluid accumulation in the abdominal and thoracic cavities (562). Severely affected pups usually die shortly after birth. Mildly affected animals that recover should not be used for breeding, and parents of affected individuals should be considered possible carriers of the trait.

CALCINOSIS CIRCUMSCRIPTA

Calcinosis circumscripta, or *tumoral calcinosis*, is a subgroup of *calcinosis cutis*, a condition characterized by dystrophic mineralization of tissue not associated with systemic disorders or kidney disease (768). The cause is not known at this time, and a mode of inheritance has not been determined. Occasionally dystrophic mineralization is the result of underlying renal failure, parathyroid hyperplasia, or metastatic visceral calcification.

The condition occurs predominantly in young, large-breed dogs, such as German shepherd dogs (but also in Boston terriers, boxers, dachshunds, and many other breeds), and presents as well circumscribed, nonpainful subcutaneous swellings with occasional ulceration and fistulation (768, 900). In the largest retrospective study done to date, German shepherd dogs accounted for almost half of all cases documented (932). Although lesions are usually found on the dorsum and extremities, they can occur anywhere, including the footpads, pressure points, and even in the oral cavity. Calcinosis circumscripta has been associated with renal dysplasia in a Lhasa apso (394).

Diagnosis is confirmed by histopathologic findings of dystrophic mineralization in the deep dermis and panniculus in the absence of systemic disease. Treatment includes only surgical excision because the cause of the dystrophic mineralization is unknown. Until more is known about the genetics of the condition, affected animals should not be used for breeding.

COLLAGENOLYTIC GRANULOMA

Collagenolytic granuloma, also known as *eosinophilic granuloma*, is believed to be an immune-mediated disorder with some resemblance to Well's syndrome in people. The condition is seen most commonly in Siberian huskies, in which it is believed to be a familial trait (848). Clinically, the condition appears as nodules and plaques, often in the mouth or on the underside or flanks. Affected dogs are otherwise healthy, and the lumps are neither painful nor itchy.

The diagnosis is confirmed by biopsies for histopathologic evaluation, in which collagen breakdown is associated with an influx of eosinophils, lymphocytes and histiocytes, and the development of palisading granulomas (927). The condition responds to anti-inflammatory to immunosuppressive therapy. Though collagenolytic granuloma possibly represents an inherited susceptibility to collagen injury, there are no scientific grounds on which to base breeding recommendations.

COLOR-DILUTION ALOPECIA

Synonyms for color-dilution alopecia include *color mutant alopecia*, *blue Doberman syndrome*, *fawn Irish setter syndrome*, and *blue dog disease*. This condition describes the patchy, poor haircoat that can develop in animals bred for unusual hair color, especially those described as "blue" and "fawn." The blues are diluted forms of the normal black and tan color, and fawns are diluted forms of red coloration. The main breeds affected are the Bernese mountain dog, Chihuahua (blue), chow chow (blue), dachshund (blue), Doberman pinschers (blue, red), Great Dane (blue), Irish setter (fawn), Italian greyhound (blue), miniature pinscher (blue), saluki, schipperke (blue), Shetland sheepdog (blue), standard poodle (blue), whippet (blue), and Yorkshire terrier (gray-blue) (42, 105, 694, 695, 768, 891). Another manifestation of color-dilution alopecia may be the follicular lipidosis of "mahogany" points reported in rottweilers (396).

The specific genetic basis of the disease is unknown. Defects in melanization and structure of hair cortex have been described. The condition is believed to be associated with the interplay of different factors with the double-recessive allele on the D locus. The affliction, however, cannot be determined only by the *dd* homozygous recessive, as not all color-diluted dogs develop associated haircoat problems. In dachshunds, pedigree analysis has suggested an autosomal recessive mode of inheritance (42). There is considerable breed variability. Whereas 90% of blue Doberman pinschers develop color-dilution alopecia, the condition does not seem to occur in color-diluted Weimaraners. Incidence data are not available for most breeds.

Dogs with color-dilution alopecia are born with normal coats but later suffer from hair loss, dry skin and bacterial infections. In most cases, by the time the animal is 6 months of age, the owner notices a sparse haircoat that is bluish-gray in color if the normal color is black, blond in color if the normal color is fawn, and liver-colored if the normal color is red. The lesions usually are fully manifested by 2 years of age, although the age of onset is occasionally up to 6 years.

Diagnosis is confirmed with biopsies for histopathologic assessment or by carefully examining plucked hairs microscopically. Direct microscopic examination of plucked hairs typically reveals the presence of clumped melanin in the cortex and medulla. With histopathologic evaluation, common findings are distorted hair follicles, follicular hyperkeratosis, abnormal melanin pigmentation, clumping of melanin in the epithelium, and hypergranulosis. The histopathologic findings are similar to that seen with black hair follicular dysplasia. With follicular lipidosis, abnormal clumping of pigment is mild; predominant findings include swelling of follicular matrix cells and lipid staining by oil-red-O. Interpretation of Weimaraner skin biopsies must be done cautiously, as even normal skin tends to have histologic similarity to dogs with color-dilution alopecia.

Treatment is strictly symptomatic because the abnormal hairs are not replaced by normal fur. Antiseborrheic shampoos and oil rinses are usually helpful. If bacterial folliculitis is observed, appropriate antibiotics and/or topical antiseptics should be administered.

Owners are advised not to breed affected animals, their siblings, or their parents. Dogs that have produced any pups with the condition must be considered as carriers for the trait. The condition can be entirely avoided if owners select dogs with non-diluted colors. It must be reiterated, however, that some breeds with color-dilute alleles have little problem with CDA, so breeding recommendations must vary with the incidence in specific breeds. No screening tests are currently available for carriers.

CONGENITAL HYPOTRICHOSIS

Hairlessness from birth can occur in different breeds, and the genetics are not necessarily identical. These cases have to be distinguished from the breeds purposely bred to be hairless, such as the Abyssinian sand terrier (African hairless dog), Mexican hairless (Xoloitzcuintli), Chinese crested dog, and Turkish naked dog (190, 524, 797, 882). Hairlessness in these breeds represents the heterozygous state (Hrhr) of an autosomal dominant trait (768). However, in the American hairless terrier (rat terrier), the hairlessness is transmitted as an autosomal recessive trait (802, 884), with affected animals being homozygous (haha).

In breeds not intended to be hairless, hypotrichosis is a congenital, and probably hereditary, problem. Congenital hypotrichosis is a rare disorder in which fur is partially absent since birth. A subgrouping of ectodermal defects, it may occur alone or with other manifestations, such as abnormal dentition or tear production. An elaborate system of nomenclature has been proposed, to classify ectodermal dysplasias in animals based on the classification in humans (321).

The genetics of hypotrichosis may differ with each breed-specific entity. Some are more common in males and may indicate sex-linked inheritance. Breeds reported with hypotrichosis include the basset hound, beagle, Belgian shepherd, bichon frisé, cocker spaniel, French bulldog, Labrador retriever, Lhasa apso, rottweiler, toy poodle, whippet, and Yorkshire terrier (176, 191, 387, 465, 554, 635, 768). Congenital hypotrichosis has been reported in a female Labrador retriever and a rottweiler (465).

Separating this disorder from ectodermal defects (below) is arbitrary. Congenital hypotrichosis is distinguished by its suspected mode of inheritance, and biopsies revealing a decrease in density of hair follicles and adnexa, not necessarily a complete absence such as seen in ectodermal defects. Clinically, the condition appears as patches of complete alopecia ranging from focal alopecia to complete lack of fur (alopecia universalis), evident since birth (321). No curative treatment is available. In the X-linked varieties, affected males should not be bred and their dams should be considered carriers of the trait. No screening tests are available to detect carriers.

CUTANEOUS ASTHENIA

Also known as *Ehlers-Danlos syndrome* and *dermatosparaxis*, this condition refers to a group of related biochemical disorders that affect the strength of collagen, the fibrous connective tissue of the body. In humans, there are several different subgroupings, but these conditions have not been studied extensively in dogs. New classifications in human medicine also include, as collagen diseases, Marfan syndrome, Menke's syndrome, and osteogenesis imperfecta (853). Several gene-encoding peptides form procollagen molecules and several encoding enzymes remove excess amino acids from procollagen to form collagen (332, 853). Mutations in any of these genes can give rise to one of the variants of cutaneous asthenia. One form, cutaneous asthenia resulting from improper collagen formation and packing, has been documented in the dog as an autosomal dominant trait (705).

Breeds affected include the beagle, boxer, dachshund, English setter, English springer spaniel, Garafiano shepherd dog, German shepherd dog, greyhound, Irish setter, keeshond, Manchester terrier, red kelpie, St. Bernard, schnauzer, soft-coated wheaten terrier, Welsh corgi, and cross-breeds (768, 797, 887). In general, mutation in collagen structural genes results in dominant forms of the disorder, whereas gene mutations for enzymes that process procollagen are typically recessive.

Affected dogs have skin that stretches excessively and can rip with even minimal trauma and the tensile strength of the skin is only $^{1}/_{27}$th that of nonaffected littermates.

A clinical diagnosis can be made by measuring stretched skin and creating a skin extensibility index. It is calculated by dividing the maximal extension of the dorsal skin fold by the length from the base of the tail to the occipital crest and multiplying by 100 (332). Affected dogs have values above 14.5%. Histopathologic findings are variable. The collagenous fibers in the affected skin are small and sparse compared to control sections. Electron microscopic and biochemical analysis of the dermal collagen is needed for definitive diagnosis. No successful therapies for affected animals are available.

To give appropriate breeding advice, the form of cutaneous asthenia involved should be documented. For autosomal recessive forms, affected animals should not be bred, parents should be considered obligate carriers, and siblings should be suspected carriers. When the problem is clearly a dominant trait, affected animals and the parent carrying the trait should not be bred, but the nonaffected parent can be used for breeding.

DALMATIAN BRONZING SYNDROME

Dalmatian bronzing syndrome may be an inherited defect of uric acid metabolism, similar to gout in people. Although the mode of inheritance has not been determined with certainty, the condition is limited to the Dalmatian. Excessive uric acid excretion and the tendency to form uric acid uroliths (stones) are presumed to be autosomal recessive, but this does not explain the incidence of Dalmatian bronzing syndrome when all Dalmatians have excessive uric acid excretion.

One of the manifestations of high uric acid levels conceivably is a patchy, poor haircoat and change in skin color to a bronze hue. It is also possible, though, that the clinical manifestations are entirely a result of bacterial folliculitis and mild furunculosis and have nothing whatsoever to do with uric acid levels.

Diagnosis involves skin biopsies for histopathologic assessment and careful scrutiny of blood uric acid levels. The uric acid level in most Dalmatians is several times higher than uric acid levels in other breeds. Thus, screening based on uric acid levels is tempting but is quite difficult to rely on with any certainty.

Treatment involves controlling superficial folliculitis with antibiotics and topical antiseptics and, potentially, feeding a vegetarian-based diet low in purine content, and/or using drugs such as allopurinol. Managing the folliculitis with systemic antibiotics and antibacterial shampoos often results in temporary resolution of the coat changes.

The value of restricting purine has not been completely explored. Broccoli, kale, mustard greens, carrots, and tomatoes are low in purines. Asparagus, cauliflower, beans, peas, mushrooms, spinach, and whole grains are high in purines. Cheese, milk, and eggs are low in purines, but most fish (e.g., herring, mackerel, sardines), organ meats (e.g., liver, kidney, sweetbreads), poultry (chicken, duck, turkey), and meats (beef, lamb, pork, veal, game) are high in purines. The worst offenders are organ meats, fish, and wild game. Liver treats should not be given to Dalmatians. The best treats include fruits, cottage cheese, and breakfast cereals (not whole grain). Care must be taken when giving table scraps (especially liver, fish, beef and pork) to Dalmatians. Because the rate of absorption and excretion of allopurinol varies significantly among Dalmatians, as does the extent of hyperuricosuria, an oral dose must be titrated to the needs of each dog (598).

This defect in purine metabolism seems to be present in almost all Dalmatians. Therefore, to offer convincing genetic advice is difficult. Dogs that continually develop problems despite being on low-purine diets should not be bred.

DEMODECTIC MANGE

Demodectic mange, *demodicosis*, or *red mange*, is an inflammatory disease of the hair follicles that appears to be attributable in part to the presence of *Demodex* mites and in part to an inherited or acquired immune defect (580, 768) (Figure 3-2). The mites are transmitted from the bitch to the nursing pups in the first few days of life (580). Although the specifics have not yet been demonstrated conclusively despite years of research, the condition is thought to involve a defect in the cell-mediated immune system. Lymphocytes from dogs with juvenile-onset demodicosis have impaired stimulation and significantly decreased CD4:CD8 ratios (159), although neither seems to correspond well with clinical severity (116). Dogs with demodectic mange have impaired lymphocyte blastogenesis, fewer cells expressing interleukin-2 (IL-2) receptors, and decreased production of IL-2 (581).

The mode of inheritance is unknown, but there are breed predilections. Breeds overrepresented with juvenile demodicosis include the Afghan hound, beagle, Boston terrier, boxer, bull terrier, Chihuahua, Chinese shar pei, collie, dachshund, Dalmatian, Doberman pinscher, English bulldog, English pointer, German shepherd dog, Great Dane, Lhasa apso, Old English sheepdog, pug, rottweiler, and Staffordshire terrier (411, 527, 572, 582, 699, 768). Adult-onset demodicosis may be seen more commonly in the English bulldog, miniature poodle, shih tzu, and West Highland white terrier (572).

When young animals are affected, we are most likely to suspect an immune deficit. When older animals are affected, we most often suspect any underlying disease that interferes with resistance to disease, such as Cushing's syndrome and hypothyroidism, and perhaps cancer and diabetes mellitus (269, 768). Thus, demodicosis is typically divided into juvenile and adult-onset varieties, although the distinction is not always clear-cut.

Diagnosis is confirmed by skin scrapings in most cases. Biopsies are indicated only occasionally, especially in dogs with thick skin (e.g., Chinese shar pei). Immunopathologic evaluation of cases suggests that CD3+ lymphocytes are prevalent within interface infiltrates, and IgG_4 is found in lesions of perifolliculitis (160, 234).

Treatment is aimed at supportive care to overcome any immune deficit, correcting any underlying conditions (e.g., internal parasites, heartworm), and using medicated shampoos to cleanse the skin surface and hair follicles. About 90% of cases of juvenile demodicosis will self-cure without miticidal therapy (580). Specific treatment to kill mites, such as amitraz (527, 768), ivermectin (815, 875), or milbemycin oxime (643, 698), is reserved for cases that fail to self-cure or those that are getting progressively worse despite conservative therapy.

Although a mode of inheritance has not been determined, it is recommended not to breed animals with juvenile demodicosis (580). While this position is not always easy to defend, animals with a congenital or inherited immune deficiency may indeed contribute this undesirable trait to future generations if breeding is allowed. In addition, females have been observed to develop worsening clinical signs during estrus, so ovariohysterectomy is a very real consideration. Older animals that develop demodectic mange most likely have acquired the disease and are therefore not a threat to the gene pool. No screening tests are available

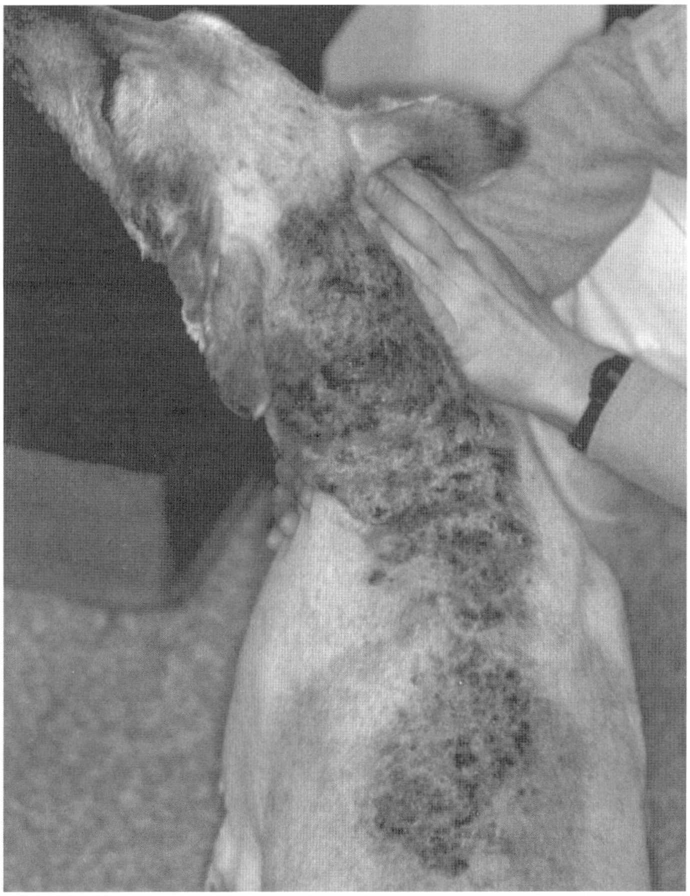

Figure 3-2 Demodicosis
Courtesy of Dr. Thomas Lewis, Mesa Veterinary Hospital, Mesa, Arizona

for carriers of the disease. Animals that self-cure have a much better prognosis than those requiring miticidal therapy.

DERMATOMYOSITIS

Dermatomyositis is an inflammatory disease of the skin, muscle, fat, and sometimes blood vessels. The genetics were once thought to be straightforward, but more recent investigations have painted a more complicated picture. The mode of inheritance is still believed to be autosomal dominant with variable expressivity in the collie (421, 433) and Shetland sheepdog (469). It has been proposed that the full-blown condition is seen only in genetically prone animals triggered by a viral infection (553). This, in turn, triggers an immune reaction that results in the damage to the skin and muscle (919).

Breeds affected include the Australian cattle dog, basset hound, Beauceron shepherd, chow chow, collie, German shepherd dog, kuvasz, Pembroke Welsh corgi, and Shetland sheepdog, (48, 400, 419, 768, 1117). Ulcerative dermatosis, as seen in Shetland sheepdogs, may be a subset of dermatomyositis in dogs.

Most affected collies begin to show signs at about 12 weeks of age. They develop what look like scrapes on the face, ears, elbows, hocks, and other friction points (433). The tip of the tail may also lose its hair. Muscle wasting is most profound over the top of the head and on the hindquarters. The clinical presentation differs somewhat between breeds. In Shetland sheepdogs, the myositis component develops later and is most profound on the face and lower extremities (421). In Pembroke Welsh corgis, the dermatitis is confined primarily to the face and ears (1117).

Biopsy of the skin and/or muscle for histopathologic assessment, or electromyographic (EMG) studies of affected muscle, can usually support a diagnosis. Evaluation of skin biopsies often reveals a diffuse mononuclear cell dermal infiltrate (418), but one may also find an interface dermatitis with some similarities to lupus erythematosus.

Muscle biopsies in severely affected dogs may reveal inflammatory cell infiltrates, muscle fiber degeneration, regeneration, and atrophy (420). Spontaneous needle electromyogram abnormalities include fibrillation potentials, positive sharp waves, and bizarre high-frequency discharges (433).

Treatment is experimental at this time. Vitamin E and pentoxifylline have both been used, the latter of which is the treatment of choice among verterinary dermatologists despite not being licensed for this purpose. Systemic antibiotics and topical antiseptics are often helpful in controlling the secondary pyoderma.

Although it has become more complicated to offer breeding recommendations, all affected individuals clearly should be removed from any breeding program. If the parent carrying the trait can be determined, that individual also should not be bred. Siblings of the affected individual should be screened carefully for evidence of even minor involvement. This would be sufficient grounds to remove those animals from breeding programs.

DERMOID SINUS

Dermoid sinus refers to an abnormal tunnel that forms between the skin surface and the spinal column. The mode of inheritance is unknown and is variably described in the literature as dominant with inconsistent penetrance (452) and recessive (630). The Rhodesian ridgeback is affected most often, but the condition is sporadically seen in other breeds such as the boxer (768), Chow chow (68), Kerry blue terrier (768), Siberian husky (189), Yorkshire terrier (303), and shih tzu (943).

The diagnosis can be confirmed by injecting dye into the tunnel and demonstrating a spinal attachment via radiography. Surgical excision of the tract is the only successful therapy. Affected animals should not be bred. If one of the parents is clearly affected, the other parent may be unaffected and can still be used for breeding. If neither parent has clinical evidence of dermoid sinus, both probably should be removed from the breeding program. In that case, siblings of the affected animal should be considered to be suspect carriers.

ECTODERMAL DEFECT

Ectodermal defect is a hereditary congenital alopecia observed from birth. This defect has been reported in the beagle, Belgian shepherd, cocker spaniel, Lhasa apso, miniature poodle, and whippet breeds (768, 797, 946). Hair follicles are totally absent, and associated adnexa in the alopecic skin and abnormal dentition are commonly reported.

Clinical signs of alopecia from birth suggest an ectodermal defect. Biopsies for histopathologic assessment are necessary to confirm the diagnosis. No specific treatment is available for ectodermal defect. Affected animals should not be bred.

EPIDERMAL DYSPLASIA

Epidermal dysplasia refers to a serious form of keratinization disorder (seborrhea) that reflects a defect in development of skin cells (keratinocytes). Although the mode of inheritance in unknown, the West Highland white terrier is the breed affected most often and it is believed to be a genetically determined disorder complicated by secondary microbial infections (696). The skin becomes dark, scaly, and thickened, and pups are often quite itchy. Most cases are noticed in the first 3 months of life. It is unusual for affected pups to reach 6 months of age without displaying evidence of the condition. This is important because the condition resembles allergies, which usually don't initially appear until after 6 months of age.

Diagnosis is made by biopsy. Treatment is symptomatic and intensive and is directed at both the keratinization disorder and the secondary bacterial and yeast surface infection. Until more is known about the genetics of the condition, affected animals, their siblings, and their parents should not be bred. No screening tests are available for carriers. This recommendation may seem overly rigid, given that the genetics of the condition are not known. Because affected pups suffer significantly, however, it is best to err on the side of caution.

EPIDERMOLYSIS BULLOSA (EB)

Epidermolysis bullosa (EB) refers to a group of mechanobullous diseases of unknown etiology and involves structural defects at various levels of the basement membrane zone. Congenital and acquired forms have been described in people. Early cases described as epidermolysis bullosa simplex (EBS) were probably actually dermatomyositis, given current information. Epidermolysis bullosa is actually much rarer than dermatomyositis and has a different classification system. The three major categories, based on the location of blistering within the basement membrane zone, are:

Epidermolysis bullosa simplex (epidermolytic EB). Epidermolysis bullosa acquisita has been described in a Great Dane, with evidence of circulating autoantibodies targeting collagen VII epitopes (793).

Junctional epidermolysis bullosa. Junctional epidermolysis bullosa has been documented in a toy poodle (276). A milder form (mitis junctional epidermolysis bullosa) has been well-documented in a mongrel dog (752, 753). A subtype of junctional epidermolysis bullosa—epidermolysis bullosa junctionalis progressiva (non-lethal localized JEB)—has been described in German shorthaired pointers and is believed to be inherited as an autosomal recessive trait (401, 779). It primarily affects the footpads and pinnae.

Dystrophic epidermolysis bullosa. An epidermolysis bullosa-like syndrome similar to dystrophic epidermolysis bullosa in humans has been described in the Beauceron (Berger de Beauce) and the Akita (754, 794).

The condition most often involves oral mucosa, footpads, pinnae, and frictional sites. Specific diagnosis requires electron microscopic demonstration of cleft formation and indirect immunofluorescence of antibodies directed against collagen and basement membrane proteins. In German shorthaired pointers, collagen XVII is deficient, suggesting that the condition may be caused by a mutation on the COL17A1 gene (401, 779, 795). Therapy for most cases is symptomatic, and there are no curative treatments.

Too few cases have been reported in dogs to make any reasonable breeding recommendations. An exception is the German short-haired pointer, in which affected animals should not be bred, parents are considered obligate carriers, and siblings are suspect carriers.

FAMILIAL BENIGN PEMPHIGUS

Also known as *Hailey-Hailey disease*, this is a rare condition that starts in young pups, usually only a few months of age. It is presumed to be autosomal dominant with variable expressivity (1015). It has been reported in English setters, and a similar case was reported in a Doberman pinscher (768). Small bumps evolve into large, hairless areas with profound crusting.

Diagnosis is confirmed by biopsies for histopathologic assessment. No treatment is available at present. Discovering which parent passed along the trait is possible in many cases, and affected animals should not be bred. Normal-appearing individuals are likely clear of the trait, although some animals may have mild forms of the disease that aren't clinically apparent.

FAMILIAL VASCULOPATHY

Familial vasculopathy is a rare and poorly understood condition of German shepherd dogs that often starts in pups 6 to 8 weeks of age (868). Studies suggest an autosomal recessive mode of inheritance (1103). Affected dogs are lethargic and develop fever and swollen joints. There is swelling of the nose, crusting and ulceration of ear margins and tail tip, and swelling and ulceration of the footpads. The condition often worsens following vaccination. It is presumed to be a disorder of immune responsiveness but has not been fully characterized.

Diagnosis is confirmed by biopsies for histopathologic assessment. Tests for platelet factor-3 are positive in most cases but must be evaluated carefully because most normal pups have transient increases in platelet factor-3. Platelet numbers are normal in affected individuals. Although most treatments are ineffective, some animals get better on their own. Affected animals should not be bred, even if they recover completely, and their parents should be considered as obligate carriers. Siblings are suspect carriers. No screening tests are available to detect carrier status.

FOLD DERMATITIS

Skin-fold pyodermas involve folds of skin that are continually traumatized by friction and do not have adequate ventilation. There are many different varieties, including whole-body folds (e.g., Chinese shar pei), facial folds (e.g., pug), lip folds (e.g., spaniels), vulvar folds (e.g., older bitches), and tail folds (e.g., Boston terriers). In most cases the condition is a direct result of a dog's preponderance to have wrinkles. The pattern of inheritance is considered autosomal dominant because the wrinkles are often a distinguishing feature of the breed. Breeds predisposed to skin-fold pyoderma include the bloodhound, Boston terrier, boxer, Chinese shar pei, cocker spaniel, English bulldog, English springer spaniel, French bulldog, Pekingese, and pug (768).

Diagnosis can be made visually. Management requires regular cleansing of the skin folds to combat infection. Permanent correction requires surgical removal of the skin fold (1132).

Fold dermatitis occurs because many breeders consider wrinkles desirable. Breeding animals with few or no wrinkles is the best way to eliminate fold dermatitis from the purebred dog population but is unlikely to be an option with either breeders or pet owners.

FOLLICULAR DYSPLASIA

Follicular dysplasia refers to a collection of clinical entities associated with abnormal hair loss or defective follicle formation that doesn't have a specific etiology (Figure 3-3). This classification

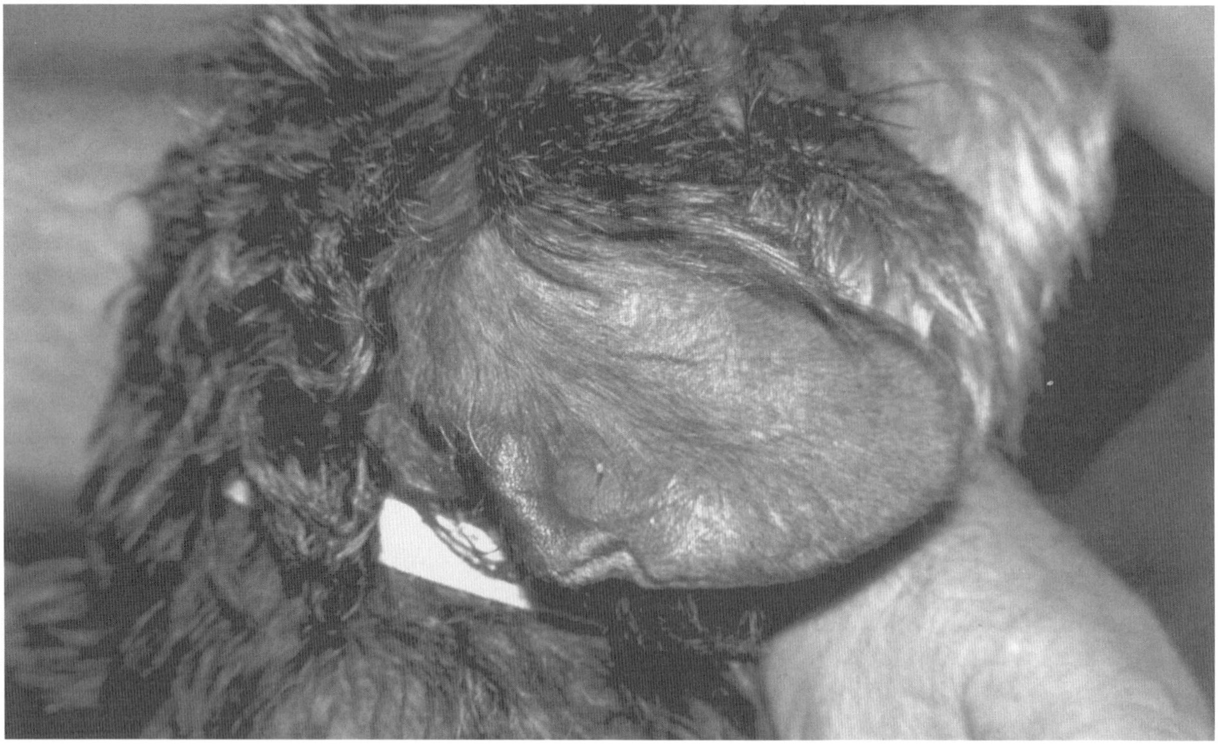

Figure 3-3 Follicular dysplasia
Courtesy of Dr. Thomas Lewis, Mesa Veterinary Hospital, Mesa, Arizona

represents several unrelated conditions that share certain clinical features. Because many different entities are involved in this clinical grouping, no uniform pathogenesis should be anticipated. Given the striking breed predilections for the individual subgroups, however, a genetic connection should reasonably be inferred.

Follicular dysplasia cases have clinical signs that are relevant in specific breeds, but generalizations aren't of much help to practitioners. In most cases, the conditions tend to spare the face and distal extremities in favor of the dorsal trunk. Consistent findings are selective loss of primary hairs, changes in coat quality, and often hyperpigmentation of the skin in affected areas.

- Black hair follicular dysplasia is a tardive (not apparent at birth) hereditary alopecia in dogs that have at least some black fur (945). The condition is inherited as an autosomal recessive trait (922). It has been observed in the American cocker spaniel, basset hound, beagle, bearded collie, dachshund, Gordon setter, Jack Russell terrier, papillon, pointer, saluki, and schipperke, as well as mongrels (531, 768, 1007). The puppies are normal at birth. As the dog matures, hair on several of the black patches of skin fails to grow. Sparse, fragile hair and scales are seen. The hair on the adjacent white skin grows normally. Dysplasia of the follicle in the alopecic areas of black skin occurs, with resulting abnormal hair development and shedding. The white skin is not affected. In all likelihood, the condition represents a localized expression of that seen in color dilution alopecia. Affected animals should not be bred and parents should be considered likely carriers of the trait.
- Woolly syndrome is seen most commonly in Siberian huskies, but similar presentations have been reported in Alaskan malamutes and English springer spaniels (768, 847). There is a loss of primary hairs, and the secondary (undercoat) hairs are dry and crimped, like wool. Complete alopecia may be present in areas of friction and wear, such as pressure points and under collars. The skin tends to hyperpigment in affected areas, and the undercoat assumes a more reddish hue. Use of animals in breeding programs is considered a breeder option.
- Saddle alopecia is seen primarily in Airedale terriers and Portuguese water dogs (697), in which there is hair loss on the dorsum in a

saddle-like distribution. Occasionally, islands of normal hair growth appear within the large patches of alopecia. The alopecic pattern tends to wax and wane, but without the seasonality seen with cyclic flank alopecia. Use of animals in breeding programs is considered a breeder option.

- Cyclic flank alopecia is discussed in more detail in Chapter 4, which deals with endocrine disorders. There is loss of both primary and secondary hairs on the flank and lateral trunk, and associated hyperpigmentation of the skin. This condition is assumed to have some relationship to photoperiod, because hair loss and regrowth tend to be seasonal. With time, however, hair loss is progressive, with less than complete hair regrowth.
- Waterline disease is a poorly understood condition that affects black Labrador retrievers. It is characterized by pruritus, a keratinization disorder, and alopecia of the ventrum and legs. The condition is named for the abrupt absence of fur, often appearing as a linear pattern, parallel with the topline. Use of animals in breeding programs is considered a breeder option.
- Coat-dilution alopecia is seen primarily in Irish water spaniels, Portuguese water dogs, and curly-coated retrievers. Some primary hairs are lost, and the undercoat assumes a lighter hue. Portuguese water dogs have abnormal melanization of the pilosebaceous units (697). The condition generally starts at 2 to 4 years of age, with hair loss attributable to fracture of the hair shafts.
- Irish water spaniels develop a unique form of follicular dysplasia that involves the skin on the neck, flanks, dorsum, rump, and thighs. Preliminary genetic investigation suggests an autosomal dominant mode of inheritance (164). Preliminary clinical research on these dogs indicates that some respond to hypoallergenic diets and some have disturbances of the steroidogenic pathway similar to adrenal sex-hormone dermatosis.

The diagnosis of follicular dysplasia can be suspected on the basis of history and clinical signs and is confirmed with biopsies for histopathologic assessment. Samples should be taken from the most profoundly affected areas. Not surprisingly, biopsy findings tend to differ with the individual clinical condition. The clinical signs of alopecia limited to the black patches of skin on a spotted black and white dog are suggestive of black hair follicular dysplasia. Biopsies for histopathologic assessment can be used for confirmation. Changes noted are the same as for color-dilution alopecia.

Woolly syndrome is characterized by hair follicles arrested in the catagen stage and the appearance of "flame follicles"; the flame follicles—follicles with abundant tricholemmal keratinization and a pronounced glassy membrane—are also seen in growth hormone/castration-responsive dermatoses. Similar changes are seen with saddle alopecia. Follicular dysplasia in Portuguese water dogs is associated with prominent apoptosis of keratinocytes in the inner and outer root sheath and dissolution of the hair matrix of anagen hair follicles.

In seasonal flank alopecia, both primary and secondary follicles are distorted and may appear dwarfed in appearance. During recovery, diagnostic changes may be difficult to find. To date, hormonal profiles of dogs with seasonal flank alopecia have not detected any irregularities.

For most cases of follicular dysplasia, the coat changes are permanent, and only symptomatic treatment (shampoos, moisturizing rinses, fatty acid supplements) for dry, scaly skin is entertained. Antibiotics are employed to control pyoderma if it is problematic. Synthetic retinoids are sometimes used to treat a poorly responsive exfoliative dermatosis. Successes with etretinate have been reported for some cases of color-dilution alopecia and seasonal flank alopecia; improvement is typically evident within 30 days. In seasonal alopecia, the hair loss waxes and wanes; treatment may also be contemplated with oral or injectable melatonin, with the injectable product (1 to 3 implants with 12 mg melatonin, depending on the dog's size) giving the most consistent results. Oral melatonin dosage is not standardized, but the product is being used anecdotally at 5 mg BID-TID for 30 to 60 days. For waterline disease complicated by *Malassezia* yeasts, treatment with ketoconazole can be beneficial. Otherwise, the condition doesn't respond well to the therapies described above.

Genetic counseling for owners of dogs with follicular dysplasia is complicated in that the disorder is likely to be different in every breed represented. Until more is known, affected animals should not be bred. To make suggestions regarding the parents, siblings, and other close relatives is tougher.

GREYHOUND ALOPECIA

The pathogenesis of greyhound alopecia is poorly understood. No endocrine abnormalities have been reported, and greyhound alopecia possibly is a variant of follicular dysplasia. Because the condition is more prevalent in working dogs (racers and blood donors), and it may clear spontaneously when these dogs are adopted into homes, stress is thought to have some role (976).

A bilaterally symmetrical regional alopecia involves the outer aspects of the thighs, and occasionally the ventrum. For the most part, the alopecia seems to be completely asymptomatic. The diagnosis is confirmed with biopsies for histopathologic assessment. There is no specific treatment for Greyhound alopecia, because it causes no health consequences. Conscientious neglect is recommended. Anecdotally, melatonin has been used in treatment, in doses similar to those used for recurrent flank alopecia.

Because no information on the heritability of the condition is available, and because it is entirely cosmetic in nature, breeding restrictions are probably not necessary at this time.

ICHTHYOSIS

Ichthyosis is a condition in which the surface of the skin becomes covered with thick, tenacious scale. In people, ichthyosis has several genetic mechanisms and several different variants (1131). It is not known if all of these same variants are found in dogs. On a basic level, the ichthyoses are divided into epidermolytic and non-epidermolytic forms. The epidermolytic ichthyoses are attributable to mutations in keratins, and non-epidermolytic ichthyoses are associated with defects in formation of the cornified envelope or the intercorneocyte lipid layers (794).

The three major forms of epidermolytic ichthyoses are epidermolytic hyperkeratosis, ichthyosis bullosa of Siemens, and epidermolytic palmar/plantar hyperkeratosis. Breeds affected with ichthyosis include the Cavalier King Charles spaniel, Doberman pinscher, golden retriever, Jack Russell terrier, soft-coated wheaten terrier, standard poodle, and West Highland white terrier (5, 439, 591, 768). Epidermolytic palmar/plantar hyperkeratosis has been reported in Yorkshire terriers and Rhodesian ridgebacks (794). Likely, several different mechanisms and modes of inheritance are evident, similar to the situation in people. The condition is sufficiently rare that generalizations are difficult to make. In only one instance has a true familial pattern been apparent (5). An autosomal recessive mode of inheritance is considered likely in most cases (591).

Diagnosis is confirmed by biopsies for histopathologic assessment. Electron microscopy is typically necessary to document the specific form of ichthyosis (5). Treatment is symptomatic only, with moisturizing agents and, potentially, with retinoids. Affected animals should not be bred, and parents should be considered carriers of the trait. Siblings are suspect carriers. No screening tests are currently available to detect carriers.

JUVENILE CELLULITIS

Juvenile cellulitis, also known as *juvenile pyoderma* and *puppy strangles*, is a disease of young dogs (usually younger than 6 months) that likely has an immunologic pathogenesis. It is reported most commonly in dachshunds, golden retrievers, yellow Labrador retrievers, Gordon setters, Lhasa apsos, and pointers (552, 768, 1116). Clinically, the condition involves swelling and inflammation of the face and submandibular lymph nodes. Multiple animals in a litter may be involved. Although the condition resembles a pyoderma, bacterial infection is not a primary component.

This condition responds to a short course of immunosuppressive therapy with little chance of recurrence. Not enough is known about the heritability of this condition to make recommendations regarding breeding.

LENTIGO

Lentigo is a relatively rare condition in which black spots appear on the skin. The mode of inheritance is not known with certainty but is suspected to be autosomal dominant (768). The breed affected most often is the pug (104, 768). To date, none of these lesions has later turned into malignant cancers such as melanoma. The dogs remain in good health but cannot be shown because of the abnormal pigmentation.

No treatments are available, although dermabrasion and electrodesiccation have been used in people who have the same condition. It is best not to breed affected animals, even though the condition is more cosmetic than medical. No screening tests are available to detect carriers, but if the condition is truly autosomal dominant, one of the parents should display evidence of the condition. The other parent is likely to be free of the problem and can be used for breeding.

LETHAL ACRODERMATITIS

Lethal acrodermatitis is a fatal disorder seen in white bull terriers. It is inherited as an autosomal recessive trait (480). Thymic hypoplasia, as well as an underlying defect in trace mineral metabolism, may be involved. There is a marked deficiency of T-cells and impaired cell-mediated immune responsiveness. Serum zinc and copper levels tend to be diminished, and an association with ion deficiency (1058), though not proved, is believed to be a cause.

Affected animals normally are presented at about 1 to 3 months of age with splayed toes, lighter than normal pigmentation, pododermatitis, mucocutaneous crusting, and hyperkeratotic footpads. Concurrent paronychia, diarrhea, abnormal behavior, and bronchopneumonia are often present. The dogs develop a stilted gait, and interdigital dermatitis and footpad lesions are common. Most patients succumb to pneumonia. The majority of cases involve a secondary *Malassezia* infection.

Unfortunately, the diagnosis is often confirmed only on post-mortem examination, when a markedly hypoplastic or absent thymus is evident. Neither skin biopsies nor blood tests are diagnostic. Biopsies, however, are characterized by parakeratotic hyperkeratosis, moderate epidermal hyperplasia, leukocytic exocytosis, and serocellular crusting. Blood profiles may reveal lowered plasma zinc levels, decreased serum alkaline phosphatase (ALP) and alanine aminotransferase (ALT), a nonregenerative anemia, and impaired lymphocyte blastogenesis. Cytological preparations from skin lesions often demonstrate the presence of *Malassezia* yeasts. Suspicions can be verified by post-mortem examination, if necessary. As stated, these dogs have smaller thymus glands than normal.

Lethal acrodermatitis has no successful treatment, and animals do not seem to benefit from administration of zinc or any other symptomatic therapy. Most dogs die of overwhelming infection. Some anecdotal reports document success with ketoconazole therapy, although this treatment is directed primarily at the secondary *Malassezia* infection. Etretinate therapy is also being evaluated.

Affected animals should not be bred, and their parents should be considered as carriers of the trait. Siblings are suspect carriers. No screening tests are available to detect carriers of the condition.

LICHENOID-PSORIASIFORM DERMATITIS

This is a harmless condition in which wart-like bumps appear on the skin, usually on the inner ear flaps or the abdomen, or both. The mode of inheritance is unknown, but the condition is seen almost entirely in the English springer spaniel (4, 768). Most dogs are younger than 3 years of age when they are first affected. The condition tends to wax and wane and doesn't respond reliably to any medications. Biopsies will confirm the diagnosis; and there is severe epidermal hyperplasia with pegs extending into the dermis, superficial dermal inflammation, and Munro microabscesses (395, 640). Although the recommendation is not to breed affected dogs, the condition is merely cosmetic and not likely to affect the health and well-being of future generations.

LUPOID DERMATOSIS

Lupoid dermatosis is a poorly understood condition of German shorthaired pointers. It affects young dogs, usually under 4 years of age. The exact genetic nature of the condition is unknown but is thought to be familial (1112). Some circumstantial evidence points to the involvement of an immune pathomechanism (1089).

Most dogs are first affected by about 6 months of age. Thickening and scaling of the skin often starts on the head, hocks, and scrotum before becoming more generalized. The nails might also slough. Some dogs develop fever, and some shed protein in their urine.

The diagnosis is based on histopathologic assessment, and the pattern of inflammation noted bears some resemblance to the interface pattern seen in lupus erythematosus, erythema multiforme, and dermatomyositis. Treatment, though not consistently effective, has been attempted with prednisone, retinoids, and combinations of niacinamide and tetracycline. Some dogs respond to fatty acid supplements containing eicosapentaenoic acid or gamma-linolenic acid, or both (1089).

Until more is known about the genetics of this disorder, it is best not to breed affected animals, their siblings, or their parents. No screening tests are available for carriers. In this way, the trait in this breed might be eliminated before it becomes more established.

LUPOID ONYCHOPATHY

Lupoid onychopathy, also known as (symmetrical) *lupoid onychodystrophy*, is a claw disorder characterized by onychomadesis and onychodystrophy (onychorrhexis, onychomalacia, onycholysis) of multiple digits (often all 18 claws). The breeds most commonly affected seem to be boxers, Doberman pinschers, German shepherd dogs, greyhounds, Irish setters, rottweilers, and Weimaraners (919, 935). Although the pathogenesis is unknown, the histopathological similarity to lupus erythematosus and the clinical responsiveness to fatty acid supplements and other mild anti-inflammatory medications is intriguing.

In conditions such as lupoid onychopathy (symmetrical lupoid onychodystrophy), screening for underlying disorders, such as adverse food reactions, immune deficit, and hypothyroidism, is important. Radiographic evaluation of the affected digits also should be contemplated. Diagnosis is confirmed by histopathologic assessment of the entire distal digit. Analysis of mineral content of shed nails suggests possible increased concentrations of calcium, potassium, sodium, and phosphorus in cases of idiopathic onychomadesis (440).

Successful treatment of lupoid onychopathy relies on fatty acid supplements containing large amounts of eicosapentaenoic acid, combinations of eicosapentaenoic acid with gamma-linolenic acid, or anti-inflammatory doses of tetracycline (or doxycycline) with niacinamide (52, 768). Clinical improvement is typically seen in 3 to 4 months. For resistant cases, pentoxifylline has been advocated but not diligently investigated. During flare-ups, the topical application of corticosteroids for several days often gives prompt relief. As a final solution for patients that don't respond to medical therapy, onychectomy is a successful surgical option worth considering. Surgery will usually eliminate the lameness and pain associated with the onychodystrophy (67).

At this time, information on which to base breeding recommendations is insufficient. For now, it is best to advise that affected animals not be bred.

MALASSEZIA DERMATITIS

Malassezia pachydermatis is a yeast commonly found on the skin and mucous membranes of dogs. It is not considered to be infectious, although health-care workers have been known to transfer the organism from their pet dogs to children in an intensive care unit. In the vast majority of cases, the yeast infection occurs secondarily to an underlying problem such as allergy or a keratinization disorder. Breeds at increased risk include the American cocker spaniel, basset hound, English setter, shih tzu, and West Highland white terrier and many others are cited in other reports (649).

The diagnosis can be confirmed by cytologic evaluation, biopsies for histopathologic evaluation, or microbial cultures. Treatment includes killing the yeasts with appropriate topical and systemic therapy. Advice cannot be given regarding breeding strategies because a familial connection to yeast susceptibility has not been determined.

MALIGNANT HISTIOCYTOSIS

Malignant histiocytosis and systemic histiocytosis are two related histiocytic disorders most commonly reported in the Bernese mountain dog, but also seen in the coonhound, Doberman pinscher, flat-coated retriever, golden retriever, keeshond, and rottweiler (768, 1105). Although a mode of inheritance has not been determined, this condition is considered familial in the Bernese mountain dog (730, 893), perhaps polygenic (803), or perhaps autosomal recessive in nature (731). The condition is recognized more often in males but seems unlikely to be X-linked because trends are noticed in paternal as well as maternal lines.

The disease consists of cutaneous and systemic spread of histiocytic cells (730). The course of the disease is quite variable, from mild lesions with periods of remission to rapid progressive disease leading to death. The diagnosis is confirmed by biopsies for histopathologic assessment. It is important to differentiate the condition from the strictly cutaneous histiocytoses (136) in which a systemic component is absent.

Successful treatment has been reported with the human T-cell line TALL-104 (1085). The Institute for Genetic Disease Control in Animals (GDC) maintains an open registry for both histiocytosis and mastocytoma in Bernese mountain dogs, along with a research database for other tumors in this breed. Until more is known of the genetics underlying this condition, affected animals should not be bred and the parents should be considered likely carriers of the trait. Siblings should be considered suspect carriers.

MUCINOSIS

Mucinosis is a somewhat rare and confusing condition in which the supporting network under the skin is replaced in areas by mucin, which is a secretion with the texture of mucus. The mode of inheritance is unknown, but the condition has been reported in the Chinese shar pei, Doberman pinscher, Labrador retriever, and Shetland sheepdog (260, 768). All Chinese shar peis have more subcutaneous mucin than other breeds. This probably accounts, in some fashion, for their wrinkles. Females appear to be affected more often than males. The mucinosis of Chinese shar peis results from massive accumulation of hyaluronic acid and, to a lesser extent, chondroitins 4 and 6 sulfate and dermatan sulfate in the dermis and panniculus (249, 1088).

The condition is characterized by lumps and bumps. Biopsies will confirm a diagnosis by demonstrating the presence of excessive mucin in the dermis and subcutis. The mucin tends to be metachromatic with toluidine blue, alcian blue positive, and removed by hyaluronidase treatment (260). No reliable therapy is available. Rarely, spontaneous remission is reported. When excessive mucinosis interferes with breathing, triamcinolone or prednisone can be administered twice a day for 10 days and then tapered so treatment ends after 30 to 40 days. This one-time treatment is usually enough to reduce the mucin content, but some animals do require more continuous treatment (on alternate days) or periodic readministration. For resistant cases, pentoxifylline has been used anecdotally.

Until more is known about the genetics of the condition, it is important not to breed affected animals. Parents and siblings should be considered suspect carriers. No screening tests are available to detect carriers.

NODULAR DERMATOFIBROSIS

Nodular dermatofibrosis is a marker for an internal malignancy and is believed to be transmitted as an autosomal dominant trait in the German shepherd dog (711, 829). It has also been reported in the golden retriever (636), boxer (1113), and mixed-breed dogs (765, 1113). Lumps and bumps form on the skin surface, but almost always in association with a cancer affecting the kidneys (cystadenocarcinoma) or the uterus. Most dogs are over 5 years of age when they are first affected.

Diagnosis of the skin problem is made by biopsies for histopathologic evaluation. The internal cancer diagnosis may require radiography, ultrasonography, or exploratory surgery. Given the genetic nature of this condition, affected animals should not be bred and at least one of the parents should be expected to be affected. Because this condition does not become apparent until later in life, affected animals may have been bred already.

It is best to discontinue that line of breeding until assessment can reveal which animals are affected. Although no screening tests are available, computed tomography is the best way to detect early cases in dogs that are intended for breeding (710).

PANNICULITIS

Panniculitis is an uncommon inflammatory disease of the subcutaneous fat of dogs caused by a variety of underlying disorders. Although the specific causes are many and varied, some panniculitides clearly are immune-mediated and others result from microbial, nutritional, metabolic, traumatic, neoplastic, or undetermined causes (1). Many cases were thought to have an underlying alpha-1-antitrypsin deficiency (950), but this seems unlikely given the results of more recent studies (463). Genetics do not appear to play a primary role, but some evidence suggests that the dachshund and collie breeds are predisposed to nodular panniculitis, and other forms are breed-specific in the German shepherd dog and perhaps the miniature poodle (1, 768). In the largest retrospective analysis done to date, however, no age, breed, or sex predilections could be established (931).

In nodular panniculitis, multiple subcutaneous, firm nodules, 0.5 to 5 cm in diameter, are found on the trunk and neck. Fever and bacterial cellulitis are typical associated findings. In a sterile pedal panniculitis of German shepherd dogs, the panniculitis is limited to the footpads dorsal to the midline of the carpal or tarsal pads and is associated with painful, deep fistulous tracts (820). Finally, a focal panniculitis and associated alopecia can result from the subcutaneous injection of rabies vaccine (441). Poodles seem to be most commonly affected (768).

The disorder is confirmed by biopsies for histopathologic assessment, but many tests may be needed to determine the underlying cause. To be effective, treatment must be directed at the underlying cause. Many of the immune-mediated disorders are treated with immunosuppressive therapy. For animals with rabies vaccine-induced focal panniculitis, no treatment is necessary, although pentoxifylline has been used successfully on an anecdotal basis. When the next rabies vaccine is required, however, it should be administered intramuscularly. German shepherd dogs with sterile pedal panniculitis respond best to anti-inflammatory doses of prednisone combined with vitamin E. Although it is best not to breed affected dogs, a familial trend has not been determined for nodular panniculitis.

PERIANAL FISTULAE

Perianal fistula is a condition in which draining tracts form around the anus. The condition originally was thought to be caused by infection and was called perianal pyoderma and anal furunculosis. The etiology, however, is not clear-cut (235). Little evidence is available to support the contention that this is a true bacterial disease. Researchers for years have been trying to determine the cause of the condition and have proposed many possibilities, such as overproduction by local glands, poor ventilation associated with low tail carriage, anal sac disease, and hip dysplasia (129, 648, 1064). Most likely it is an inflammatory condition of the glands surrounding the anus or the tracts that drain them. An association between perianal fistulae and inflammatory bowel disease is suspected, especially in German shepherd dogs (422). The mode of inheritance is unknown, but the condition affects males twice as often as females and there are strong breed predispositions for German shepherd dogs and Irish setters (548, 768).

The clinical presentation of perianal fistulae is quite characteristic, with numerous draining tracts and ulcers immediately surrounding the rectum. The diagnosis is typically based on clinical signs alone, but confirmation requires histopathologic assessment of surgical biopsies. Although some cases respond to immunosuppressive therapy, immunologic testing has not been helpful (235). Dogs that are most likely to respond to immunosuppressive therapy are those for which biopsies reveal eosinophilic infiltration.

Management of these perianal fistulae is often disappointing because these cases do not respond consistently to antibiotics, corticosteroids, or surgery (289). Clipping the hair in the affected area and flushing with a suitable antiseptic, such as chlorhexidine or povidone-iodine, will keep the area clean but won't effect a cure (231). Immunosuppressive therapy is helpful in dogs in which eosinophilic infiltration is most profound. Cyclosporine treatment has also been reported as highly effective (644, 646). Surgery, cryosurgery, laser surgery, and treatment with vitamin A derivatives (retinoids) have all been used successfully, in select cases (289, 290, 648, 768, 1064). Because a hereditary link has not been firmly established, it is best that affected animals not be bred, but this is a cautious approach rather than one based on genetic evidence.

SCHNAUZER COMEDO SYNDROME

Also known by breeders as "schnauzer crud," this is a keratinization disorder that affects hair follicles, primarily along the topline. The mode of inheritance is not known with certainty. The condition is seen only in the miniature schnauzer.

In affected animals, bumps, scabs, and blackheads are evident on the back (949). There is typically some associated hair loss. The diagnosis is usually straightforward but can be confirmed by biopsy for histopathologic assessment.

Treatment of the blackheads and cleaning out the plugged pores are the established therapies. Benzoyl peroxide, alcohol wipes, and other acne remedies are the most successful forms of topical therapy. Sometimes, oral vitamin A derivatives (retinoids) are needed to bring the condition under control. In other cases, the condition remains refractory to conventional therapies (413). Though the recommendation is not to breed affected individuals, this is a strictly cosmetic disorder that does not affect the animal's overall health.

SEBACEOUS ADENITIS

Sebaceous adenitis is a perplexing collection of inflammatory skin diseases that have in common a destruction of hair follicle elements, especially the sebaceous glands. So many different breeds are affected, and the clinical variation so profound, that sebaceous adenitis most likely is not a single diagnosis but, rather, several different conditions that share some common clinical or pathological findings (906).

The mode of inheritance is unknown with certainty in any breed, but preliminary studies suggest that it may be autosomal recessive in the standard poodle (277). Among the many breeds affected are the Airedale, Akita, American cocker spaniel, American Eskimo, basset hound, chow chow, collie, dachshund, Dalmatian, Doberman pinscher, English springer spaniel, German shepherd dog, golden retriever, Hovawart, Irish setter, Labrador retriever, Lhasa apso, Maltese, miniature pinscher, miniature poodle, Old English sheepdog, Pomeranian, St. Bernard, Samoyed, Scottish terrier, shih tzu, standard poodle, toy poodle, vizsla, and Weimaraner (277, 768).

Most animals are in young adulthood when they are first affected (897, 928). A classification system for sebaceous adenitis divides most cases into two types.

Type I, seen in long-coated breeds, in which the condition progresses rapidly and responds to symptomatic therapy only.

Type II, seen in short-coated breeds, which progresses slowly and responds best to retinoids and cyclosporine.

This classification scheme is simplistic, though, and treatments should be formulated based on responsiveness to drugs in specific breeds. Treatment may be attempted with a variety of drugs (e.g., prednisone, cyclosporine, etretinate, Vitamin A), but responses show a lot of breed variation (151, 1115). All affected animals benefit from intensive topical therapy designed to restore moisture to the skin and remove excess surface keratin. Oil-based baths and rinses are the most successful of the topical therapies. Proper diagnosis requires biopsies for histopathologic assessment, and these should be sent to veterinary pathologists who have expertise in skin disorders.

Although we don't know the genetics of the condition with certainty, it certainly does seem to be familial in most of the breeds studied.

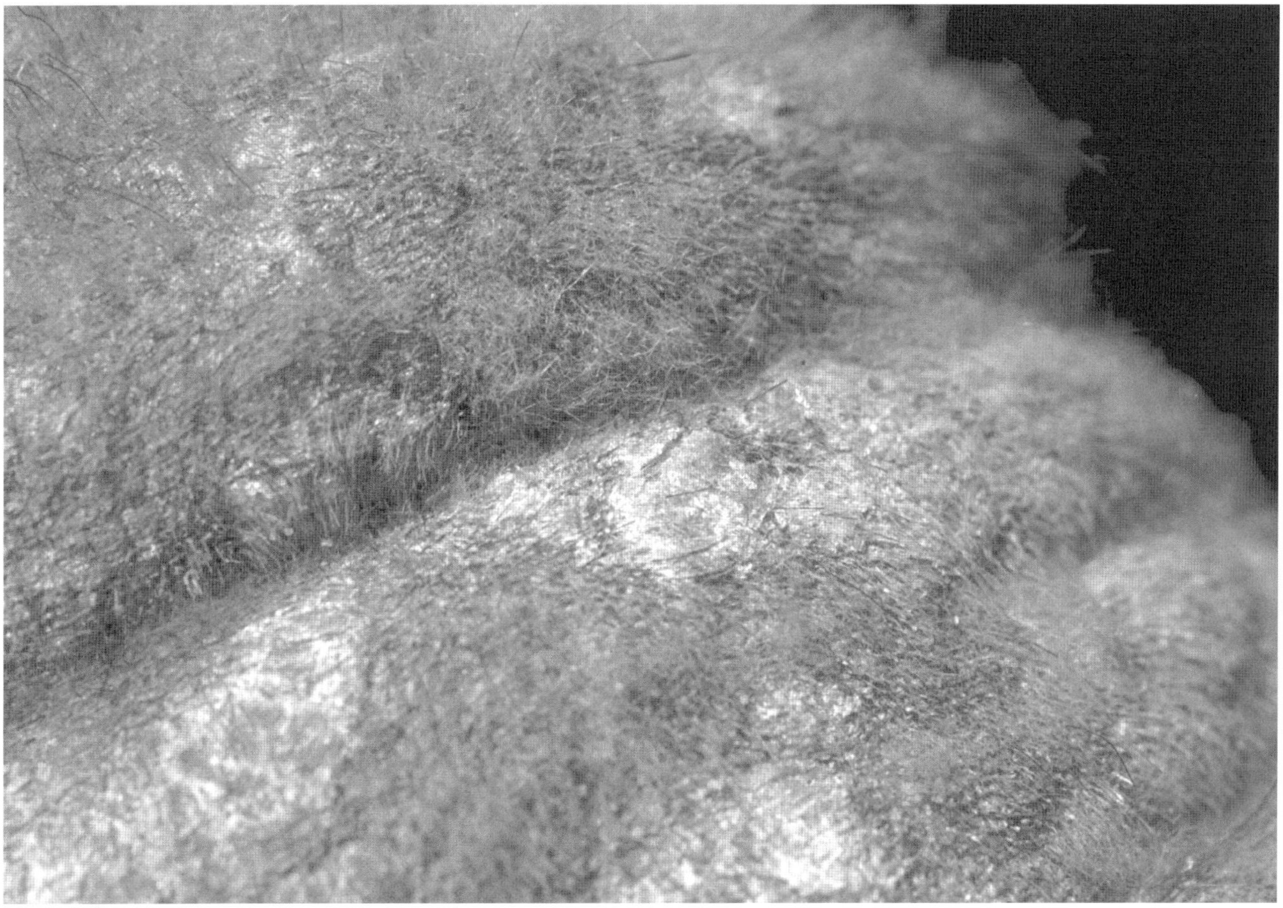

Figure 3-4 Seborrhea
Courtesy of Dr. Thomas Lewis, Mesa Veterinary Hospital, Mesa, Arizona

Accordingly, it is best not to breed affected animals, or, potentially, their siblings or their parents. No screening tests are available for carriers other than the standard poodle. In the standard poodle, normal-appearing carriers sometimes can be detected by early biopsies. Subclinically affected poodles do not seem to be carriers but actually to have a mild form of the disease (277). Animals that appear normal but have more than two hair follicles affected in two 6mm punch biopsies are classified as subclinical and should not be used for breeding. These biopsies are usually taken from the topline between the head and the shoulder blades. For breeds other than the standard poodle, two 6mm biopsies should be taken from affected areas early in the course of the disorder, when changes are most likely to be evident.

The Institute for Genetic Disease Control in Animals maintains an open registry for sebaceous adenitis in the standard poodle, and samples are judged as "affected," "questionable," or "normal." Normal does not imply that the animal is not affected but, rather, that biopsy samples showed no evidence of the disease.

SEBORRHEA

Many cases of skin disorders are diagnosed incorrectly as seborrhea. True seborrhea is an inherited defect of the skin and how it orients itself. If seborrheic skin is grafted onto a normal dog, it continues to be seborrheic. Thus, the defect is inherent in the skin itself and is not an internal disorder. Affected dogs are often scaly, greasy, and smelly (Figure 3-4). Waxy and infected ears are common. Idiopathic seborrheic dermatitis, a severe form of this syndrome, is reported almost exclusively in spaniels, especially the cocker spaniel (561).

The mode of inheritance for seborrhea is not known with certainty. It may be autosomal dominant with variable expressivity. Others favor an autosomal recessive mechanism, at least in the West Highland white terrier (802). In most breeds, the mode of inheritance remains unknown.

Breeds affected include the American cocker spaniel (949), basset hound (561), Chinese shar pei (561), Doberman pinscher (561), English springer spaniel (933, 949), German shepherd dog (949), golden retriever (949), Irish setter (561), Labrador retriever (561), poodle (561), rottweiler (592), and West Highland white terrier (561).

The disorder is typically evident by 2 years of age, and secondary bacterial and yeast (*Malassezia pachydermatis*) infections are commonly reported (66). In the rottweiler, the seborrheic dermatitis may be accompanied by other congenital anomalies (592). Biopsies are recommended so true seborrhea can be distinguished from the many look-alike (smell-alike) keratinization disorders that are more common.

Treatment is intensive and requires frequent medicated shampooing and often oral retinoids or vitamin D analogs (e.g., calcitriol) to control the rampant turnover of abnormal skin cells (768, 849). Affected animals should not be bred. Until more is learned about the genetics of the condition, it is difficult to make breeding recommendations for parents and siblings.

SPICULOSIS

Spiculosis refers to a hair follicle defect in which hairs are brittle and thickened and form nodules known as spicules. In all likelihood, the defect originates from abnormal fusion of primary and secondary hairshafts, with an onset between 6 and 12 months of age. Although the mode of inheritance is unknown, the condition is limited to male Kerry blue terriers (655).

The diagnosis is suspected based on clinical signs and can be confirmed with histopathologic assessment. If necessary, successful treatment can be initiated with isotretinoin. Even though the recommendation is to not breed affected dogs, the problem is minor and entirely cosmetic.

ULCERATIVE DERMATOSIS

Ulcerative dermatosis is a poorly understood condition seen in the collie and Shetland sheepdog. It is thought to possibly represent a variant of dermatomyositis (465) or perhaps a subset of cutaneous lupus erythematosus. Lesions may be triggered or worsened by trauma, estrus, or concurrent disease. A genetic nature for the disorder has not been proven, but a familial nature is suspected because the condition occurs only in these two breeds.

Vesiculopustular eruptions evolve into coalescing ulcers, most commonly involving the inguinal area. The diagnosis is suspected on the basis of breed predisposition and clinical signs and is confirmed by biopsies for histopathologic assessment. Some dogs have electromyographic abnormalities similar to dogs with dermatomyositis. No specific treatments are available for ulcerative dermatosis, although pentoxifylline or the combination of doxycycline (or tetracycline) and niacinamide has had the most success anecdotally. Until more is known about the condition, affected animals should not be used for breeding.

VITAMIN A-RESPONSIVE DERMATOSIS

Vitamin A-responsive dermatosis is a condition of scaling and crusting, centered on the hair follicle rather than the skin surface. It responds to supplementation with large doses of vitamin A. This is not a deficiency disease and has nothing to do with dogs being on a nutritionally deficient diet. The mode of inheritance is unknown, but it is seen in the American cocker spaniel, Cairn terrier, and Labrador retriever (768, 929, 949).

The syndrome is characterized by dandruff, hair loss, and marked crusting, especially on the topline. Diagnosis is confirmed by biopsies for histopathologic assessment, in which characteristic findings include marked orthokeratotic hyperkeratosis and follicular hyperkeratosis. Blood levels of vitamin A are invariably normal in affected dogs. By definition, the condition responds to supplementation with megadoses of vitamin A, typically within 3 to 8 weeks. Although it is recommended not to breed affected animals, little evidence is available to suggest that the disorder is truly familial.

VITILIGO

Vitiligo is a patchy loss of pigment that may be inherited or acquired. In general, it refers to white patches that appear on the surface of the skin. Whitening of the hairs is called *leukotrichia*, and graying of the hair is *poliosis*. A heritable form of vitiligo has been reported in the Belgian Tervuren, Doberman pinscher, German shepherd dog, Labrador retriever, and rottweiler (768, 930, 1137), and the condition has also been reported in Old English sheepdog littermates (934). It is not uncommonly reported in the dachshund, German short-haired pointer, and Newfoundland (12).

Anti-melanocyte antibodies have been found in the serum of affected Belgian Tervurens. Progressive leukotrichia and leukoderma have also been reported in a Newfoundland dog. A similar loss of pigment in chow chows is attributable to an inherited deficiency of tyrosinase, an enzyme important in pigment production (768). Leukotrichia has been reported in Labrador retrievers that started to show whitening of the hairs on the face, back, and legs by 8 weeks of age (1111). Apparently the condition resolved on its own by 14 weeks of age, with no need for treatment.

Some anecdotal evidence suggests that nutritional intervention may be useful in certain cases of vitiligo. To date, the most popular combination is oral folic acid and injectable cobalamin (768). Too few cases have been reported to make any definitive comments. It is recommended that biopsies and blood profiles be done on all cases of pigmentary change, to differentiate genetic and nongenetic causes. Although the genetics of most forms of vitiligo remain unknown, the recommendation is to not breed affected animals. There are no screening tests to detect carriers.

X-LINKED ECTODERMAL DYSPLASIA

X-linked ectodermal dysplasia, a rare condition seen in German shepherd dogs, is transmitted as an X-linked recessive trait (157). Fibroblasts from affected dogs have a specific decreased expression of epidermal growth factor receptors on their plasma membranes, similar to findings in human patients with X-linked anhidrotic/hypohidrotic ectodermal dysplasia (HED). There tend to be symmetrical areas of hairlessness, together with missing or misshapen teeth. Biopsies of affected areas reveal a complete absence of hair follicles and adnexa.

Affected animals should not be bred, and the dam should be considered an obligate carrier. Female siblings should be considered potential carriers of the condition.

ZINC-RESPONSIVE DERMATOSIS

Zinc-responsive dermatosis is a scaling and crusting disorder that does not result from a dietary deficiency of zinc. Some dogs seem to require higher doses of zinc in their diet than others, perhaps because of some problem with absorption of zinc from the digestive tract. There is a clear breed predisposition for Alaskan malamutes, American Eskimo dogs, Samoyeds, and Siberian huskies, but Doberman pinschers and Great Danes may also be affected (768, 949).

The mode of inheritance is currently unknown. Alaskan malamutes have a genetic defect that interferes with intestinal zinc absorption (164). It is thought that a transient zinc deficiency might develop in rapidly growing Doberman pinschers and Great Danes, making their zinc-responsive dermatosis different from that seen in the northern-breed dogs (164, 768). Some ingredients in dog foods can also interfere with zinc absorption; these ingredients include calcium, fiber, iron, tin, and copper.

Most affected dogs have crusting on the nose, periocular areas, footpads, elbows, and hocks as a result. Itchiness is seen in about half of affected dogs. Diagnosis can be confirmed with biopsies for histopathologic evaluation. By definition, the condition responds to supplementation with zinc, which must be continued daily for life. Recurrence is common if zinc dosing is missed or the frequency is decreased (164).

Until more is known about the genetics of this condition, it is best not to breed affected animals. Although no screening tests are available to detect actual carriers, parents and siblings should be considered suspect carriers.

CHAPTER 4

Endocrine Disorders

The profession has made great strides in studying the genetics of endocrine disorders so that meaningful genetic counseling can be accomplished. This includes unraveling the mystery of adrenal sex hormone imbalance in the Pomeranian, creating a registry for hypothyroidism, and documenting the genetic basis for diabetes mellitus in at least one breed of dog.

ADRENAL SEX-HORMONE DERMATOSES

Adrenal sex-hormone imbalance may occur in intact or neutered males and females. The condition, sometimes called alopecia X, has been reported as a familial dermatosis in the chow chow, keeshond, Pomeranian, poodle, and Samoyed (768, 898). The specific pathogenesis of adrenal sex-hormone imbalance is not known. The condition is postulated to have become more common as breeders consciously select for animals that grow a thick hair coat (hirsutism) (921). Abnormal adrenal steroidogenesis may result in adrenocortical hyperprogestinism and hyperandrogenism (921).

Based on the similarity of the canine dermatosis to the syndrome in people, a partial deficiency of an adrenal enzyme, 21-hydroxylase, is suspected, at least in the Pomeranian. This partial enzyme defect reduces cortisol, which subsequently stimulates excess adrenocorticotrophic hormone (ACTH) secretion, adrenal hyperplasia, and excess adrenocortical androgen production.

Hair follicles have sex hormone receptors that can convert one sex hormone to another. Therefore, elevated adrenocortical sex hormones could bind to the follicle hormone receptors and create the haircoat changes observed in the adrenal sex-hormone syndrome. Growth hormone-responsive dermatosis actually may be a subset of this disorder, as sex hormones have both stimulatory and inhibitory effects on the secretion of growth hormone (920).

Clinically, the disorder is similar to growth hormone-responsive dermatosis in that it affects animals in young adulthood and they develop a bilaterally symmetrical alopecia, often with pronounced hyperpigmentation (Figure 4-1). The primary hairs are lost first, followed eventually by secondary hairs. The diagnosis is confirmed by assessing sex hormone levels before and after an injection of ACTH. In most dogs, progesterone and 17-hydroxyprogesterone are elevated. Other hormones that are usually elevated include 17-β-estradiol, dehydroepiandrosterone (DHEA), androstenedione, and testosterone (768).

The treatment of choice for intact animals with adrenal sex-hormone imbalance is neutering. This resolves the situation in most cases and stops the animal from passing on the trait to future generations. If neutering fails to resolve the problem, methyltestosterone, o,p-'DDD (mitotane), and ketoconazole have all been used to treat the condition (768).

Until the genetics of the condition are better understood in the different breeds affected, all affected animals should be removed from breeding programs. More far-reaching restrictions are not warranted at this time, especially because the condition is more of a cosmetic than a medical concern.

DIABETES MELLITUS

Diabetes mellitus is traditionally divided into four subgroups:

1. Insulin-dependent diabetes mellitus (IDDM)
2. Non-insulin-dependent diabetes mellitus (NIDDM)
3. Gestational diabetes
4. Diabetes attributable to other disease processes.

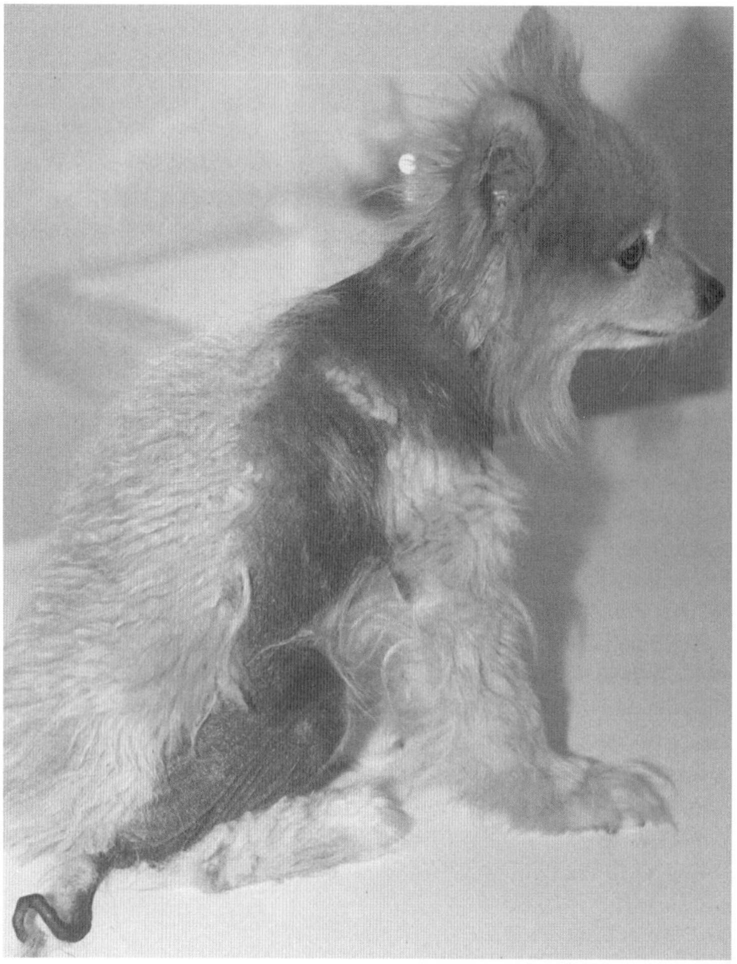

Figure 4-1 Adrenal sex hormone dermatosis
Courtesy of Dr. Lowell Ackerman, Mesa Veterinary Hospital, Mesa, Arizona

IDDM seems to involve a genetic predisposition to developing an autoimmune process, resulting in destruction of beta cells in the pancreatic islets of Langerhans (451). Diabetes has been proven to be hereditary in a line of keeshonden, likely as an autosomal recessive trait (*dmdm*), causing islet cell hypoplasia (549). Also at greater risk are the Alaskan malamute (637), chow chow (175), Doberman pinscher (384), English springer spaniel (175), Finnish spitz (637), golden retriever (384), Labrador retriever (384), miniature schnauzer (384), Old English sheepdog (175), poodle (451), schipperke (637), and West Highland white terrier (175).

Although many cases of diabetes mellitus are believed to be familial, only in keeshonden has the mode of inheritance been determined. A recessive mode of inheritance has been suggested in the golden retriever (175).

Diabetes mellitus usually becomes clinically evident when 75% of the pancreatic beta cells are destroyed and hyperglycemia results. In keeshonden, this is typically evident by 6 months of age. Diagnosis is based on consistent clinical signs (e.g., polyuria, polydipsia, polyphagia, weight loss), persistent hyperglycemia, and glucosuria. About 50% of diabetic dogs have beta cell-specific autoantibodies (451).

Treatment is initiated with insulin in most cases. Feeding diets high in dietary insoluble fiber may aid in glycemic control (767). Measuring fructosamine (81) or glycosylated hemoglobin (288) concentrations may aid in determining the extent of glycemic control.

Prevention may become easier as autoantibody testing becomes more refined. It may then be possible to test close relatives of diabetic dogs to determine relative risk. In keeshonden, both parents of affected dogs should be considered as obligate carriers of the trait and should not be used in future matings. Until more is learned about the condition and its heritability, it is advisable not to include affected individuals in breeding programs. Parents and siblings should be considered potential carriers of the trait.

GROWTH HORMONE-RESPONSIVE DERMATOSES

Growth hormone, also known as somatotropin, is secreted by the adenohypophysis (anterior pituitary gland) and acts either directly on tissues or by intermediaries, known as somatomedins. Like most of the body's hormones, growth hormone is controlled by a negative feedback loop. Growth hormone-releasing factor stimulates release of growth hormone, and somatostatin inhibits its release. In the adult dog, growth hormone deficiency does not affect stature. Growth hormone is necessary for hair growth and the development of elastic fibers in the skin.

A putative growth hormone-responsive alopecia has been described in the American water spaniel, chow chow, keeshond, miniature and toy poodles, Pomeranian, and Samoyed (611, 920, 937). A mode of inheritance has not been determined. There is a clinical overlap between animals being diagnosed with growth hormone-responsive dermatosis or hyposomatotropism and those being described as adrenal sex-hormone dermatosis, castration-responsive dermatosis, and alopecia X.

Clinically, the condition is distinctive. Young adults, predominantly males, develop a bilaterally symmetrical alopecia that affects only the trunk. Often, the skin becomes extremely hyperpigmented in the hairless areas. Otherwise, the condition is entirely asymptomatic and the dogs remain in good health.

Skin biopsies for histopathologic assessment are suggestive, and the diagnosis is confirmed by a growth hormone response test in which growth hormone and insulin-like growth factor 1 (IGF-1) are measured before and following an injection of a growth hormone stimulant, such as xylazine, medetomidine, clonidine, or growth hormone releasing factor (147, 324, 768, 920). These drugs can drastically lower blood pressure, and severe hypotension has been reported in small breeds. In most cases, even though growth hormone levels may be low, IGF-1 levels tend to be normal, suggesting that the lack of growth hormone response to stimulation is not a primary event (895). No treatment is necessary for this strictly cosmetic disorder, but some dogs respond to castration (556), melatonin (768), or growth hormone (611, 768, 937).

To make any recommendations regarding breeding strategies is difficult because so much remains unknown about this perplexing disorder. It is best to avoid using animals from affected families in breeding programs.

HYPERADRENOCORTICISM (CUSHING'S SYNDROME)

Hyperadrenocorticism, also known as Cushing's syndrome, results when the body produces too much cortisol, its own form of cortisone. In 85% of cases, the condition results from a tumor (not usually malignant) in the pituitary gland (pituitary-dependent hyperadrenocorticism) of the brain. About 70% of these pituitary tumors are located in the pars distalis, and 30% in the pars intermedia. The remaining 15% of non-pituitary hyperadrenocorticism cases arise from tumors (half are malignant) on the adrenal glands (adrenal-dependent hyperadrenocorticism), located near the kidneys.

Pituitary-dependent hyperadrenocorticism (PDH) is usually caused by a small pituitary corticotrophic adenoma that secretes excess adrenocorticotropic hormone (ACTH). The cause of adenoma formation is either overstimulation of the adenohypophysis, resulting from a defect in the hypothalamus, or a genetic disorder in one adenohypophyseal cell line (1071). In one study screening canine pituitaries for mutations of the Gs-alpha, H-ras, K-ras, and N-ras genes, no mutations were found in any of the codons tested; this suggests that gene mutation is not often involved in the tumorigenesis of corticotrophic adenomas in dogs (1071).

The condition is typically seen in middle-aged to old animals, not pups. Although a mode of inheritance has not been proposed, pituitary-dependent hyperadrenocorticism is reported most often in the boxer (768, 775), Boston terrier (768, 775), dachshund (768, 775), Dandie Dinmont terrier (768), poodle (768, 775), and Yorkshire terrier (768).

Cushing's syndrome has many different clinical manifestations, the most common of which are an increase in thirst, hunger, and the need for urination. Other clinical signs include hair loss, susceptibility to infection, muscle atrophy, and lack of energy (Figure 4-2).

Several different screening tests for Cushing's syndrome are available, including systemic arterial blood pressure and urine protein/creatinine ratios (799). A normal urinary cortisol:creatinine ratio (UCCR) is presumptive evidence that the dog does *not* have Cushing's syndrome. Final confirmation usually relies on a low-dose dexamethasone suppression test or ACTH stimulation test (405). The ACTH stimulation test has a higher positive-predictive value when studies take into consideration the prevalence of the disease in the population (1069).

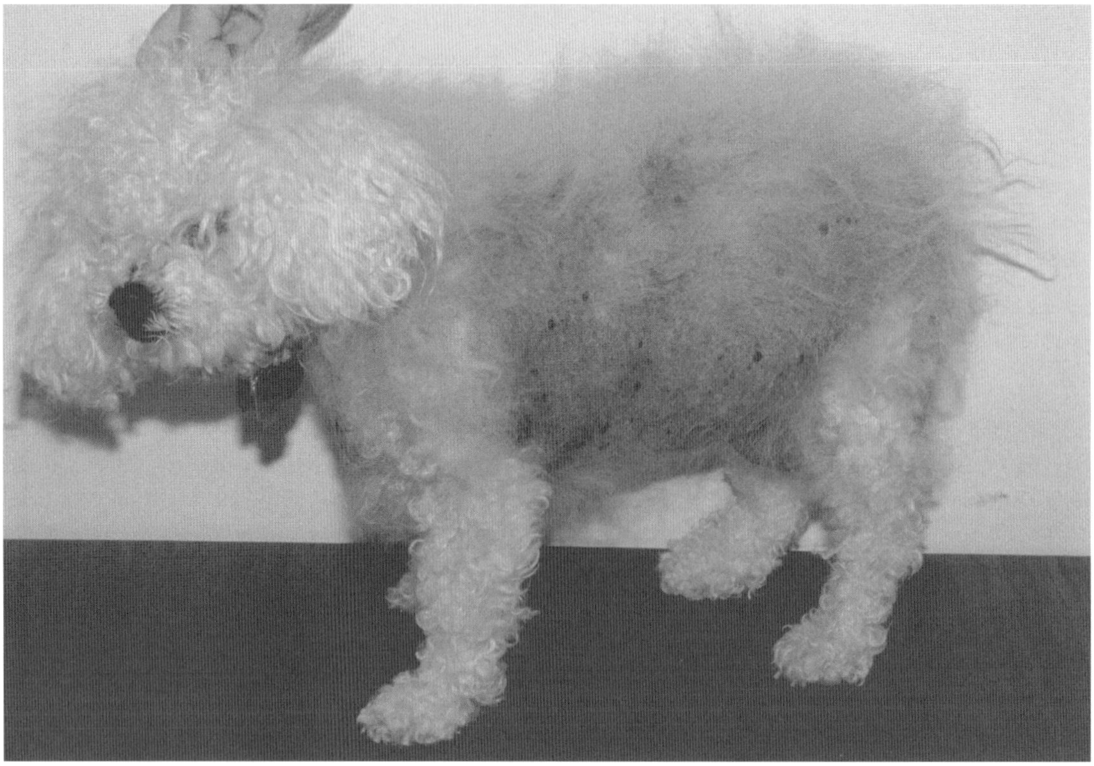

Figure 4-2 Hyperadrenocorticism
Courtesy of Dr. Lowell Ackerman, Mesa Veterinary Hospital, Mesa, Arizona

The low-dose dexamethasone suppression test can help distinguish dogs with pituitary tumor from those with adrenal tumor, unless there is no adrenal suppression (305). In that instance, differentiating pituitary and adrenal forms of the disease is made on the basis of high-dose dexamethasone-suppression testing, endogenous ACTH testing, or adrenal ultrasonography. Ultrasonography is an effective method for localizing adrenal lesions but not for differentiating benign and malignant processes (53).

Treatment for the pituitary disease is most often attempted with mitotane (44, 253, 830), ketoconazole (44, 768), or selegiline (44, 124). For large pituitary tumors (at least 8 mm), radiotherapy can help shrink the tumor, but it is not adequate for controlling clinical signs in most cases (381). ACTH stimulation testing is the preferred method of monitoring response to therapy and is superior to urine cortisol-creatinine ratios (UCCR) (22, 274). The UCCR fails to predict post-ACTH cortisol concentration during mitotane treatment sufficiently to be a clinically reliable indicator of treatment control (860). For adrenal tumors, the treatment used most often is surgery or large doses of the medicines mentioned above.

ACTH Stimulation Testing

- Collect baseline sample
- Inject 5 mcg/kg synthetic ACTH IV (maximum 250 mcg)
- Collect post-stimulation sample in 1 hour

Cushing's syndrome is more prevalent in the breeds mentioned, but a specific genetic connection has not been determined. Thus, the best means of prevention is to select dogs from families with no history of the disease.

HYPERPARATHYROIDISM

Juvenile hyperparathyroidism is a primary hyperplasia of the parathyroid glands that is inherited as an autosomal recessive trait in the German shepherd dog (384). It leads to stunted growth, polyuria, polydipsia, and muscle weakness. Laboratory abnormalities include hypophosphatemia with increased fractional clearance of phosphorus, increased plasma levels of PTH, hypercalcemia, and radiographic evidence of decreased bone density (384). Affected dogs should not be used for breeding, and the parents are

Handling of Cortisol Samples

If EDTA-treated plasma is obtained for cortisol assay, no cooling is necessary. If a serum sample is obtained, however, it should be shipped in an insulated container with cool packs (45)

considered obligate carriers of the trait. Siblings are suspect carriers.

HYPOADRENOCORTICISM (ADDISON'S DISEASE)

Hypoadrenocorticism is not an uncommon endocrine disorder in dogs that can occur as primary atrophy of the adrenal cortex or secondary to pituitary insufficiency. The most common cause in the dog is believed to be an immune-mediated destruction of the adrenal gland. Familial hypoadrenocorticism has been described in the leonberger (971), Nova Scotia duck tolling retriever (134), Portuguese water dog (46), and standard poodle (515, 775, 831, 947). Other breeds suspected to be at increased risk include the Great Dane (515, 775, 831), rottweiler (775, 831), soft-coated wheaten terrier (775, 831), and West Highland white terrier (515, 775, 831). There also seems to be a predilection for females (134, 664, 775, 831), some quoting a female preponderance of 70% (46, 515). A condition known as type II polyglandular autoimmune syndrome, or Schmidt's syndrome, has been described in dogs that have deficiencies of both adrenal and thyroid hormones (971).

The clinical presentation is extremely diverse, and many cases are misdiagnosed initially as something else until enough clinical signs become apparent. Typical signs of the disorder are weakness, depression, vomiting, diarrhea, and abnormal cardiac function (594). Basic laboratory tests may be suggestive, with characteristic electrolyte disturbances of hyponatremia and hyperkalemia. The diagnosis is confirmed with ACTH stimulation tests or actual ACTH levels. It is also important to assess thyroid function concurrently, as some animals develop the polyglandular syndrome mentioned above.

Treatment must be directed against the adrenal deficiency, as well as at the clinical conditions, such as hypotension, hypovolemia, hyperkalemia, and acidosis. Replacement therapy with both glucocorticoid and mineralocorticoid hormones is usually required, but cases with glucocorticoid deficiency may be controlled without mineralocorticoids (594). Either desoxycorticosterone pivalate (DOCP) or fludrocortisone acetate may be considered for initial treatment of mineralocorticoid deficiencies (525). It is best not to breed affected animals, especially those with familial hypoadrenocorticism.

HYPOTHYROIDISM

Hypothyroidism is a complex syndrome associated with a progressive deficiency of thyroid hormone. It is the most common of the endocrine disorders seen in dogs, yet a true incidence is not known with certainty. Most cases are attributable to idiopathic atrophy of the thyroid gland or lymphocytic thyroiditis (918). Based on a variety of studies, several breeds have been cited as being predisposed to the condition:

Afghan hound (768)
Airedale terrier (704)
Alaskan malamute (768)
American cocker spaniel (704, 814)
beagle (814)
boxer (769, 814)
borzoi (181)
Chinese shar pei (699, 745, 768)
chow chow (768)
dachshund (704, 814)
Doberman pinscher (704, 769, 814)
English bulldog (768, 814)
golden retriever (704, 814)
Great Dane (769, 814)
Irish setter (704, 769, 814)
Irish wolfhound (768)
miniature schnauzer (704, 769, 814)
Newfoundland (768)
Pomeranian (704)
poodle (769, 814)
Shetland sheepdog (704, 814).

Unfortunately, most breed surveys have not been completed with definitive diagnostic testing, so true breed associations are not known with certainty. There are no true incidence rates or prevalence estimates for hypothyroidism in the canine population (912). Congenital canine hypothyroidism has also been reported (383) but is rare.

Canine hypothyroidism is a diagnostic challenge because of the wide variations in clinical signs. It is a progressive disease that may be classified as early (compensated) or late (advanced) disease. Most dogs do not develop clinical signs until young adulthood. Even then, the manifestations are vague and a diagnosis may not be confirmed until years later. Increased susceptibility to infection and

Table 4-1 OFA Hypothyroidism Certification Program

Conclusion	FT_4D	cTSH	TgAA
Normal	Normal	normal	negative
Autoimmune thyroiditis	Decreased	increased	positive
Compensated autoimmune thyroiditis	Normal	increased	positive
Idiopathic reduced thyroid function	Decreased	increased	negative
Equivocal		all other results	

lower energy levels are common early manifestations. Bilaterally symmetrical alopecia, weight gain, seborrhea, intolerance to cold, reproductive failure, anemia, and poor hair regrowth following clipping are usually not seen until later in the progression of the disorder (812).

Systemic diseases (euthyroid sick syndrome) and drug therapies have significant effects on thyroid hormone levels and can complicate diagnosis. In addition, many different assays and function tests have been developed in an attempt to identify the most sensitive and specific thyroid tests for hypothyroidism. On basic blood profiles, the most common abnormality is elevated cholesterol, but this is a nonspecific finding. Until recently, serum thyroxine (T_4) and triiodothyronine (T_3) have been used as thyroid screening tests. These were often followed by a thyrotropin-stimulating hormone (TSH) response test as a confirmatory test. Now, however, three new tests have made correct diagnosis of hypothyroidism a more routine matter:

1. Free T_4 (FT_4) by equilibrium dialysis (832)
2. Canine thyroid-stimulating hormone (cTSH) (1138)
3. Thyroid autoantibody levels—namely, thyroglobulin autoantibodies (TgAA), T_3 autoantibodies (T_3AA), and T_4 autoantibodies (T_4AA) (1032)

The combination of FT_4 and cTSH assays is the screening test of choice for primary hypothyroidism (768, 832). Though antibodies against microsomal antigen and antinuclear substance can also be evaluated, only anti-thyroglobulin antibody seems to be correlated with lymphocytic thyroiditis (1064). False-positive results (elevated cTSH) occur in 10% to 15% of dogs with nonthyroidal illness; and several hounds (Afghan hound, Irish wolfhound, saluki, Scottish deerhound) have higher levels of cTSH than dogs of other breeds (768). Preliminary reports suggest that elevated TSH is found in 60% to 80% of hypothyroid dogs (811). In dogs with hyperadrenocorticism, approximately 25% have a serum FT_4 concentration below normal (811). Based on preliminary research, TgAA levels seem to be a useful predictor of lymphocytic thyroiditis, seen in perhaps 50% of hypothyroid dogs (768). TgAA levels have the potential for aiding early diagnosis of thyroiditis in dogs and identifying dogs likely to perpetuate hypothyroidism in breeding programs (751).

The diagnostic accuracy of cTSH combined with FT_4D makes this two-test combination the diagnostic assessment of choice. Autoantibodies, specifically TgAA, are useful for early recognition of lymphocytic thyroiditis and for genetic counseling on a breed-by-breed basis.

A certifying registry is available through the Orthopedic Foundation for Animals, in which cTSH, FT_4D, and TgAA are assessed. The information is useful to breeders in determining the best dogs for a breeding program relative to the incidence of lymphocytic thyroiditis. A certificate and breed registry is available for dogs found to be "normal" at 12 months of age. Reevaluation is recommended at 2, 3, 4, 6, and 8 years of age. Dogs with equivocal test results should be reevaluated 3 to 6 months later. Table 4-1 summarizes the OFA certification program for hypothyroidism.

The standard treatment for primary canine hypothyroidism is replacement therapy with levothyroxine (T_4). A minimum of 2 to 3 months of treatment is usually required to elicit a good clinical response. Thyroid levels should be monitored periodically and the dosage modified accordingly (813). Given the potential for inheritance, it is difficult to justify breeding affected individuals (518). It is harder to render advice applicable to parents, siblings, and other close relatives.

PITUITARY DWARFISM (HYPOPITUITARISM)

Pituitary dwarfism is inherited in German shepherd dogs and Karelian bear dogs as a simple autosomal recessive trait (920). The most common pathological finding is a cystic Rathke's cleft (283). The condition also has been reported in the spitz,

Weimaraner, and toy pinscher, but a mode of inheritance has not been determined in these breeds (384, 774). A second presentation of hypopituitarism was reported in a litter of inbred Weimaraners that had concurrent absence of the thymic cortex and growth hormone deficiency.

Pituitary dwarfism is uncommon. The owner's early observations in the pituitary dwarf are failure to grow and retention of a puppy coat compared to littermates. The clinical signs are variable depending upon the extent of impairment of function of the pituitary gland. Progressive symmetrical bilateral alopecia and hyperpigmentation are observed. The skin may become thin and scaly. Behavioral abnormalities (aggression) and variable gonadal abnormalities (atrophic gonads, anestrus) may also be apparent. The other hormones that may be deficient in hypopituitarism are thyroid, adrenocortical, and gonadal. In the immunodeficient Weimaraner puppies, a wasting syndrome was observed at a few weeks of age. Emaciation, lethargy, and persistent infections preceded death.

Diagnosis of a pituitary dwarf is presumptive based on failure to grow. Radiographs will detect skeletal and organ abnormalities. The diagnosis is confirmed by documenting a growth hormone deficiency. Because dwarfism may be associated with hypothyroidism and hypoadrenocorticism, full endocrine profiles should be done with all suspected pituitary dwarfs.

Symptomatic treatment may include antiseborrheic shampoos and rinses. Administration of growth hormone may resolve dermatologic manifestations but will not result in reversal of the dwarfism unless it is instituted early. Because growth hormone is not available commercially, it is not a valid option for treatment in most cases. Medroxyprogesterone acetate also can be used for the long-term treatment of congenital growth hormone deficiency, as an alternative for heterologous growth hormone (556).

In the German shepherd dog and Karelian bear dog, in which the mode of inheritance has been determined to be autosomal recessive, affected individuals should not be bred. Parents of these dogs should be considered as obligate carriers of the trait, and siblings as potential carriers.

RECURRENT (SEASONAL) FLANK ALOPECIA

The cause of recurrent flank alopecia, also known as seasonal flank alopecia, has yet to be determined. It may be a follicular dysplasia or a pineal endocrinopathy. Disorders of sex hormones or growth hormone also have been considered. The breeds primarily affected are the Airedale terrier (689), bearded collie (768), boxer (689), English bulldog (899), and miniature schnauzer (899). The condition, however, has been reported in many breeds, including the affenpinscher, Bouvier des Flandres, briard, bullmastiff, dachshund, Doberman pinscher, German shorthaired pointer, golden retriever, Griffon Korthal, Labrador retriever, Lhasa apso, rottweiler, and Scottish terrier (323, 768, 1092). A hereditary nature has not been confirmed.

In most cases, bilaterally symmetrical truncal hair loss begins in the fall and starts to remit in the spring. Many reports, however, describe the opposite seasonal pattern of hair loss and regrowth. The hair loss is confined primarily to the lateral trunk, and there is associated hyperpigmentation of skin in the area. The fur grows back spontaneously in 3 to 4 months in most cases, but the new hair may be coarser, finer, or of a slightly different color.

The diagnosis of recurrent flank alopecia is confirmed by biopsies for histopathologic assessment. Histopathologically, there are dilated and hyperkeratotic primary follicles and epidermal hyperpigmentation (689). Endocrine profiles, including tests for growth and reproductive hormones, are invariably normal (221). Despite a dearth of evidence for an endocrine etiology, the treatment of choice (in addition to conscientious neglect) is melatonin. Affected animals should not be used for breeding.

CHAPTER 5

Gastrointestinal Disorders

Even though gastrointestinal disorders are common, the genetic nature of most of these conditions remains poorly defined. At present, a genetic test is available for only one: copper hepatopathy in Bedlington terriers.

CHRONIC INFLAMMATORY HEPATIC DISEASE

Chronic inflammatory hepatic disease, also known as chronic active hepatitis, is a catch-all phrase for myriad liver diseases that result in inflammatory hepatitis, bile duct proliferation, fibrosis, and cirrhosis. Predisposed breeds include the American cocker spaniel, Bedlington terrier, Doberman pinscher, Labrador retriever, Skye terrier, and West Highland white terrier (261). In most cases, the underlying problem has to do with decreased biliary copper excretion, and this is dealt with as a separate topic—copper hepatopathy. In many other cases, no underlying cause is determined. A role for canine adenovirus type 1 (CAV-1) cannot be supported currently (178), but it is possible that the virus could cause the initial damage that eventuates in a self-perpetuating chronic liver disease.

Although elevated liver enzymes are to be expected, the diagnosis is confirmed on the basis of liver biopsy. Iron accumulation is a consistent finding (337). Most Doberman pinschers with chronic inflammatory hepatic disease have increased levels of hepatic copper, but not as high as seen with copper hepatopathy in Bedlington terriers (214, 996, 1031).

Whenever possible, underlying problems should be treated. Otherwise, symptomatic therapy consists of managing the diet, treating any secondary bacterial infections, and using drugs such as corticosteroids, ursodeoxycholate, colchicine, and zinc to address inflammatory mediators. In cases of hepatitis that seem to be familial, affected animals should not be used for breeding, and the mating that produced the affected individual should not be repeated.

CLEFT PALATE/CLEFT LIP

Congenital defects of the hard and soft palates may be an inherited trait with incomplete penetrance in the shih tzu breed, and possibly in pointers, bulldogs, and Swiss sheepdogs (198, 425, 647). An autosomal recessive mode of inheritance has been documented for cleft palate in Brittany spaniels (873). The condition is also common in the American cocker spaniel, Boston terrier, Cairn terrier, dachshund, English toy spaniel, German shepherd dog, Labrador retriever, miniature schnauzer, and Pekingese (181, 460). Breeders report cleft palate commonly in the French bulldog, but true incidence in the breed has not been determined. A syndrome in St. Bernards, purported to be autosomal recessive in nature, includes palate agenesis, anotia, incomplete bifid tongue, preaxial hind paw polydactyly, and an extra thoracic vertebra and rib (1084).

Cleft palate and cleft lip can result from either hereditary or environmental causes. The environmental causes include administration of drugs such as corticosteroids, metronidazole, or griseofulvin during pregnancy, among other possibilities. The diagnosis can be confirmed by visual inspection.

Mild problems might not require any treatment, but major defects require surgical correction. The use of folic acid to prevent cleft palate in the dog has been explored (292) and has lowered the incidence of cleft palate in Boston terriers studied, from 17.6% to 4.2%. Affected animals should not be bred.

COLITIS

Colitis refers to inflammatory disorders of the large intestine. Of the numerous variants reported, only histiocytic ulcerative colitis seems to have a strongly familial basis and is seen most commonly in boxers and French bulldogs (130). Chronic large-bowel diarrhea is the most common sign, and the diagnosis can be confirmed by colonic biopsies and histopathologic evaluation.

Several drugs are available for treatment, including sulfasalazine and immunosuppressive medications. Although it might be sensible to suggest that affected individuals not be bred, no evidence is available to suggest that the condition is truly heritable.

COPPER HEPATOPATHY

Some dogs are prone to developing liver disease in association with an inherited metabolic defect that causes copper to accumulate in the liver and lead to toxicity. This is similar to Wilson's disease in humans, but research has determined that the gene responsible for the condition in dogs is not identical to that in people, although affected dogs do have a defect in biliary excretion of copper (1149). The condition is reported in many breeds but most commonly in the Bedlington terrier, in which the frequency of the disease allele may be as high as 0.5 in both the US and British population of dogs, with 75% being either affected or carriers (103). Because the condition is spread as a recessive trait (404, 484), both parents must be carriers if a dog is found to be affected.

Other breeds reported with the presumed familial form of the condition include the beagle, Skye terrier, and West Highland white terrier (404, 436, 539, 889, 1033). Elevated hepatic copper levels have also been reported in the Airedale terrier, bulldog, bull terrier, cocker spaniel, collie, dachshund, Dalmatian, Doberman pinscher, German shepherd dog, keeshond, Kerry blue terrier, Labrador retriever, Norwich terrier, Old English sheepdog, Pekingese, pitbull terrier, poodle, Samoyed, schnauzer, and wire fox terrier (1030, 1032, 1151).

Affected dogs develop a slowly progressive form of liver disease. They are usually in young adulthood when the condition is first recognized. Normal hepatic copper concentrations are less than 400 ppm on a dry-weight basis, and hepatic damage begins to be noticeable when the hepatic copper concentration is above 2000 ppm (1030). Jaundice develops late in the course of the disease when liver function is severely compromised. The condition seems to differ somewhat in West Highland white terriers; they tend to accumulate copper in the liver early in life but seem to level out at copper levels between 400 ppm and 2000 ppm and remain asymptomatic (1030).

Researchers have discovered a genetic marker for copper toxicosis (1149) in the Bedlington terrier that can be detected by a DNA linkage test. This laboratory evaluation is an exceptionally important method for detecting carriers of the disease (455). The first test offered by VetGen used a linked marker that had two alleles (1 and 2) but required a known affected dog in the pedigree, confirmed by liver biopsy. More than 90% of dogs that were 1/1 were homozygous normal; over 90% that were 2/2 were homozygous affected; and those that were 1/2 were carriers.

That information was used to create marker typing that doesn't require the cumbersome assessment of the earlier version. With marker typing, a dog that is 1/1 is 90% likely to be homozygous normal (clear); a dog that is 2/2 is 72% likely to be affected (another 24% are carriers); and a dog that is 1/2 has a 95% chance of being a carrier. Results of the test can be formally registered with the Orthopedic Foundation for Animals.

Ideally, carriers should be removed from all breeding, to completely eliminate the trait. In breeds with a high incidence of copper toxicosis, it may be necessary to breed carrier to unaffected until enough unaffected animals are available for future breedings. This pairing produces unaffected and carrier animals but no affected individuals.

In breeds other than the Bedlington terrier, confirmation of diagnosis is still based on the results of liver biopsy and quantitative liver copper assay; carriers are not detected until they produce affected progeny (443). For dogs other than the Bedlington terrier with a family history of copper hepatopathy, it is advisable to select breeding animals that have had routine liver function screening. Although this won't pick up early cases in which no liver pathology is present, it is a less invasive method of screening. Those that have abnormal liver function tests on two occasions, one month apart, should have a liver biopsy and copper assay before being used in a breeding program.

A related condition, which has not been well characterized in the dog, is known as Menkes syndrome. In this X-linked condition, copper accumulates in the liver and is deficient in most other tissues of the body. The result is kinky hair, degenerative neurologic disease, and failure to thrive. In the dog, the Menkes gene has been identified on the X chromosome (403).

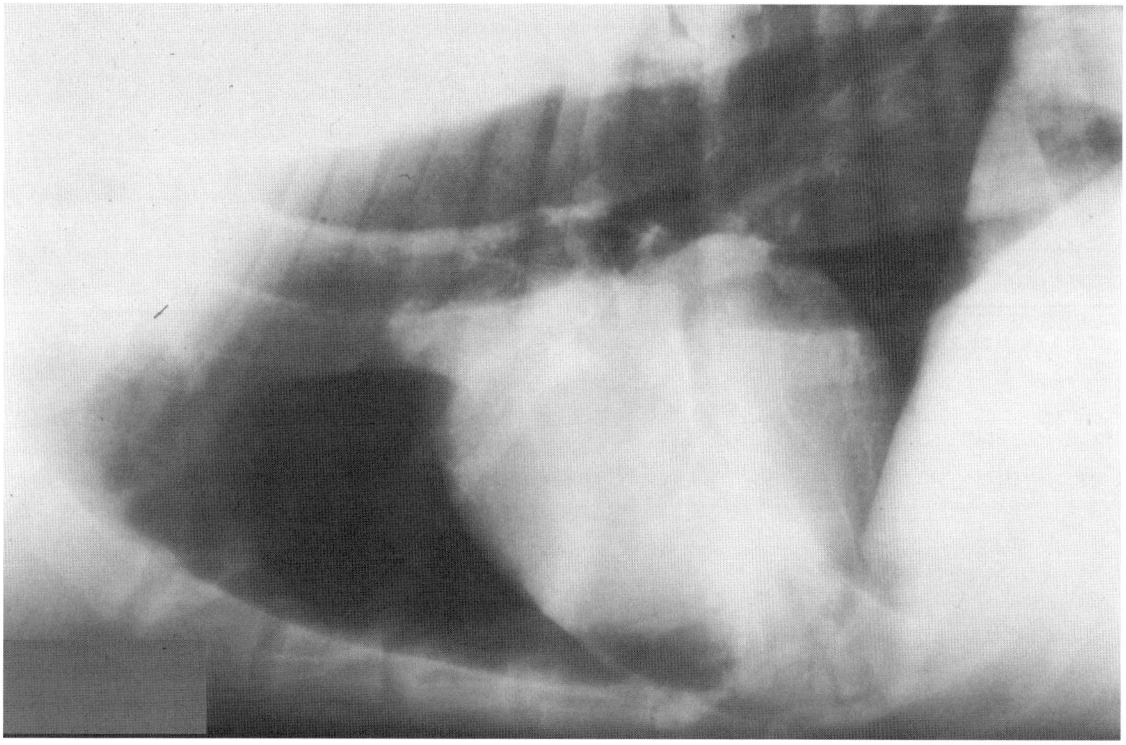

Figure 5-1 Lateral view of thorax of Labrador Retriever with megaesophagus and aspiration pneumonia
Courtesy of Jonathan T. Shiroma, Veterinary Radiologist, MedVet, Columbus, Ohio

ESOPHAGEAL MOTILITY DISORDERS

Esophageal motility disorders consist of congenital megaesophagus, esophageal hypomotility, and esophageal dysfunction. Congenital megaesophagus is inherited in the wire fox terrier as an autosomal recessive trait, and in the miniature schnauzer as an autosomal dominant trait (404, 479). There is also increased incidence in the Bouvier des Flandres, Chinese shar pei, German shepherd dog, Great Dane, greyhound, Irish setter, Labrador retriever, and Newfoundland (83, 187, 479). Esophageal dysfunction in the Chinese shar pei may also result from segmental hypomotility and esophageal redundancy (479).

A familial form of dysphagia associated with megaesophagus has been reported in young Bouviers des Flandres (82). This entity is believed to be a possible subset of muscular dystrophy. Onset of clinical signs is often first seen in puppies, although veterinary attention is typically not sought until the dogs are young adults. The clinical signs are attributable to dysphagia, although the prognosis is affected more by the aspiration pneumonia, which is a common sequel. Plasma creatine kinase (CK) levels are often increased, but histopathologic assessment of pharyngeal and esophageal muscle is needed to confirm the diagnosis. Affected dogs should not be used for breeding.

Clinically, esophageal motility disorders are characterized by regurgitation in puppies. Dogs fail to thrive, may produce excess saliva, and may develop respiratory distress as a consequence of aspiration pneumonia. The diagnosis can be suspected on the basis of plain radiographs and confirmed with contrast studies (Figure 5-1). Treatment includes feeding animals from an elevated platform and experimenting to see which consistency of food they tolerate best. Medical and surgical alternatives have been disappointing.

In the wire fox terrier, in which the condition is transmitted as an autosomal recessive trait, affected animals should not be bred and parents should be considered obligate carriers. Siblings are suspect carriers. In the miniature schnauzer, not breeding affected animals should eventually eliminate the trait from breeding lines.

EXOCRINE PANCREATIC INSUFFICIENCY

Exocrine pancreatic insufficiency (EPI) is typically attributable to pancreatic acinar atrophy; it rarely results from pancreatic hypoplasia or chronic pancreatitis. Although it has been reported in many breeds, it is seen most commonly in the German shepherd dog, in which there seems to be a genetic predisposition (40, 1106), possibly as an autosomal recessive trait (409). The collie (1107) and English setter (64) breeds also seem to have a hereditary form of the disorder.

Clinically, the condition is progressive and results in weight loss and semi-formed feces in the face of a ravenous appetite. The condition becomes clinically apparent with the loss of 85% to 90% of the exocrine pancreatic mass. Overgrowth of bacteria in the proximal small intestine follows in about 70% of cases. Coprophagia, pica, and occasional vomiting are also reported.

The diagnosis of EPI warrants a battery of tests for malassimilation, but the condition is typically confirmed with the assay for serum trypsin-like immunoreactivity (TLI). This test is very specific and requires just a single sample for analysis. The only difficulty in interpretation arises when the result falls borderline between obvious EPI and low normal. In these cases, it is best to retest in 1–2 months. Treatment is relatively straightforward and involves the dietary replacement of pancreatic enzymes, which are readily available commercially. Response, however, can vary significantly depending on the treatment product selected (1123).

Because the exact mode of inheritance for EPI is not known, it is best to eliminate from breeding programs individuals that are affected or have a family history of the condition. For the German shepherd dog, in which pancreatic insufficiency is believed to have an autosomal recessive mode of inheritance, parents should be considered carriers of the trait and siblings must be considered suspect carriers.

GASTRIC DILATATION-VOLVULUS (BLOAT)

Gastric dilatation (bloat) occurs when the stomach becomes distended with air. The air gets swallowed into the stomach when susceptible dogs exercise, gulp their food or water, or are stressed. Although bloat can occur at any age, it becomes more common as susceptible dogs get older. The breeds most vulnerable are those with a deep chest, such as boxers, Gordon setters, Great Danes, Irish setters, St. Bernards, standard poodles, and Weimaraners (109, 368). Also considered to be at increased risk are basset hounds, bloodhounds, borzois, Bouviers des Flandres, briards, collies, Doberman pinschers, German shepherd dogs, German shorthaired pointers, Irish wolfhounds, Labrador retrievers, Newfoundlands, and Scottish deerhounds (109, 133, 181). Purebreds are three times more likely than mutts to suffer from bloat.

Advice to Owners

Although bloat can't be completely prevented, you can do some easy things to greatly reduce risk.

- Don't leave food down for dogs to eat as they wish. Divide the day's meals into three portions, and feed morning, afternoon, and evening.
- Try not to let your dog gulp its food; if necessary, add some chew toys to the bowl so the dog has to work around these to get the food.
- Add water to dry food before feeding. Have fresh, clean water available all day but not at mealtime.
- Do not allow exercise for 1 hour before and after meals.

Following this feeding advice may actually save your dog's life. On the other hand, no studies have been done to support the contention that soy in the diet increases the risk of bloat. Soy is relatively poorly digested and can lead to flatulence, but the gas accumulation in bloat comes from swallowed air, not gas produced in the intestines.

Although bloat on its own is uncomfortable, the possible consequences are what make it life-threatening. As the stomach fills with air like a balloon, it can twist on itself and impede the flow of food within the stomach, as well as the blood supply to the stomach and other digestive organs. This twisting (volvulus or torsion) not only makes the bloat worse, but also results in toxins being released into the bloodstream and blood-deprived tissues dying.

Cardiac arrhythmias contribute to mortality in dogs that develop gastric dilatation-volvulus (577). These events, if allowed to progress, usually result in death in 4 to 6 hours. Approximately one-third of dogs with bloat and volvulus will die, even under appropriate hospital care, 15% within the first week (369).

A prospective study has demonstrated that physical condition at time of presentation is the most important variable in determining prognosis. The dogs that were depressed at the time of presentation were three times as likely to die as those that were alert, whereas those that were comatose at presentation were 35.8 times more likely to die (369). The same study showed that dogs treated medically had a 54.5% rate of recurrence, and those stabilized surgically with a gastropexy had a recurrence rate of only 4.3%. For those undergoing surgical management, mortality is most affected by the presence of cardiac arrhythmias, gastric necrosis, and the need for splenectomy (117).

Affected dogs will be uncomfortable, restless, depressed, and have an extended abdomen. They need veterinary attention immediately or they will suffer from shock and die. A variety of surgical procedures can be used to correct the abnormal positioning of the stomach and organs. Intensive medical therapy is also necessary to treat for shock, acidosis, and the effects of toxins.

A mode of inheritance has not been determined for gastric dilatation, although breeds with a deeper and narrower thorax have an increased risk (367). A study in Irish setters suggested that inbreeding itself does not profoundly affect risk, but genetic influences may be linked to thoracic depth/width ratios (916, 918). If thoracic conformation is linked to gastric dilatation-volvulus, at least in the Irish setter, this may provide an opportunity for selecting breeding stock to decrease the risk.

Another study done in Irish setters found that the most significant predisposing risks for developing gastric dilatation included aerophagia, a single food type, and feeding once daily, and that precipitating risks included recent kenneling and a journey by car (291). Interestingly, intensity or duration of exercise, temperament, appetite, and speed of eating did not contribute significantly to risk.

GLUTEN-SENSITIVE ENTEROPATHY

Gluten-sensitive enteropathy, also known as wheat-sensitive enteropathy, is a hereditary defect in small intestinal mucosal function associated with a sensitivity or intolerance to gluten. The condition is reported in Irish setters (1128) and appears to be familial (227, 844). Clinically, the condition presents as chronic diarrhea, starting when animals are 4 to 7 months of age.

The diagnosis can be suspected on the basis of folate/cobalamin levels, absorption studies, and biopsy, but is confirmed when the clinical problems resolve following institution of a gluten-free diet. Intestinal permeability testing, specifically urinary lactulose to rhamnose ratios, may be an adequate screening test during oral gluten challenge (342). Characteristic ultrastructural changes, such as stunted or irregular microvilli, are typically evident by 4 months of age (631).

Jejunal biopsies exhibit partial villous atrophy with intra-epithelial lymphocytes. Assessment of microvillar membrane proteins reveals an intense 85kDa protein spot. Both can be corrected by feeding a gluten-free diet (828). Dogs typically improve within 4 to 6 weeks after commencing the gluten-free meal, and treatment consists of feeding a nutritionally balanced gluten-free diet on a lifelong basis. Affected dogs, and those with a family history of gluten-sensitive enteropathy, should not be bred.

IMMUNOPROLIFERATIVE ENTEROPATHY

Immunoproliferative enteropathy is a poorly understood disorder of basenjis characterized by chronic intermittent bouts of diarrhea, anorexia, and weight loss (623). It seems to run in families, but the precise mode of inheritance has not yet been determined. Immunoproliferative enteropathy is really a syndrome, associated with an immune-mediated intestinal condition (lymphoplasmacytic enteritis), protein loss through the intestines (protein-losing enteropathy), abnormal digestion of nutrients (maldigestion), poor absorption (malabsorption), and increased concentrations of immunoglobulin A in the bloodstream.

Clinically, most affected dogs are in young adulthood when they are first affected, and some are even middle-aged. Diarrhea is severe and intermittent, and may be preceded by loss of appetite. The condition improves, only to recur again and again. This is associated with weight loss, and there may be bilaterally symmetrical alopecia. Despite all these ailments, most affected dogs appear bright and alert. Episodes of diarrhea may be prompted by stressful events such as boarding, dog shows, "heat," and vaccination.

The diagnosis isn't simple because so many other disorders can cause intermittent diarrhea in dogs. These include enteritis, exocrine pancreatic insufficiency, histoplasmosis, parasites, lymphosarcoma, and metabolic disorders, among others. The hallmark of diagnostic changes in immunoproliferative enteritis is elevated levels of IgA with characteristic changes noted on endoscopic biopsy. With an ultrasound examination, the generalized thickening of the intestinal wall is usually apparent.

Immunoproliferative enteritis has no cure, but clinical manifestations are sufficiently variable that some animals will do well despite a long-term poor prognosis. The small intestinal bacterial overgrowth (SIBO) associated with immunoproliferative enteritis is best controlled by special diets (low in sugars, starches, and fats) and antibiotics. Good quality protein sources and rice usually make up the basis of a therapeutic diet. Dietary protein source does not seem to be a factor in the pathogenesis of immunoproliferative enteropathy (99). Fructo-oligosaccharides (FOS), natural compounds found in various plants, make an excellent alternative to starch when they are used in diets for dogs with SIBO. Antibiotics such as metronidazole, tylosin, and oxytetracycline seem to be most effective. The immunological component is treated with immunosuppressive drugs such as prednisone, alone or with azathioprine.

Affected dogs should not be used for breeding. Until the pattern of inheritance for this disorder is better understood, giving meaningful advice regarding selection of "clear" individuals is difficult.

PANCREATITIS

Acute pancreatitis is commonly encountered in dogs, and there is a clear breed predisposition in dogs, if not evidence for outright inheritance. High-fat diets, abnormal lipid profiles, hypercalcemia, ischemia, and drug administrations (e.g., corticosteroids, L-asparaginase, azathioprine) have all been implicated as initiating causes of pancreatitis (961). Intercurrent diseases—especially diabetes mellitus, hyperadrenocorticism, obesity, hypothyroidism, chronic renal failure, neoplasia, congestive heart failure, and autoimmune disorders—are also commonly reported, although they may not be actual risk factors (192). Breeds at increased risk include the Airedale, Cairn terrier, Lhasa apso, miniature poodle, miniature schnauzer, and schipperke (192).

Vomiting, anorexia, depression, and acute abdominal pain are characteristic clinical signs of pancreatitis (913). Diagnosis can be rendered based on radiographic or ultrasonographic findings and elevated serum levels of the pancreatic enzymes lipase and amylase. Therapy involves restricting oral food intake and providing adequate parenteral fluids. Surgery is considered if pancreatic abscess or pseudocyst is suspected, the patient has hemorrhagic necrotic pancreatitis that doesn't respond adequately to medical management, or bile-duct obstruction or bowel ischemia is suspected (913).

To make recommendations regarding breeding affected dogs is difficult because no data are available to substantiate a familial link. In families where acute pancreatitis is prevalent, the dogs should not be bred. This can prove troublesome, as most cases are reported in dogs older than 7 years of age (192), which most likely would have been used in breeding programs already.

PORTOSYSTEMIC SHUNTS

Congenital portosystemic shunts (PSS) are vascular anomalies that divert portal venous blood directly to the systemic venous circulation, bypassing the liver. Intrahepatic shunts occur when the fetal ductus venosus fails to close at or following birth. Extrahepatic PSS occurs when a congenitally anomalous blood vessel leaves the portal circulation, bypasses the liver, and connects directly with the systemic venous circulation. Although the hereditary nature of portosystemic shunts has not been proven (482), these are most commonly reported in the American Cocker spaniel (404, 857), Australian cattle dog (585, 1041), Cairn terrier (404), dachshund (585), Irish wolfhound (404, 678), Maltese (585), miniature schnauzer (404, 638, 1041), and Yorkshire terrier (126, 404, 638), and may be associated with other congenitohereditary defects, such as cryptorchidism.

A less severe form, hepatoportal microvascular dysplasia, may be inherited in Cairn terriers (585). With microscopic shunting, the small volume of blood shunted away is the only difference between this and the macroscopic varieties. Dogs with microvascular dysplasia alone tend to be older and have higher values for mean corpuscular volume (MCV) and serum total protein albumin, creatinine, cholesterol, urea, and blood glucose, while those dogs with both portosystemic shunting and microvascular dysplasia tend to have higher values for pre- and postprandial serum bile acid concentrations, leukocyte counts, and serum alkaline phosphatase and aspartate aminotransferase activities (14). Recently, a condition resembling idiopathic or noncirrhotic portal hypertension of humans has been reported in Doberman pinschers (250). These dogs lack evidence of intrahepatic arteriovenous fistulae, portal vein atresia, or intrahepatic fibrosis.

Clinically, portosystemic shunting is evident in young animals (under 1 year of age) and tends to be progressive, yet intermittent. Affected pups tend to be thin and smaller than nonaffected littermates. It is important to be aware that more than one individual in a litter may be affected by PSS. Although gastrointestinal signs are often nonspecific, most diagnoses are suspected when the liver impairment results in hepatic encephalopathy. Urinary tract disease is also evident at times, associated with crystals (ammonium biurate) and calculi that form in the presence of high blood ammonia levels.

The diagnosis is suspected with laboratory alterations reflecting mild liver disease, elevated bile acids, ammonium biurate crystalluria and abnormal sulfobromophthalein (BSP) retention and ammonia tolerance testing. If necessary, the diagnosis can be confirmed by portography or Technetium scans, which also provide information on the anatomical location of the shunt (Figure 5-2).

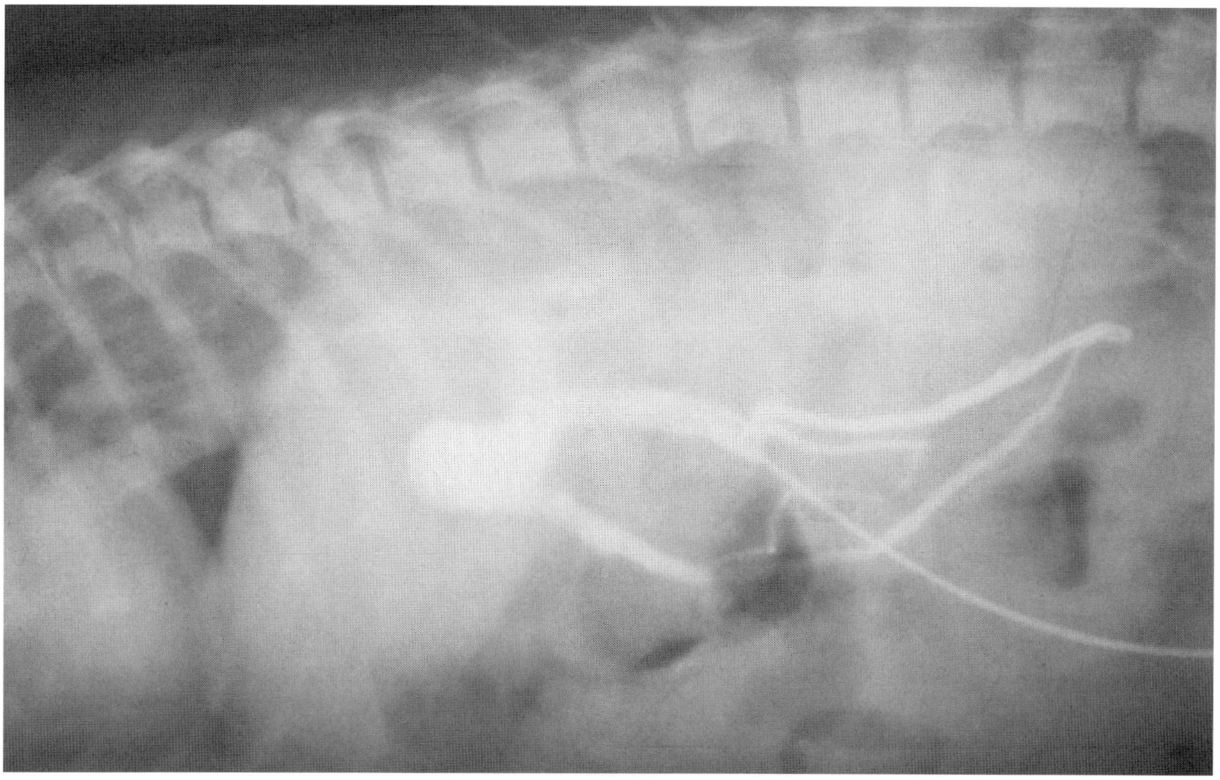

Figure 5-2 Intra-operative mesenteric portogram
Courtesy of Jonathan T. Shiroma, Veterinary Radiologist, MedVet, Columbus, Ohio

Doberman pinschers with idiopathic noncirrhotic portal hypertension usually have erythrocyte microcytosis, increased concentrations of bile acids, and a small liver on ultrasonography.

Treatment is directed at using medical therapy to stabilize the patient with neurologic signs and surgery aimed at shunt occlusion. A significant proportion of dogs with portosystemic shunts managed medically have a reasonably good quality of life (1098). Gradual vascular occlusion with an instrument such as the ameroid constrictor is a good method for treating single extrahepatic shunts (1087). For dogs with intrahepatic portosystemic shunts that survive surgery, about 75% become clinically asymptomatic and require no further medication or diet control (1109). Because the exact genetic nature of congenital portosystemic shunting is not known, it is best to exclude from breeding programs animals from families with a history of this condition.

PROTEIN-LOSING ENTEROPATHY

Protein-losing enteropathy refers to a collection of small intestinal diseases that result in the loss of plasma and proteins into the gastrointestinal tract. For example, one cause is congenital intestinal lymphangiectasia, reported to be common in the Norwegian lundehunde (404, 1128) and the basenji (460). Whereas the condition in the Norwegian lundehunde is a primary condition, in the basenji it occurs secondary to immunoproliferative enteropathy. In the soft-coated wheaten terrier, protein-losing enteropathy and nephropathy appear familial, perhaps autosomal recessive. Adverse food reactions are believed to be involved with the condition in this breed (1057). Other causes, which may or may not have a hereditary component, include eosinophilic gastroenteritis, plasmacytic-lymphocytic enteritis, and granulomatous enteritis.

Typically, the conditions are associated with chronic diarrhea and possibly weight loss, ascites, and anorexia, but not in all cases. Measurement of fecal alpha-1-protease inhibitor with a canine ELISA assay may be a sensitive indicator of the condition but is not yet routinely available from veterinary laboratories. The underlying problem should be identified by endoscopic biopsies. Treatment should be directed at the underlying problem, and feeding low-fat or MCT-based diets to minimize lymphatic absorption.

Until more is known about the genetics of the condition, it is difficult to make informed breeding recommendations. For the time being, and assuming the condition does turn out to be an autosomal recessive trait, affected animals should not be bred and parents should be considered carriers. Normal-appearing siblings should be considered suspect carriers.

PYLORIC STENOSIS

Pyloric stenosis is a narrowing of the pyloric canal, resulting in partial or complete obstruction to the outflow of ingesta from the stomach to the small intestines. Congenital antral hypertrophy, caused by hypertrophy of pyloric circular smooth muscle or mucosa, is most commonly reported in the Boston terrier and boxer (478). The principal clinical feature of the condition is vomiting, starting immediately after weaning, with the introduction of solid food.

The diagnosis can be confirmed with contrast radiographic studies or gastroscopy. Mild cases can be treated with small, frequent feedings of highly digestible foods and medications such as metoclopramide and cisapride. Surgery is the treatment of choice for long-term management, and 80% of dogs do well post-operatively (478). It is best not to breed affected dogs, even though the mode of inheritance has not been determined.

SMALL INTESTINAL BACTERIAL OVERGROWTH (SIBO)

Small intestinal bacterial overgrowth (SIBO) is often considered to be an important cause of chronic diarrhea in the dog. The German shepherd dog is the breed affected most often. Beagles are occasionally affected (1127). The reasons for this condition are unclear. In fact, some researchers are not convinced that primary SIBO has been adequately documented in the dog. It is known that German shepherds are prone to a variety of other intestinal ills, as well as IgA deficiency. It is hypothesized currently that the combination may be the trigger for development of SIBO. This is just a hypothesis; however, and the whole story is far from complete. Other assertions suggest links to achlorhydria (lack of stomach acid), excessive antibiotic therapy, stagnant loop syndrome, and exocrine pancreatic insufficiency.

Regardless of the initiating cause, the proliferation of bacteria in the small intestine affects the absorption of nutrients from this region of bowel. Affected dogs may have difficulty digesting starch; fats may be broken down to hydroxy fatty acids; and bile salts may be deconjugated. All can result in diarrhea.

The diagnosis is not straightforward. One of the first screening tests to run is blood levels of the vitamins folate and cobalamin. Typically, serum levels of folate are elevated and levels of cobalamin are depressed. Confirmation may require quantitative bacterial culture of intestinal fluids (248). Blood levels of lactulose/rhamnose and xylose/3-O-methylglucose, measured before and 2 hours after oral administration of these compounds, seem to be a valid method of assessment (994). Biopsies usually don't reveal changes that can confirm the diagnosis, but characteristic findings include jejunal villous atrophy with increased numbers of lymphocytes and plasma cells within the lamina propria and the surface epithelium (63). Researchers are looking at a hydrogen breath test for dogs similar to the one used with people (58). Initial results are encouraging.

Treatment for SIBO involves administration of an antibiotic (e.g., tetracycline) and feeding a diet low in carbohydrates (sugars and starches) and fats. Good quality protein sources and rice usually make up the basis of a therapeutic diet. Fructo-oligosaccharides (FOS), natural compounds found in various plants, make an excellent alternative to starch when used in diets for dogs with SIBO (1126). Eventual relapse likely means that the underlying condition was never addressed. Affected dogs should not be used for breeding. Until more is learned about the genetics of the condition, it is difficult to make informed breeding recommendations.

CHAPTER 6

Hemolymphatic Disorders

Diseases of the hemolymphatic system have been studied intensively, and definitive diagnosis is becoming more routine. Now we can identify carriers in many instances, and this gives us the tools needed for effective genetic counseling.

CUTANEOUS AND RENAL GLOMERULAR VASCULOPATHY

Cutaneous and renal glomerular vasculopathy is a poorly understood ulcerating disease that affects racing greyhounds. It has variably been referred to as "Alabama rot" and "Greenetrack disease." Restriction of this syndrome to greyhounds, and in some cases to littermates or closely related litters, suggests a genetic predisposition (152). The ultimate cause remains elusive, but infectious and immune-mediated causes are being considered. A dietary microbial toxin, possibly from *E. coli*, could be involved, especially considering that most racing greyhounds are fed a raw-meat diet. Because episodes have been reported in dogs that have never eaten raw-meat diets, though, more than one cause is likely.

Clinical signs are the result of a vasculopathy of deep arterioles in the dermis and subcutis (208). Glomerular vessels are similarly affected, and ultrastructural changes suggest that glomerular endothelial damage is an important early event in the pathogenesis of the condition (444).

The disease is one of multiple well-demarcated ulcers, principally involving the legs but occasionally including the trunk and inguinal region. Most affected dogs remain active and alert, but some suffer from systemic illness and kidney disease. Biopsies for histopathologic assessment confirm the diagnosis.

The only treatment indicated for cutaneous and renal glomerular vasculopathy to date is excellent supportive care, which includes feeding a nutritious and easily assimilated commercial diet, topical wound therapy, subcutaneous or intravenous fluids, and coverage with a bactericidal antibiotic (e.g., cephalexin) for 7 to 10 days. Until more is learned about the condition, information on which to base breeding recommendations is lacking.

FACTOR I DEFICIENCY

Fibrinogen is the substrate for thrombin and the precursor of fibrin. Afibrinogenemia has not been conclusively documented in dogs (502), but dysfibrinogenemia has been seen in borzois (407) and collies (320), and hypofibrinogenemia has been seen in St. Bernards (320) and vizslas (75). Dysfibrinogenemia is suspected when the activated coagulation (clotting) time (ACT), activated partial thromboplastin time (aPTT), prothrombin time (PT), and thrombin time (TT) are prolonged. The result is typically mild bleeding. With hypofibrinogenemia, the clotting profiles are similar but fibrinogen levels are reduced.

Because most case reports have not provided sufficient information to distinguish between dysfibrinogenemia and hypofibrinogenemia, it might be best to categorize the clinical severity as mild to severe rather than to worry about distinctions of terminology. Bleeding diathesis can be severe and require infusions of plasma or cryoprecipitate.

Too few cases have been documented to predict a mode of inheritance or offer meaningful advice regarding genetic counseling. Both autosomal recessive and autosomal dominant forms have been described in other species.

FACTOR II DEFICIENCY

Prothrombin is synthesized in the liver and is converted to thrombin by the action of the prothrombinase complex. Prothrombin deficiency is extremely rare in dogs. Too few cases have been reported to make any breed-related associations, but it has been reported in the English cocker spaniel, boxer, and otterhound (263). The condition is suspected when the activated partial thromboplastin time (aPTT) and prothrombin time (PT) are prolonged and the thrombin time (TT) is normal. The diagnosis is confirmed by analysis of factor II activity.

Treatment may be attempted with transfusions of plasma or whole blood. Too few cases have been documented to predict a mode of inheritance (other than in the boxer) or offer meaningful advice regarding genetic counseling. In the boxer, hypoprothrombinemia is inherited as an autosomal recessive trait (320). In this breed, affected animals should not be bred and parents are considered obligate carriers. Siblings are suspect carriers.

FACTOR VII DEFICIENCY

Factor VII deficiency is relatively rare but has been reported in the Alaskan malamute, beagle, boxer, bulldog, and miniature schnauzer (70, 703). It is believed to be transmitted either as an autosomal recessive trait (70) or as an autosomal dominant trait (320), depending on whose research one chooses to believe. Animals rarely suffer from spontaneous hemorrhage but, rather, display easy bruising or postsurgical oozing.

The diagnosis is suspected when the prothrombin time (PT) is slightly prolonged and the activated partial thromboplastin time (aPTT) and thrombin time (TT) are normal, and is confirmed by analysis of factor VII activity. Treatment is rarely indicated, but transfusions with plasma can be attempted, if needed.

Ideally, affected animals should not be used for breeding and parents and siblings should be considered as potential carriers and tested for the trait. Because the clinical significance of this condition is controversial, however, the ultimate decision regarding inclusion or exclusion in a breeding program should be a breeder option.

FACTOR VIII DEFICIENCY (HEMOPHILIA A)

Factor VIII deficiency is one of the most common inherited coagulopathies of dogs, reported in almost all breeds. It is transmitted as an X-linked recessive trait and is most commonly reported in the German shepherd dog (320, 706, 1025), German shorthaired pointer (499), and Siberian husky (706). It is also seen with some frequency in the beagle, Cairn terrier, Chihuahua, collie, English setter, French bulldog, greyhound, Irish setter, Labrador retriever, poodle, St. Bernard, Samoyed, Shetland sheepdog, vizsla, and Weimaraner (46, 281, 322, 673). This list is far from complete. Hemophilia A has been reported in nearly all breeds, and in mongrels as well.

> **Factor VIII Deficiency (Hemophilia A)**
>
> Hemophilia A is one of the most common inherited coagulopathies in dogs, being reported in almost every dog breed and in mongrels as well. While DNA testing is likely to become available for hemophilia in the not-too-distant future, such tests are likely to be breed-specific since it is anticipated that there are likely many different mutations at work in the different breeds.

As an X-linked trait, the condition is transmitted by females and manifested primarily in males. Females develop hemophilia only when the sire is a hemophiliac and the dam is either a carrier or a hemophiliac. A gene defect has been documented in dogs (144), but in people hundreds of different mutations can result in hemophilia A. The same situation is believed to be true for dogs. Regardless of the actual gene defect, the result is absent or reduced factor VIII activity.

Depending on the actual activity level of factor VIII in the blood, hemophilia A can cause neonatal deaths. Although some cases can be subclinical, with sufficient factor VIII activity to avoid spontaneous hemorrhage, most dogs become lame as a result of bleeding into the joints and muscles. Even minor surgeries can result in profound bleeding episodes in the hemophiliac dog. Hemophilia A should be considered as having numerous presentations in young male dogs, including excessive or pronounced bleeding, swelling, lameness, and even neurologic disorders.

In general coagulation screening profiles of hemophiliac dogs, the activated partial thromboplastin time (aPTT) is prolonged while the PT (prothrombin time) and thrombin time (TT) are normal. The diagnosis is confirmed by measuring factor VIII activity. Levels between 5% and 10% of normal may be tolerable, less than 3% may be associated with spontaneous hemorrhage, and levels less than 1% of normal typically cause severe clinical signs, including neonatal mortality. Small dogs seem to tolerate lower levels better than larger dogs, presumably because of less weight bearing on capillaries.

Factor VIII coagulant antigen (fVIII:CAg) assay can determine if the defect is quantitative or qualitative in nature, but this assay is available only for human hemophiliacs. In dogs, the factor VIII coagulant (FVIII:C) activity, rather than the antigen, is measured. The stabilization and activity of factor VIII coagulant requires complexing with von Willebrand factor (vWF) in the blood.

Current tests do not conclusively detect carriers of the trait. A combination of FVIII:C and vWF measurement may be helpful for purposes of genetic counseling, but misclassification is still a major limitation of this approach (726). The aPTT is a good screening test for hemophilia and for monitoring response to therapy. Studies have shown that the DNA polymorphisms in the human factor VIII gene can be used to detect carriers of hemophilia in the dog (180). A commercial DNA linkage test should be available in the near future. Direct DNA tests will likely be extremely breed-specific, however, and have yet to be developed.

Factor VIII deficiency has no cure. Treatment includes transfusions with fresh-frozen plasma or, preferably, cryoprecipitate. An inhibitor of factor VIII:C may be present (1038). In these cases, it is best to consider increased transfusion therapy. Some clinicians add corticosteroid treatment to the therapeutic regimen, but this is controversial.

Affected dogs should not be used for breeding, and the dam of any affected dog is an obligatory carrier and should also be removed from the breeding population. Siblings of the affected dog and its dam are assumed to be potential carriers. All siblings of the affected dog and its dam should be screened for factor VIII:C and vWF activities. Also, any daughters of an affected dog are obligate carriers and should not be bred.

FACTOR IX DEFICIENCY (HEMOPHILIA B)

Hemophilia B, also known as Christmas disease, is presumed to be the second most common severe coagulopathy affecting dogs, and at least three mutations have been characterized at the gene level (70, 115). Therefore, hemophilia B in different breeds may result from different mutations in the factor IX gene.

Preliminary research suggests that the occurrence of hemophilia B within each breed or line represents a spontaneous and unique mutation event (399). Thus, in the Lhaso apso, there is a deletion and a base transition (650), whereas in Labrador retrievers, the entire gene is deleted (115). These changes render the final factor IX molecule nonfunctional. The disorder is transmitted as an X-linked recessive trait, regardless of the actual gene mutation present. Breeds reported with hemophilia B are the following:

> **Factor IX Deficiency (Hemophilia B)**
>
> Hemophilia B affects many breeds of dogs, and different gene mutations have been documented. While still in the experimental stages, it is possible that gene therapy will become a viable treatment option.

- Airedale terrier (263)
- Alaskan malamute (263, 320, 673)
- American cocker spaniel (263, 320, 673)
- Bichon frisé (263)
- Black and tan coonhound (216, 263, 320, 673)
- Cairn terrier (216, 263, 320, 673)
- French Bulldog (263, 673)
- German shepherd dog (263, 304)
- German wirehaired pointer (263)
- Labrador retriever (115, 263, 320, 1078)
- Lhasa apso (650)
- Old English sheepdog (263)
- St. Bernard (216, 263, 320, 673)
- Scottish terrier (263, 320)
- Shetland sheepdog (263)

Depending on the actual activity level of factor IX in the blood, hemophilia B can be life-threatening. Although some cases are subclinical, with sufficient factor IX activity to avoid spontaneous hemorrhage, most dogs develop lameness as a result of bleeding into the joints and muscles. Even minor surgeries can result in profound bleeding episodes in the hemophiliac dog.

In general coagulation screening profiles of affected dogs, the activated partial thromboplastin time (aPTT) is prolonged and the PT (prothrombin time) and thrombin time (TT) are normal. The diagnosis is confirmed by measuring factor IX activity. Levels between 5% and 10% of normal are usually tolerable; less than 3% may be associated with spontaneous hemorrhage; and levels less than 1% of normal typically cause severe clinical signs, including neonatal mortality. Small dogs seem to tolerate lower levels than larger dogs.

A factor IX antigen (FIX:Ag) assay is used to determine if the defect is quantitative or qualitative in nature, but in most cases a FIX activity assay is all that is available from commercial laboratories. Current tests do not conclusively detect carriers of the trait, although a combination of FIX activity and FIX:Ag is likely to be predictive.

Factor IX deficiency has no cure. Treatment includes transfusions with fresh-frozen plasma, cryo-poor plasma, cryosupernatant, or whole blood. If more than one transfusion is needed (as in most cases), it is best to measure not only factor IX antigen (fIX:Ag) but also inhibition of factor IX activity. If an inhibitor is present, increased transfusion therapy, or possibly concurrent treatment with corticosteroids, will likely be required.

Recently, a new gene therapy called chimeraplasty has been used experimentally in dogs with hemophilia B. Chimeraplasty is a novel gene repair technology designed to correct genetic mutations or to inactivate genes implicated in specific physiological and disease processes. The term *chimera* is used because the treatment employs a combination of DNA and RNA. The RNA/DNA sequence in these oligonucleotide compounds aligns with the DNA sequence in the gene that carries the mutation and replaces the mutation with the correct base pair. This experimental technology is being developed and marketed by Kimeragen, Inc., Newtown, Pennsylvania. Recombinant Factor IX is available for use in humans (e.g., BeneFix™), but inhibitor formation seems to preclude its use in dogs.

Affected dogs should not be used for breeding, and the dam of any affected dog should also be removed from the breeding population. All siblings of the affected dog and its dam (and her siblings) should be screened for factor IX activity. A commercial DNA test for hemophilia B is currently not available. Because several different defects seem to be associated with the condition, the test likely will have to be breed-specific. Gene therapy will likely be a treatment option at some time in the future (107, 639, 715) and, experimentally, hepatic gene transfer has been utilized in the dog (508).

FACTOR X DEFICIENCY

Factor X deficiency is rare but has been reported in the American cocker spaniel (70, 263) and Jack Russell terrier (70, 263). It is transmitted as an autosomal dominant trait, with variable penetrance (320). Individuals homozygous for the gene are usually stillborn or die within the first weeks of life with massive hemorrhage (75). In human medicine, this condition has been referred to as Stuart-Power trait (407).

The diagnosis is suspected when the activated partial thromboplastin time (aPTT) and prothrombin time (PT) are prolonged and the thrombin time (TT) is normal. The diagnosis is confirmed by specific analysis of factor X activity. Levels of 70% or less may be associated with hemorrhage; animals with less than 5% activity are at most risk; levels below 5% of normal are usually lethal. Stillbirths are common to parents carrying the trait. Affected animals should not be bred, and both parents and all siblings should be carefully evaluated for evidence of the disorder.

FACTOR XI DEFICIENCY

Factor XI deficiency, also known as plasma thromboplastin antecedent deficiency, or Rosenthal syndrome, is rare in dogs. The mode of inheritance in this species has not been confirmed, but it is autosomal dominant in people and autosomal recessive in cattle. It is presumed to be autosomal incompletely dominant in the dog (322), but it has also been reported in the literature as autosomal recessive (320). Factor XI deficiency has been reported in the English springer spaniel (263, 320, 407), Great Pyrenees (263, 320, 407), Kerry blue terrier (75, 320, 532), and Weimaraner (263).

Spontaneous hemorrhage is rare in affected dogs, but they typically show protracted bleeding following surgery or trauma. The diagnosis is suspected when the activated partial thromboplastin time (aPTT) is prolonged and the prothrombin time (PT) and thrombin time (TT) are normal. The diagnosis is confirmed by specific analysis of factor XI activity. An inhibitor to factor XI may be present.

Treatment for specific bleeding episodes is attempted with transfusions of fresh-frozen plasma. Affected animals should not be bred, and parents and siblings should be carefully evaluated for evidence of the disorder.

FACTOR XII DEFICIENCY

Factor XII deficiency (Hageman trait) is rare in dogs. The mode of inheritance in at least one family of miniature poodles was determined to be autosomal dominant (70), but it has also been reported in the literature to be autosomal recessive in poodles (320). Other breeds affected include the Chinese shar pei, German shorthaired pointer, and standard poodle (114, 263). The condition is known to be autosomal recessive in cats and is discovered relatively frequently on coagulation screening of cats with bleeding tendencies. Hageman trait is not typically associated with a bleeding diathesis or thrombosis.

The diagnosis is suspected when the activated partial thromboplastin time (aPTT) is markedly prolonged and the prothrombin time (PT) and thrombin time (TT) are normal. The diagnosis is confirmed by specific analysis of factor XII activity. Treatment is usually not required. Ideally, affected animals should not be bred and parents and siblings should be evaluated carefully for evidence of the disorder. Because the clinical significance of this condition is controversial, however, the ultimate decision regarding inclusion or exclusion in a breeding program should be a breeder option.

HEREDITARY MACROCYTOSIS/STOMATOCYTOSIS

Hereditary macrocytosis/stomatocytosis is a poorly defined entity that may reflect an erythrocyte membrane defect. It is characterized by macrocytosis (and/or stomatocytosis) and a mild reticulocytosis, without evidence of anemia. It has been reported in the Alaskan malamute and the miniature schnauzer (802). In the malamute, it has been associated with chondrodysplasia (75).

A form of familial stomatocytosis, similar to Menetrier's disease in people, is associated with hypertrophic gastritis (867, 922). Familial macrocytosis and dyshematopoiesis has been reported in poodles, in which the macrocytosis is also associated with hypersegmented neutrophils. Animals affected with the disorder should not be bred, and parents and siblings should be carefully evaluated for evidence of the disorder.

HEREDITARY NONSPHEROCYTIC HEMOLYTIC ANEMIA

Hereditary nonspherocytic hemolytic anemia, resulting from a shortened life span of red blood cells, has been reported in beagles and is presumed to have an autosomal recessive mode of inheritance (624). A more severe nonspherocytic hemolytic anemia has also been reported in poodles, associated with hemosiderosis, myelofibrosis, reticulocytosis, hepatosplenomegaly, and osteosclerosis (461, 858). Whereas the condition in beagles results in a moderate anemia, the disorder in poodles is severe and can be fatal. Affected animals should not be bred, and parents are suspect carriers of the trait.

METHEMOGLOBIN REDUCTASE DEFICIENCY

Methemoglobin reductase deficiency results in methemoglobinemia, which can cause brown mucous membranes, weakness, and, potentially, hypoxia. Fortunately, most dogs with methemoglobin reductase deficiency are asymptomatic. Breeds recognized with the disorder include the borzoi (426, 677), Chihuahua (426, 677), English setter (426, 677), Pomeranian (315, 426, 677), poodle (426, 677), toy Eskimo (427, 677), Welsh corgi (426, 677), and some mixed-breed dogs (677).

Although this is presumed to be a genetic disorder, no family studies have been completed. A diagnosis can be confirmed by measuring erythrocyte methemoglobin reductase (cytochrome-b5 reductase) enzyme activity. Even though affected dogs have a normal life expectancy, excluding them from breeding programs is prudent.

LYMPHEDEMA

Primary lymphedema has been reported in the Belgian Tervuren, borzoi, English bulldog, German shepherd dog, German shorthaired pointer, Great Dane, Labrador retriever, Old English sheepdog, poodle, and rottweiler (75, 232, 461, 579, 673, 1022). It is presumed to be caused by developmental defects in the lymphatics and lymph nodes. The condition is characterized by pitting edema, typically on the limbs, and a generalized form has been reported as a heritable condition in bulldogs (75).

The diagnosis can be confirmed by lymphangiography. Surgery may be an option, but spontaneous recovery with advancing age has been reported in some cases. Insufficient information is available on the condition on which to base breeding recommendations, other than that affected animals should not be bred.

MICROCYTOSIS

Microcytosis can be associated with portosystemic shunts or with deficiencies of iron, pyridoxine, or copper, and a presumed inherited microcytosis also has been reported in Akitas and Shiba Inus (380). The animals are clinically normal and have a low mean corpuscular volume (MCV), without concurrent anemia. Thus, it is important to recognize microcytosis in Akitas and Shibas as a variant of normal.

Breeding recommendations are difficult to make because the condition is asymptomatic. Breeders will have to decide if they wish to rid their lines of this trait.

PELGER-HUET (PH) ANOMALY

PH anomaly is a hereditary defect of white blood cells. The mode of inheritance is not known for certain, but it is presumed to be autosomal dominant (75). Animals that are carriers of the trait have neutrophils that are poorly segmented (and eosinophils, basophils, etc.), but otherwise they are not immune-compromised or predisposed to infection (566). Dogs that receive a PH gene from both parents usually die before they are born, and survivors are considered immune cripples.

The condition in reported in the Australian blue heeler, Australian shepherd, black and tan coonhound, basenji, border collie, Boston terrier, cocker spaniel, foxhound, German shepherd dog, redbone hound, Samoyed, and in mongrels (530).

The importance of determining the carrier state of PH is that the white blood cell changes may lead clinicians to suspect an ongoing infection when, in reality, it is just a serendipitous finding. The diagnosis is typically made when toxic changes cannot be found to accompany the presumed "left shift," so that PH anomaly rather than infection is suspected.

No therapy is needed for PH anomaly because there is no associated clinical disease. Animals with PH anomaly, however, should not be bred so the trait can be removed from the gene pool. Parents are considered to be obligate carriers, and siblings to be suspect carriers. If two animals with PH anomaly are inadvertently bred, the litter size will be reduced because pups receiving PH genes from both parents will likely die *in utero*.

PREKALLIKREIN DEFICIENCY

Prekallikrein deficiency, also known as *Fletcher trait*, is rare in dogs but is presumed to be an autosomal recessive disorder (70). It has been described only in the poodle (75, 177) and in association with factor XII deficiency (801). The condition rarely results in a bleeding diathesis.

The condition is suspected when the activated partial thromboplastin time (aPTT) is prolonged and the prothrombin time (PT) and thrombin times (TT) are normal. The diagnosis is confirmed by analysis of prekallikrein activity. Specific treatment is not usually required, but transfusion with plasma remains an alternative, if necessary.

Affected animals should not be bred, and parents should be considered as obligate carriers of the trait. Siblings are suspect carriers. Because the clinical significance of this condition is controversial, the ultimate decision regarding inclusion or exclusion in a breeding program should be a breeder option.

PSEUDOHYPERKALEMIA

Hyperkalemia refers to elevated levels of potassium in the blood (a potentially fatal disorder), and pseudohyperkalemia is a false elevation of potassium caused by some peculiar blood cell properties in the Akita, and potentially other Japanese breeds (e.g., Shiba Inu, Tosa Inu) as well. Most blood cells contain potassium, but some Akitas (and others) have higher cellular levels of potassium than other breeds. The increased red cell potassium content seems to be quite common in these breeds.

The condition causes a problem only because it can induce laboratory errors. If a blood sample is drawn to perform biochemical tests and the sample is not evaluated promptly or separated (removing the cells from the serum) within a few hours, the intracellular potassium will be released and the laboratory may report that the patient has hyperkalemia. Whether the increased plasma potassium content results from spontaneous erythrocyte hemolysis from red cell fragility or whether the sodium/potassium pump of these breeds is more susceptible to failure is unknown (241).

As an aside, this red cell peculiarity also makes these breeds more susceptible to onion toxicity, so client counseling should include cautions about feeding onions to the breeds in question. Because hyperkalemia can lead to heart irregularities and the cause (e.g., hypoadrenocorticism, to which the Akita is also prone) can be difficult to pinpoint, this *false* disorder absolutely has to be recognized before extensive and expensive tests are conducted. In addition, affected dogs should not be used as blood donors because life-threatening hyperkalemia could potentially result from stored blood. Because the condition is medically innocuous, it is unclear whether breeding intervention is warranted.

Pseudohyperkalemia

Pseudohyperkalemia is of primary importance, not because of any adverse effects in dogs, but because it can result in laboratory findings that might be suggestive of other disease processes. The increased red cell potassium content may make these animals more susceptible to onion toxicity, but otherwise has few clinical repercussions.

PYRUVATE KINASE DEFICIENCY

Pyruvate kinase (PK) deficiency is an inherited trait associated with the shortened life span of red blood cells. Pyruvate kinase (PK) is an enzyme necessary for energy metabolism in red blood cells. When it is deficient, the red blood cells have a shortened survival time in the bloodstream, and the bone marrow attempts to compensate but spills out immature red blood cells (reticulocytes) into the blood, resulting in reticulocytosis. The red blood cells of normal dogs have only R-type PK, whereas PK-deficient dogs have both R-type and M(2)-type PK (1121). The M(2) type is the isoenzyme that typically predominates in fetal erythrocytes.

The condition is most prevalent in the basenji (360, 1122) but has also been reported in the American Eskimo dog (426), beagle (359, 428, 1122), Cairn terrier (914, 1122), and West Highland white terrier (168, 1122). The gene defect has only been characterized in the basenji and West Highland White terrier and the mutations differ by breed. Pyruvate kinase deficiency has an autosomal recessive mode of inheritance (426).

The ultimate result of pyruvate kinase deficiency is macrocytic, hypochromic, hemolytic anemia, as the body's immune system targets the defective red blood cells for destruction. The anemic dog may demonstrate exercise intolerance, pale gums, increased heart rate, and an enlarged liver and spleen. In some cases, affected dogs may appear smaller than their normal littermates.

The diagnosis is suspected when hemolytic anemia is detected in a breed at risk. Suspect dogs should also be tested for evidence of erythrocyte autoimmunity (e.g., Coombs' test, presence of spherocytes), parasites, Heinz bodies, and heartworm. The PK-deficient dog invariably tests "normal" and tends not to lose hemoglobin in the urine, such as seen with English springer spaniels affected with phosphofructokinase deficiency. Diagnosis is now much simpler since DNA tests have become available that will, with virtual certainty, detect affected, unaffected and carrier animals in the basenji breed.

PK deficiency has no cure, and most affected dogs die by 4 years of age as a result of bone marrow or liver failure. The liver failure results from iron overload, which in turn is brought about by destruction of iron-rich, hemoglobin-containing red blood cells in the liver. Iron-chelating drugs such as deferoxamine mesylate might prolong the life expectancy of affected animals by postponing liver failure, but it has no effect on the bone marrow.

Fortunately, PK deficiency now can be completely prevented by screening all breeding animals of susceptible breeds. If both parents are clear of the defect, the pups will not be affected. If the status of the parents is not known, it is best to screen the pups before purchasing them. The Orthopedic Foundation for Animals (OFA) maintains a PK deficiency genetic registry.

THROMBOPATHY

Basset hound hereditary thrombopathy (or thrombopathia) is an autosomally inherited intrinsic platelet disorder in basset hounds, with some similarity to Glanzmann's thrombasthenia in people (407, 492, 823). It is an inherited disease of platelets in which the platelets fail to aggregate properly and do not form effective hemostatic plugs. The underlying dysfunction is related to defective stimulus-response-coupled platelet activation (75).

Most commonly, clinical signs include mucosal bleeding, bruising, and prolonged bleeding from surgery or trauma but also include more prolonged bleeding and aural hematomas, such as seen with hemophilia or other bleeding disorders (161). The condition may be associated with hypothyroidism in the basset hound. The diagnosis is suspected following platelet aggregation and clot retraction assays, or when platelets of normal morphology fail to aggregate to all physiologic stimuli except thrombin. Thrombopathy seems to be an autosomal dominant trait with variable penetrance (75).

The diagnosis is not straightforward because platelet numbers are usually unaffected and specialized platelet aggregation and release assays are needed to pinpoint the defect. Nevertheless, thrombopathy and von Willebrand disease are the two most common bleeding disorders in the breed, so any bleeding tendency would require these conditions to be at the top of the differential diagnostic list.

Thrombopathy has no cure, and treatment is instituted during bleeding episodes. This is accomplished with either whole blood transfusions or, preferably, platelet-rich plasma. All relatives should be screened for this disorder, and carriers and affected animals should be removed from breeding programs.

A similar condition has been described in the spitz (72, 75). Affected dogs were anemic and suffered from chronic epistaxis and gingival bleeding. Platelets aggregate in response to thrombin in a manner similar to that described for basset hounds with thrombopathia. Affected animals should not be bred, and parents and siblings should be evaluated carefully for evidence of the disorder.

Thrombopathy—Macrothrombocytopenia

An asymptomatic thrombocytopenia associated typically, but not always, with large to giant platelets has been reported in the Cavalier King Charles spaniel (287, 973). The etiology remains unknown, but the fact that it has been reported only in the Cavalier King Charles spaniel suggests a genetic tendency. The diagnosis should be suspected when thrombocytopenia and large platelets are reported in this breed, without evidence of bleeding diathesis. No treatment is necessary. Despite the fact that this disorder appears to be asymptomatic, it would seem prudent not to use affected animals for breeding.

Thrombopathy—Platelet δ-Storage Pool Disease

Platelet δ granule deficiency, also known as platelet δ-storage pool disease, is an inherited platelet disorder, suspected to be autosomal recessive in nature, that has been reported in American cocker spaniels (137, 677) and perhaps collies (112). Platelet storage pool diseases are bleeding disorders resulting from deficiency of platelet δ (dense) granules or a depletion of granule contents.

Dogs with this disorder have normal δ granule morphology but are unable to store adenosine diphosphate (ADP). Affected dogs have moderate to severe bleeding episodes after minor trauma, venipuncture, and surgery. Studies suggest that the bleeding disorder results from a deficient δ-granule storage pool of ADP, perhaps a selective defect in δ-granule ADP transport (137).

The diagnosis is suspected on the basis of prolonged bleeding time, and normal prothrombin time (PT), von Willebrand factor (vWF) levels, activated partial thromboplastin time (aPTT), and platelet count. The diagnosis, however, can be confirmed only by determining the presence of a high platelet ATP:ADP ratio (137). Affected animals should not be bred, and parents should be considered as obligate carriers of the trait. Siblings are suspect carriers.

THROMBASTHENIC THROMBOPATHIA

Canine thrombasthenic thrombopathia is an autosomally inherited platelet function defect seen in otterhounds (71, 407). It is believed to be inherited as an incomplete dominant trait (673). Although previous reports have linked the condition to Glanzmann's thrombasthenia in people, the two conditions are different in several important ways. Clinical signs are associated primarily with mucosal surface bleeding and are exacerbated by surgery, trauma, and stress. The defect is distinguished by the occasional presence of bizarre giant platelets and reductions in membrane glycoproteins IIb and IIIa (also known as glycoproteins α_{IIb} and β_3) (75).

Another condition, which has been reported in the Great Pyrenees, actually bears the most resemblance to Glanzmann's thrombasthenia type I in people (73, 677). This condition is characterized by a severe quantitative reduction in glycoproteins α_{IIb} and β_3, collectively known as the fibrinogen receptor. The most common presentation is epistaxis and self-limiting gingival bleeding when an affected dog chews rawhide or other abrasive objects.

The diagnosis can be confirmed with quantitative clot retraction tests. Diligent screening has made this clinical disease rare in the otterhound population, and it is hoped that the same will become true for the disorder recognized in the Great Pyrenees. Affected animals should not be bred, and parents and siblings should be evaluated carefully for evidence of the disorder.

VASCULITIS

Cutaneous vasculitis is a collection of disorders in which the underlying problem includes destructive and inflammatory changes in the blood vessels. Cutaneous vasculitis can occur secondary to a number of processes, but most vasculitis syndromes are associated with immune complex deposition in the walls of blood vessels (213). Beagles (116, 941), dachshunds (768), greyhounds (208), Jack Russell terriers (818), and rottweilers (768, 939) seem to be at increased risk. Also, miniature poodles are believed to be at increased risk (1124). A hereditary link has not been determined.

The vasculitis of greyhounds, known as cutaneous and renal glomerular vasculopathy, is discussed as a separate topic, as is beagle pain syndrome, a form of meningitis associated with juvenile polyarteritis syndrome. Vasculitis has also been reported in the sites of rabies vaccination. Vasculitis is a reaction pattern and, therefore, likely has very different causes and manifestations in the different breeds affected.

Vasculitic lesions are most frequent on the dependent parts of the body—feet and ears. The most common lesion visualized and felt is an elevated bruise, so-called "palpable purpura." The involvement also may be systemic. In Jack Russell terriers, lesions are found on the distal extremities (toes, eartips, footpads), face, and over bony prominences (818). In beagles with systemic necrotizing vasculitis (juvenile polyarteritis syndrome), clinical signs most often include fever, anorexia, and cervical neck pain (116, 941). Amyloidosis has been reported in beagles that have experienced repeated acute episodes of necrotizing vasculitis (989). A similar condition has been reported in the Bernese mountain dog and boxer (352). Dachshunds with leukocytoclastic vasculitis most often present with notched pinnae (768).

Diagnosis is based on histopathologic and immunopathologic evaluation, but many tests may be warranted to unearth the underlying cause (for example, antinuclear antibody, circulating immune complexes (CIC), C1q assay, Coombs' test, cold agglutinins, rheumatoid factor, hypoallergenic food trial, bacterial or fungal culture, infectious disease titers). In beagles, elevated levels of interleukin-6 (IL-6) are detected during the acute phase of juvenile polyarteritis syndrome (453).

Biopsies for histopathologic assessment are important diagnostic tools for better categorizing the type of vasculitis present. The results of biopsies differ depending on the subtype of vasculitis. Treatment should be directed at the underlying cause if it is known. If no cause has been determined, therapy is often initiated with anti-inflammatory or immunosuppressive doses of corticosteroids or dapsone. In some cases, the vasculitis will go into remission and prednisone can be discontinued, but in most cases treatment is prolonged, often life-long. Pentoxifylline is another option. If the cause is not clearly immune-mediated, antibiotic therapy should be considered as a first-order treatment to minimize the risk of sepsis.

Because a mode of inheritance has not been determined, it is difficult to offer reliable breeding recommendations. In any case, it seems prudent to recommend that affected animals not be used for breeding.

VON WILLEBRAND DISEASE (vWD)

This disease, also known as von Willebrand's disease, pseudohemophilia, and vascular hemophilia, is by far the most common inherited bleeding disorder of dogs (242). The von Willbrand factor (vWF) is a glycoprotein that circulates in the plasma, complexed to factor VIII. Both vWF and the vWF portion of the factor VIII complex are required for platelet adhesion and for preventing the rapid clearance of factor VIII from the circulation (1027). A variety of disorders have been attributed to vWF, either for deficient synthesis of the factor or production of dysfunctional or unstable forms of the compound. The result is a platelet function defect and prolonged bleeding times.

> **Von Willebrand Disease**
>
> Von Willebrand disease (vWD) is the most common inherited bleeding disorder of dogs and has been reported in over 60 breeds. DNA testing is now available for several of these breeds. It is suspected that the mode of inheritance may not be the same for all variants of the disorder.

Many cases are subclinical or are associated with a bleeding tendency following surgery or trauma. Bleeding problems may be worse in dogs with concurrent hypothyroidism. The diagnosis is suspected when the prothrombin time (PT) and activated partial thromboplastin time (aPTT) are both normal in the face of a bleeding problem. The aPTT occasionally is abnormal when vWF is severely deficient. The diagnosis is suspected by measuring specific levels of vWF. Von Willebrand disease has been reported in more than 60 breeds of dogs and is autosomal in nature, although several different genetic defects are associated with the disorder. Reports of von Willebrand disease are on the increase (113), either because of actual prevalence or because testing has become more routine.

The genetic mutation for von Willebrand disease has been studied in several breeds of dog, although none has been published in the scientific literature to date. In the Doberman pinscher, a splice site mutation has been proposed, such that an abnormal gene still produces normal von Willebrand factor about 5% to 10% of the time. Thus, a homozygously affected Doberman with two defective genes still produces about 10% to 20% of the vWF of a normal dog. This is meant to explain the confusion in considering the disorder autosomal incompletely dominant rather than autosomal recessive. If the mutant gene has a frequency of about 0.6, about one-third of Dobermans are homozygously affected and close to half are carriers of the trait. Significantly, that means that only about 15% to 20% of the purebred Doberman pinscher population are clear of the trait and preferred for breeding.

This matter, however, is controversial, as some researchers are not convinced that a single recessive gene defect can explain the blood test results seen in tens of thousands of Doberman pinschers that suggest dominance with incomplete penetrance. Based on assessment of vWF, the condition seems to be autosomal incompletely dominant with most affected animals being heterozygotes, and most homozygotes dying during fetal development or shortly after birth (264).

In the Scottish terrier, the situation is clearer, as it results from a mutation in a single autosomal gene, with a gene frequency estimated to be 15% of the Scottie population. In the Shetland sheepdog, type-1 and type-3 vWD have been reported. A causative mutation has been proposed for the type-3 form. It has also been suggested that those with type-3 disease are actually doubly heterozygous recessive for the type I defect (265), which occurs in some humans with vWD. This remains to be proven. Perhaps 10% to 20% of Shetland sheepdogs are carriers for the severe type-3 vWD trait. The classification of vWD types is given in Table 6-1.

Von Willebrand's disease is an autosomal trait with different forms of clinical and genetic expression. In the most common form (Type-1 vWD), the gene can be inherited from either or both parents, depending on the breed or specific defect involved. Not all pups will be equally affected; it is highly variable. Carriers of the trait inherit a mutated gene from one parent but are clinically normal. Type-2

Table 6-1 Classification of vWD Types

Type	Characteristics	Breeds affected
1	low levels of vWF, but all multimers detected	Doberman pinscher, German shepherd dog, Pembroke Welsh corgi, poodle (especially standard), Airedale, Manchester terrier, some Shetland sheepdogs
2	selective depletion of certain multimers	German shorthaired pointer, German wirehaired pointer
3	severe deficiency; undetectable multimers	Scottish terrier, Chesapeake Bay retriever, most Shetland sheepdogs

vWD is clinically severe and quite rare; it occurs in German wirehaired pointers and German shorthaired pointers (114). The parents are clinically normal, but if they are both carriers, the pups may be affected. Type-3 vWD is recessive and has been recognized in Scottish terriers, Chesapeake Bay retrievers, and Shetland sheepdogs (shelties). Although shelties can be affected by either type-1 or type-3 vWD, most are prone to the more severe type-3 disease.

An accurate genetic test for vWD has been developed for certain breeds, specifically the Scottish terrier, Doberman pinscher, Manchester terrier, Pembroke Welsh corgi, poodle, and Shetland sheepdog. The test can be run on dogs of any age, even young pups. Ongoing research should make the test available for additional breeds. A sample can be easily collected by scraping the inside of the dog's mouth with a special brush and submitting it to a genetic-testing laboratory. If all breeding animals test clear, screening the puppies should not be necessary. Even if the test results appear unequivocal, it is important to remember that some controversies remain among researchers, especially related to inheritance of the condition in the Doberman pinscher and Shetland sheepdog. In these breeds, both the DNA test and the vWF assay should be done. In fact, though the DNA test is a marvelous medical advancement, vWF testing still addresses the likelihood of which animals are at risk for bleeding.

For breeds in which a DNA test for vWD is not available, the disease is diagnosed by measuring levels of von Willebrand factor (vWF) in the blood. Some significant differences are found between breeds with respect to age and vWF concentration. Most Doberman pinschers are older (about 5 years of age) when they are affected, compared to Scottish terriers and Shetland sheepdogs (younger than 2 years of age). Affected Dobermans also have more residual vWF in their blood (15%), compared to Shetland sheepdogs (8%) and Scottish terriers (0%). Affected Airedales have a prevalence rate close to that of Doberman pinschers, but vWF:Ag seldom falls below 15% and most cases are subclinical (485).

In the most common form (vWD Type-1), levels are usually 1% to 60% of normal. Animals with the recessive type-3 disease have no or negligible levels of vWF, whereas their carrier parents have reduced levels of this protein (15% to 60% of normal). Dogs with 35% or less of the normal level of vWF are at increased risk of hemorrhage. Whereas vWF tests can identify homozygously affected animals, they are less precise at characterizing carriers.

Many environmental factors can affect the protein factor assay (739, 741, 1008), making it less satisfactory for basing a breeding strategy. Because some researchers believe that hypothyroidism can be linked with vWD, thyroid profiles also can be a useful part of the screening procedure.

Many clinical cases of vWD are mild and require no specific treatment, unless some other concomitant problem further compromises hemostasis. Transfusions with cryoprecipitate or fresh-frozen plasma are indicated in some cases, and before elective or other surgeries (243). In fact, for breeds with a high prevalence of vWD, such as the Doberman pinscher, it could be argued that no surgery should be attempted without first assessing hemostatic potential with a quick test such as a mucosal or toenail bleeding time, if not vWF specifically. Drugs that interfere with platelet function, such as aspirin, phenothiazine tranquilizers, and anti-inflammatory agents, are contraindicated in all affected animals. Some dogs benefit from supplementation from thyroxine and/or desmopressin acetate (679). Recombinant von Willebrand factor may slow the rate of blood flow but has not seemed to be a dependable corrective measure (1053). Breeds that are most typically affected with von Willebrand disease are shown in Table 6-2.

Table 6-2 Breeds Predominantly Affected with von Willebrand Disease

Breed	Classification	Mode of Inheritance	Reference
Airedale terrier	1	AD, VE?	265, 485, 537
Akita	1	AD, VE?	112
Bassett hound	1	AD, VE?	265, 485, 537
Bernese mountain dog	1	Autosomal?	24
Chesapeake Bay retriever	3	Autosomal recessive	263, 485
Dachshund	1	AD, VE?	265, 485, 537
Doberman pinscher*	1	Autosomal recessive?	113, 485, 537, 740
German shepherd dog	1	AD, VE?	265, 485, 537
German shorthaired pointer	2	Autosomal recessive	112, 263, 485
German wirehaired pointer	2	Autosomal recessive	112, 114
Golden retriever	1	AD, VE?	265, 485, 537
Greyhound	1	AD, VE?	112
Irish wolfhound	1	AD, VE?	74
Keeshond	1	AD, VE?	265, 537
Kooiker	3	Autosomal recessive?	112
Manchester terrier*	1	Autosomal recessive	537
Miniature poodle*	1	Autosomal recessive	265, 485
Miniature schnauzer	1	AD, VE?	265, 485, 537
Pembroke Welsh corgi*	1	Autosomal recessive?	265, 485, 537
Rottweiler	1	AD, VE?	265, 485, 537
Shetland sheepdog*	1, 3	Both autosomal recessive?	113, 485, 537, 864
Scottish terrier*	3	Autosomal recessive	113, 485, 493, 537
Standard poodle*	1	Autosomal recessive	265, 485, 537

*Breeds for which a DNA detection test for vWD is available
AD, VE = Autosomal dominant, variable expressivity

Other breeds in which vWD is reported include the following (112, 265, 485, 991)

Afghan
Australian cattle dog
Alaskan malamute
American cocker spaniel
Azawakh
Bearded collie
Bichon frisé
Boxer
Bulldog
Cairn terrier
Collie
English cocker spaniel
English springer spaniel
English setter
Great Dane
Great Pyrenees
Smooth fox terrier
Wire fox terrier
Irish setter
Italian greyhound
Kuvasz
Labrador retriever
Lakeland terrier
Lhaso apso
Old English sheepdog
Papillon
Samoyed
Shih tzu
Siberian husky
Soft-coated wheaten terrier
Skye terrier
Swiss mountain dog
Tibetan terrier
Vizsla
Whippet
Yorkshire terrier

Carriers of vWD should not be used for breeding, even if they appear clinically normal. Although predicting carriers based on standard tests of vWF may be difficult, newer DNA tests should allow affected, carrier, and clear animals to be identified with virtual certainty. In Doberman pinschers and Shetland sheepdogs, assessment should also include vWF assays. If only clear animals are included in breeding programs for some breeds, the trait can be eliminated. In breeds such as the Doberman pinscher, however, in which less than 20% of dogs can be expected to be clear, it may be necessary to breed clear to carrier for one or two generations until enough breeding animals are available to permit matings of clear animals only.

The Orthopedic Foundation for Animals (OFA) maintains a registry for animals evaluated with the DNA test. It must also be appreciated that some breeds may have low vWF assays yet have no clinical evidence of a bleeding disorder. These animals sometimes are referred to as having canine von Willebrand trait rather than von Willebrand disease.

Recommendations regarding breeding of animals with von Willebrand trait but no evidence of bleeding disorders are not straightforward. Breeder input is required to determine how significant the problem is within the line, as well as the breed in general.

CHAPTER 7

Immunologic Disorders

Immunologic disorders represent states of both deficiency and hyperactivity. Although hypersensitivity disorders tend to have complicated modes of inheritance, most immunodeficiency disorders are simple monogenic traits. For one severe immunodeficiency disorder, X-linked combined immunodeficiency, a DNA test has been developed, so eradication of this condition from the affected breed lines should be possible.

ALLERGIC INHALANT DERMATITIS (ATOPY)

The canine version of hay fever, atopy is an extremely prevalent condition. It is believed to be a heritable predisposition to produce reaginic antibody to ordinary environmental substances such as pollens, molds, and house dust (167). As in people, the mode of inheritance is not clear-cut. If the parents are allergic, however, the pups are highly likely to be allergic as well.

The list of breeds prone to inhalant allergies is long, but this reflects local populations and gene pools. Animals are predisposed when their parents are allergic. The breeds cited most often as being susceptible to atopy include:

- bichon frisé (768)
- Boston terrier (167)
- boxer (167)
- Cairn terrier (167)
- Chinese shar pei (167, 699)
- cocker spaniel (167)
- Dalmatian (167)
- English setter (167)
- German shepherd dog (167)
- golden retriever (167)
- Irish setter (167)
- Labrador retriever (167)
- Lhasa apso (167)
- miniature poodle (768)
- miniature schnauzer (167)
- pug (768)
- Scottish terrier (167)
- shih tzu (768)
- Skye terrier (768)
- West Highland white terrier (167)
- wire fox terrier (167).

Affected animals often lick and chew at their feet and have generalized itchiness. Some breeds, such as the Dalmatian, are more likely to sneeze as an allergic manifestation; otherwise, respiratory symptoms are seen in about 15% of cases.

Diagnosis is made most precisely with an intradermal allergy test (skin test). Blood tests may aid in diagnosis but are not as precise as skin tests. Treatment may involve antihistamines, immunotherapy (allergy shots), special fatty acid supplements, itch-relieving topicals, and corticosteroids. Corticosteroids such as prednisone are effective in relieving itchiness but also have many side effects.

Until more is known about the inheritance of atopy, affected animals, and potentially their siblings or their parents, probably should not be bred. Because allergies are not life-threatening, however, breeders do not always find the argument compelling if the dog has other attributes worth preserving in progeny.

No screening tests are currently available for carriers. When they become more refined, blood tests likely will be able to predict carriers. Today's tests, based on the detection of allergen-specific IgE, are not specific enough to determine which pups will later develop inhalant allergies, and certainly not which animals carry the trait. Some anecdotal evidence, based on studies in people, indicates that allergic bitches supplemented with gamma-linolenic acid and/or eicosapentaenoic acid during pregnancy and lactation will produce pups with less susceptibility to developing allergies. This has not been substantiated by actual clinical studies in either people or dogs.

CHINESE SHAR PEI IMMUNODEFICIENCY

Chinese shar pei immunodeficiency is a poorly described entity characterized by defects in both cell-mediated and humoral immune responses (357). Immunoglobulin levels (especially IgA and IgM) tend to be low, lymphocytes fail to stimulate adequately during *in vitro* studies (876), and there is reduced synthesis of IL-6 by monocytes (357). Whether this is associated with selective IgA deficiency, which is also common in the breed, is unknown.

Clinically, young dogs are affected from a few months to several years of age. They develop an intermittent fever and a variety of systemic disorders, including ulcerative colitis, pyoderma, and demodicosis. Demonstrating defective IL-6 synthesis and low immunoglobulin levels allows for a presumptive diagnosis. Treatment is supportive, and the prognosis is guarded. Until more is known about the mode of inheritance, parents and all siblings should be considered as potential carriers, and affected animals should not be bred.

COMPLEMENT (C_3) DEFICIENCY

C_3 deficiency is a rare autosomal recessive disorder that has been reported in Brittany spaniels (357, 486, 677). Affected animals are prone to recurrent bacterial infections and to renal amyloidosis (204) or Type 1 membranoproliferative glomerulonephritis (19). The third component of complement is required to opsonize bacteria, and deficiencies lead to impaired phagocytosis of bacteria by neutrophils. Because C_3 is involved in phagocytosis, immune adherence, chemotaxis of neutrophils, anaphylatoxin generation, and leukocyte mobilization, an absence of C_3 should logically result in increased susceptibility to infections (402). The condition is the result of a frameshift deletion that generates a premature stop codon (19).

The diagnosis can be confirmed by a serum complement C_3 determination. Dogs that are homozygous for the trait have little detectable C_3 (less than 10%), whereas dogs that are heterozygous have C_3 concentrations approximately 30% to 50% of normal (308). Treatment is supportive with antibiotics but is not curative. Affected animals should not be bred. The parents of affected dogs should be considered as obligate carriers. Other family members intended for breeding should be screened first for serum C_3 levels and plasma complement activity.

CYCLIC HEMATOPOIESIS

Cyclic hematopoiesis, originally known as gray collie syndrome, involves a regulatory defect of hematopoietic stem cells in the bone marrow. The condition has been reported most often in silver-gray collie pups (357) but occasionally has been reported in other breeds, including the American cocker spaniel (461, 768), border collie (13), and Pomeranian (461, 768).

Affected collie pups are born with a silver-gray haircoat, and they may be smaller and weaker than their normal littermates. Also, the nose may be more lightly pigmented. In the collie, the trait seems to be transmitted with an autosomal recessive mode of inheritance (15, 325). In affected dogs, neutrophils exhibit impaired killing of bacteria because of metabolic abnormalities including myeloperoxidase deficiency and a defect in iodination (309).

By 8 to 12 weeks of age, affected pups start to develop problems such as fever; diarrhea; eye infections; arthralgia; microcytic, normochromic anemia; and abnormalities of their white blood cells. Nearly 100% of gray collie pups have evidence of amyloidosis by 24 weeks of age (146).

When blood samples are collected over a 2-week period, the neutrophil numbers tend to fluctuate from high to low over an 11- to 14-day-cycle. When the neutrophils are at their lowest point, these pups are highly susceptible to overwhelming infection and usually die during these periods.

Diagnosis can be confirmed by sequential blood counts over a 14-day period. Most animals succumb during periods of low neutrophil counts. Concurrently, serum levels of immunoglobulins tend to be elevated (146). Lithium carbonate temporarily corrects the cycling. Long-term treatment with recombinant canine stem cell factor (rc-SCF) and potentially canine granulocyte colony-stimulating factor (rcG-CSF) have been successful (225). Bone marrow transplantation is a potentially corrective therapeutic alternative.

Both parents should be considered as obligate carriers, and normal siblings should be considered as potential carriers of the trait. Because experienced collie breeders typically do not try to raise gray pups, the condition has become rare.

GERMAN SHEPHERD DOG PYODERMA (GSP)

GSP is an aggressive, deep pyoderma observed in the German shepherd dog and German shepherd crosses (768). Similar conditions have been reported in Dalmatians and bull terriers. A familial predisposition has been documented, and an autosomal recessive inheritance is suggested (768). Studies have suggested that GSP can be associated with flea allergy dermatitis, atopic dermatitis, food allergy, cell-mediated immunodeficiency, or hypothyroidism, or it could be an idiopathic disease (895, 896). Abnormalities in both B and T lymphocytes have been documented.

The immunological imbalance is presumed to be associated with defective T-helper cells. Analysis of B-cell populations demonstrates a striking decrease in the level of CD21+ lymphocytes, compared to controls (166). The ratio of CD4 to CD8 cell populations becomes unbalanced, with abnormal elevations of CD8 and decreases in CD4 (252). Most cases occur in the middle-aged dog, are chronic and recurring in nature, and often respond poorly to empirical antibiotic therapy. Concurrent pruritus and pain may be present and resolve after antibiotic therapy is initiated. The lesions, predominantly on the lateral thighs, dorsal back, rump, and ventral abdomen, consist of papules, pustules, ulceration, and pyogranulomatous inflammation with fistulous tracts and, occasionally, cellulitis. Lymphadenomegaly, fever, anorexia and lethargy are commonly noted.

Therapy must be directed at the underlying problem, as well as the bacterial component. Long-term systemic antibiotics, especially the potentiated penicillins, cephalosporins, and fluoroquinolones, are required to bring the condition into remission. In at least one study, enrofloxacin was listed as the drug of choice (503). Some cases never totally resolve, even with aggressive long-term treatment, and relapse is common.

Affected animals should not be bred. Until the mode of inheritance has been confirmed, both parents should be considered as potential carriers of the trait. Any family members considered for breeding programs should be evaluated for immune function by screening both B-cell and T-cell processes.

LEUKOCYTE ADHESION DEFICIENCY

Also known as granulocytopathy syndrome, Hagemoser-Takahashi syndrome, and β_2 integrin adhesion molecule deficiency, this condition is a rare, autosomal recessive disorder seen in Irish setters (308, 357, 1050). The condition results from an inherited lack of certain leukocyte integrins that are critical for leukocytes adhering to, and migrating through, endothelial cells.

Profound immunodeficiency is evident from a young age, with recurrent infections including gingivitis, oral ulcers, periodontitis, chronic pneumonia, poor wound healing, and stunted growth (677). Diagnosis is suspected with the clinical signs and persistent severe leukocytosis, and confirmed by documenting a deficiency of leukocyte-surface glycoproteins CD11a-c/CD18 β subunit and a lack of neutrophil-to-monocyte adhesion (677). The expression of CD16 also tends to be decreased in affected animals (1051). The literature includes references to an absence of the surface glycoprotein Mo1 and lymphocyte function-associated antigen 1, LFA-1 (308, 309).

Treatment is supportive with chronic antibiotic therapy, and overwhelming infection will result in death otherwise. Both parents of affected pups are considered to be obligate carriers. Other normal family members should be considered as potential asymptomatic heterozygous carriers. Prospective breeding animals should be screened for expression of CD11a-c/CD18, and carriers tend to have intermediate levels. A DNA test is available for the condition in cattle (1023), and a suitable test for dogs should be available at some point in the future.

LUPUS ERYTHEMATOSUS

Lupus erythematosus is a spectrum disorder with different variants recognized in the dog. The two accepted designations currently are *systemic lupus erythematosus (SLE)* and *cutaneous* or *discoid lupus erythematosus (CLE* or *DLE)*. In people, several more variants are recognized, of which many likely exist in the dog as well.

LUPUS ERYTHEMATOSUS (SYSTEMIC)

Breeds at increased risk of SLE include the collie, German shepherd dog, poodle, Shetland sheepdog, and spitz (768, 939). Breeds at increased risk for CLE include the Brittany spaniel, collie, German shepherd dog (especially whites), German shorthaired pointer, Shetland sheepdog, and Siberian husky (768, 939). A familial trend has been recognized, and female dogs may have a modest sex predisposition.

Systemic lupus erythematosus is characterized by multiple circulating autoantibodies that participate in immune-mediated tissue injury directed against the animal's own system, and evidence suggests that lupus may be associated with the interaction of a virus with a disturbed immune system in a genetically predisposed host, which can be complicated by exposure to ultraviolet light. The most common clinical findings in dogs with systemic lupus erythematosus (SLE) are polyarthritis, fever that does not respond to antibiotics, kidney disease (glomerulonephritis) with protein loss in the urine, anemia, oral ulcers, and skin disease (165, 768).

Specific diagnostic testing for SLE includes the antinuclear antibody test, the lupus erythematosus cell test, and biopsies for histopathologic and immunopathologic evaluation. Dogs produce autoantibodies to several individual histones but not DNA nor nucleosomal antigens, suggesting that the pathogenesis of the disorder is different in dogs than in people (716). Testing for autoantibodies targeting cytoplasmic antigens such as Ro may also be indicated.

Treatment of SLE must be individualized for each patient. In general, it is attempted with immunosuppressive doses of corticosteroids (for example, azathioprine, cyclophosphamide, chlorambucil), with or without chemotherapy. The course of SLE tends to wax and wane so periods of remission are interspersed with periods of fulminant disease. Disorders of skin, joints, and muscle often respond best to medication. Animals with glomerulonephritis, thrombocytopenia, and severe hemolytic anemia have the worst clinical outcomes.

Systemic lupus erythematosus seems to be familial, so affected animals should not be bred and care should be taken when including close relatives in a breeding program. Currently, no screening tests will determine carriers of the disorder, and no clear mode of inheritance has been determined.

LUPUS ERYTHEMATOSUS (CUTANEOUS)

Cutaneous (discoid) lupus erythematosus is one of the most common immune-mediated skin diseases seen in dogs, and it is believed to be a less harmful variant of SLE wherein systemic involvement is absent and autoantibodies are rarely found. The most common presenting sign is red, scaling dermatitis of the face, often including the nose and nasal mucosa. Loss of pigment from the nares often is noted. The lesions are exacerbated by exposure to sunlight in at least half of cases. Nasal and digital hyperkeratosis also may be noticed. In fact, nasal hyperkeratosis may be familial in Labrador retreivers (807) and may represent a subtype of cutaneous lupuserythatosus, or a crossover event with zinc-responsive dermatosis.

Dogs with cutaneous lupus erythematosus tend to have abnormalities that are detected only by histopathologic and immunopathologic evaluation. Tests that determine systemic manifestations are invariably negative.

Dogs with cutaneous disease should be sheltered from exposure to peak periods of sunlight, which can exacerbate the signs of disease. The medical treatment of CLE differs from that of SLE in that immunosuppressive therapy usually is not warranted. Initial therapy should consist of anti-inflammatory doses of corticosteroids and topical corticosteroid, together with vitamin E and fatty acid supplements containing eicosapentaenoic acid and/or gamma-linolenic acid. For animals that don't control entirely without appreciable doses of corticosteroid, the next treatment of choice would be to restrict exposure to sun (275) and institute supplementation with tetracycline and niacinamide (768).

Cutaneous lupus erythematosus seems to be familial, so affected animals should not be bred and care should be taken when including close relatives in a breeding program. Currently, no screening tests will determine carriers of the disorder, and no clear mode of inheritance has been determined.

MYCOBACTERIAL SUSCEPTIBILITY

Mycobacterial susceptibility has been reported in basset hounds (357) and miniature schnauzers (282). A mode of inheritance has not yet been determined. An interleukin or RAMP protein deficiency is suspected but not yet proven. Although most dogs are relatively resistant to avian mycobacteria, affected dogs are prone to developing systemic disease, including diarrhea, weight loss, lymphadenomegaly, and nasal discharge.

In most cases, *Mycobacterium avium* can be identified in tissue, on culture, or by BCG tuberculin skin testing. Treatment is quite involved and rarely successful. Affected animals should not be bred. Relatives should be introduced to a breeding program cautiously.

NEUTROPHIL BACTERICIDAL DEFECT

Neutrophil bactericidal defect is a rare condition seen in Doberman pinschers (308). It has tentatively been considered an autosomal recessive trait (356, 357). There is normal bacterial phagocytosis by neutrophils, but partially reduced bactericidal activity. Respiratory problems, which develop by a few weeks of age, include sneezing, coughing, and nasal discharge. An association with primary ciliary dyskinesia has not been completely ruled out.

No specific diagnostic tests are available, as the specific defect has not been identified. A persistent neutrophilia and evidence of reduced bactericidal activity allow for a presumptive diagnosis. Treatment is supportive with long-term antibiotic administration. Affected animals should not be bred. Relatives should be cautiously used in any breeding programs.

PNEUMOCYSTOSIS

A poorly understood respiratory infection seen in dachshunds (357, 461, 608), pneumocystosis is associated with *Pneumocystis carinii* pneumonia. Stunting of growth does not seem to be a feature of this disorder. The mode of inheritance has not yet been determined, but males are more often affected.

The diagnosis can be strongly suspected when *Pneumocystis* is detected (typically on a transtracheal aspirate) in a dachshund with clinical signs of dyspnea, exercise intolerance, and immune incompetence. Radiographically, the condition varies from a mild interstitial and bronchial pattern to an alveolar pattern (526). Immunoglobulin levels tend to be lower, and lymphocyte stimulation responses are depressed (608). Although the parasite can be treated medically, the underlying immune dysfunction persists and the prognosis must be considered grave. The immunoincompetence does not appear to be as debilitating in this disorder as it is in severe combined immunodeficiency. Affected animals should not be bred. Relatives should be introduced to a breeding program cautiously.

PEMPHIGUS

Pemphigus covers a complex of disorders characterized by autoantibody deposition within the epidermis that causes separation of epidermal cells from one another such that spaces are created. Four variants of pemphigus currently are recognized in animals:

1. Pemphigus vulgaris (PV)
2. Pemphigus foliaceus (PF)
3. Pemphigus erythematosus (PE)
4. Pemphigus vegetans (PVe).

The antigen in pemphigus foliaceus is desmoglein 1, whereas the pemphigus vulgaris antigen (likely desmoglein 3) resides on differentiating keratinocytes. This leads to conversion of plasminogen to plasmin by plasminogen activators, and acantholysis is the result. Pemphigus in dogs bears many similarities to its human counterpart and, therefore, the pathomechanisms are presumed to be similar. Of the different pemphigus variants, pemphigus foliaceus seems to be the most common and the one with the strongest breed predilections (49). There is a breed predisposition for the Akita, bearded collie, chow chow, dachshund, Doberman pinscher, Finnish spitz, Newfoundland, and schipperke (2, 768, 938). A milder variant of PF, PE has a breed predilection for the collie, Shetland sheepdog, and German shepherd dog (2, 768, 938).

Both pemphigus foliaceus and pemphigus erythematosus are characterized by a scaling, crusting, and/or pustular dermatitis that often originates on the head and ears; PF then becomes generalized (Figure 7-1). Animals usually do not become systemically ill. Diagnosis of pemphigus relies on clinical examination and biopsies for histopathologic examination, with or without immunopathologic assay. Direct immunofluorescence testing (immunopathologic examination) of normal-appearing perilesional tissue reveals autoantibodies in the intercellular spaces in about 65% of cases. About 50% of cases of pemphigus foliaceus show positive IF (indirect immunofluorence) titers on bovine esophagus; the tissue substrate seems to be important in this regard. Western blotting identifies that canine PF sera recognizes a 160 kDa band with identical mobility to the protein identified in human pemphigus foliaceus (470). Immunosuppressive therapy is typically accomplished with corticosteroids, chemotherapy (e.g., azathioprine, chlorambucil), or gold salts (chrysotherapy).

Although there is a definite breed predisposition for pemphigus, not much evidence is available to support familial transmission of the trait. Still, whenever possible, owners should not select affected animals for use in a breeding program.

PEMPHIGOID

Pemphigoid refers to a complex of blistering conditions characterized by autoantibody deposition at the junction between the epidermis and dermis, with blister formation immediately deep to the epidermis. Canine bullous pemphigoid has many features in common with human bullous pemphigoid, including similar immune deposition of IgG within hemidesmosomes and a hemidesmosome-associated 180-kD glycoprotein target for circulating autoantibodies (468).

There is a breed predisposition for the collie, Shetland sheepdog, Doberman pinscher, and perhaps the dachshund (3, 768, 938). A mode of inheritance has not been determined.

Clinically, the condition is characterized by erosions and ulcers, most commonly on the mucous membranes, neck, axillae, and ventrum. The diagnosis is confirmed on the basis of biopsies for histopathologic and immunopathologic evaluation. Treatment is attempted with immunosuppressive therapy, as for pemphigus.

To date, no solid evidence suggests that pemphigoid is transmitted as a simple genetic trait. Although breeding affected animals is not advisable, the use of close relatives should be a breeder option.

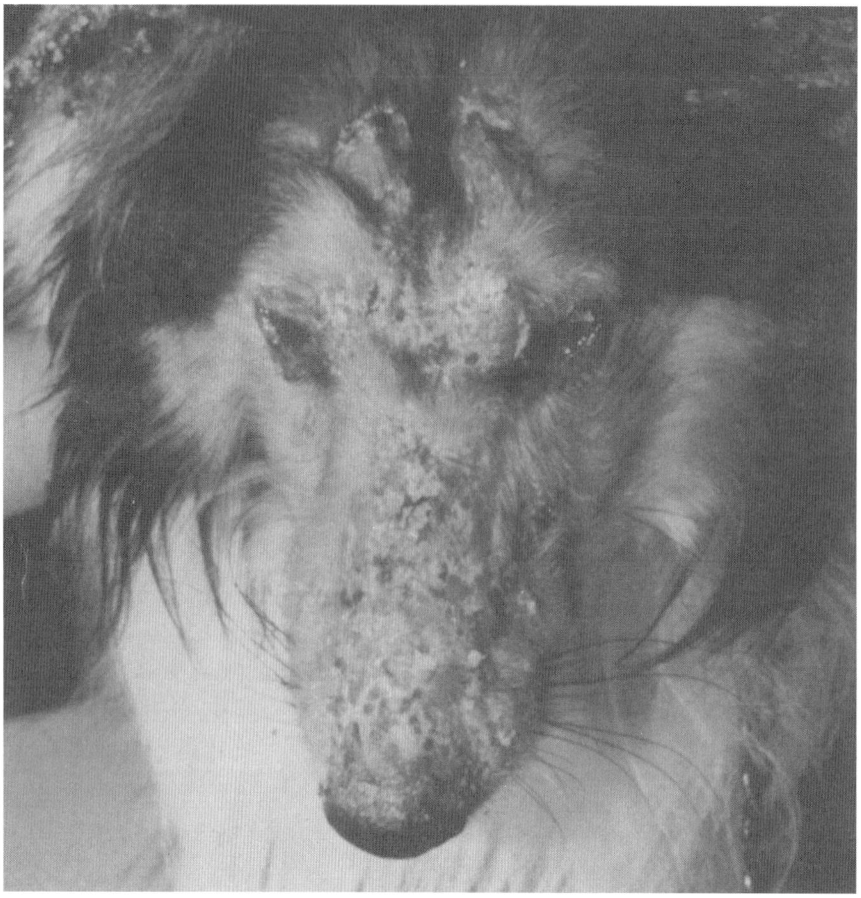

Figure 7-1 Pemphigus foliaceus
Courtesy of Dr. Lowell Ackerman, Mesa Veterinary Hospital, Mesa, Arizona

PRIMARY CILIARY DYSKINESIA

Primary ciliary dyskinesia, also known as immotile cilia syndrome and Kartagener's syndrome, refers to a condition in which the hairlike cilia in the respiratory passages, middle ear, and on the sperm, cannot perform their needed functions. The cause is abnormal function of ciliary microtubules resulting from the absence of one or both of the inner and outer dyneim arms (736).

Primary ciliary dyskinesia is believed to be inherited in people as an autosomal recessive trait, but the genetics have not been confirmed in the dog. The condition is reported most commonly in the English pointer, English springer spaniel, golden retriever, and rottweiler, and cases also have been noted in the border collie, Chinese shar pei, chow chow, Dalmatian, Doberman pinscher, Norwegian elkhound, and Old English sheepdog (737, 806).

The most common clinical manifestation of ciliary dyskinesia is recurring chronic respiratory infection in dogs 18 months of age and younger. Therefore, affected dogs often cough, may develop a runny nose, have poor exercise tolerance, and sometimes fever. The result is often bronchitis and pneumonia. The tails (flagella) of sperm are modified cilia, so many dogs with primary ciliary dyskinesia are infertile. In approximately half of affected dogs, the internal organs are transposed to the wrong side of the body. Some affected individuals also have hearing loss, middle ear infections, and dysfunction of some of the white blood cells (neutrophils primarily) needed to fight off infection.

The best ways to confirm a diagnosis of primary ciliary dyskinesia are special biopsies submitted for electron microscopic evaluation, or mucociliary clearance with a radiation counter. Both are involved procedures. In most cases, the diagnosis is suspected when a young animal gets recurrent respiratory infections that respond to antibiotics but recur soon after the drug is discontinued. With mature intact males, sperm can be evaluated for defective sperm motility. This is not an absolute test because some dogs have normal-appearing sperm and still have the condition. In about 50% of cases, chest radiographs reveal the heart on the right side of the chest.

Primary ciliary dyskinesia has no cure. Symptomatic therapy includes periodic antibiotics based on results of culture. Cough suppressants should not be used because they further impede normal defense mechanisms. If the infections can be maintained under reasonable control, affected dogs stand a chance of living a relatively normal existence. Affected dogs should not be bred and their littermates and their parents should be considered as potential carriers of the trait.

SELECTIVE IMMUNOGLOBULIN A (IgA) DEFICIENCY

IgA deficiency is the most common specific immunoglobulin deficiency in dogs. This refers to a specific lack of IgA, which is important in protecting the body surface—especially the skin, respiratory tract, digestive system, and reproductive system. IgA deficiency most likely is actually a heterogeneous collection of disorders resulting in overall IgA deficiency. It is sometimes subdivided into severe, partial, and transient subgroups. Although selective IgA deficiency seems to be most common in the beagle (308, 357, 625), Chinese shar pei (308, 357, 699, 735), and German shepherd dog (308, 357, 625), predilections have been reported in the Akita (625, 768), American cocker spaniel (625, 768), chow chow (625, 768), dachshund (625, 768), Dalmatian (625, 768), miniature schnauzer (625, 768), and West Highland white terrier (625, 768).

Clinically, IgA deficiency can manifest as surface infections, including recurrent respiratory infections, urinary tract infections, and skin infections (1040). Most dogs have a history of problems from a young age. A deficiency of IgA predisposes to infections and the development of allergies and immune-mediated diseases.

Diagnosis is confirmed by submitting serum samples for immunoglobulin analysis (IgA, IgG, IgM). Low plasma IgA concentrations, however, can also be found in clinically normal dogs. These dogs likely have normal secretory levels of IgA, but not plasma levels (362). Also, IgA levels do not reach maximal levels until 15 to 18 months of age (308). It is also possible to measure IgA levels in tears (237). Affected dogs sometimes have high levels of IgG and/or IgM in an attempt to compensate for the deficient immunoglobulin.

Blood counts and thyroid profiles should be conducted on all affected dogs to discount concurrent problems that might affect the response to treatment. The treatment of choice for IgA deficiency is nonspecific immune stimulation and judicious use of antibiotics. Although affected animals should not be bred, insufficient information is available upon which to base recommendations for selecting close family members for breeding programs.

THYMIC ATROPHY OF MEXICAN HAIRLESS DOGS

Thymic atrophy is a tardive condition in which the dogs are born with a normal thymus, which undergoes significant atrophy by several weeks of age (708). T-cell function is thus compromised in adults. The result is chronic, recurring infections.

The diagnosis is suspected on the basis of lymphocyte stimulation tests. Treatment is symptomatic only. Affected animals should not be bred. Relatives of affected animals should be used cautiously in any breeding program.

UVEODERMATOLOGIC SYNDROME

The cause of uveodermatologic (Vogt-Koyanagi-Harada-like) syndrome is currently unknown, but it may represent an autoimmune attack against melanocytes. In humans, a cell-mediated hypersensitivity reaction against melanin has been demonstrated. Thus, heavily pigmented tissues such as the uveal tract, skin, and mucous membranes are primarily involved. Unlike the condition in people, auditory and meningeal abnormalities have not been documented in the dog (732).

Breeds at increased risk include the Akita (732, 768), Alaskan malamute (768), chow chow (768), Samoyed (732, 768), and Siberian husky (732, 768). The condition has also been reported in the Ainu, white German shepherd dog, Irish setter, Shetland sheepdog, and Shiba (732, 768). Most animals are in young adulthood when they are first affected.

The condition is characterized by a serious eye disorder (granulomatous panuveitis) and concurrent loss of pigment from the nose, lips, eyelids, and occasionally the entire body. If the inflammatory process is not arrested, acute blindness can result. The diagnosis of uveodermatologic syndrome relies on biopsies of affected depigmented, erythematous, and scaling areas for histopathologic evaluation. The histopathologic presentation of skin lesions bears little, if any, resemblance to the condition seen in people. Anti-retinal antibodies may be detectable (750).

The mainstay of cutaneous therapy is topical and/or systemic corticosteroids or azathioprine. Ophthalmologists may approach the ophthalmic problems more directly, because once blindness has occurred, the return of sight is unlikely. Early therapeutic intervention usually is successful. Repigmentation may be complete, partial, or unsubstantial. The disease has a protracted course, and recurrences are to be expected. Accordingly, immunosuppressive therapy often continues for months or years to prevent recurrence.

Because the genetics of the condition have not been established, breeding recommendations are based on supposition rather than fact. Until more is learned, affected animals should probably not be used in breeding programs.

WEIMARANER IMMUNODEFICIENCY

A poorly understood entity, Weimaraner immunodeficiency is characterized by impaired phagocytic and humoral immune functions. Affected dogs are prone to suppurative and granulomatous disease processes (357). The condition is uncommon but not rare. A mode of inheritance has not been determined. Affected dogs are young and prone to high fevers, depression, and pyogranulomatous disease, mainly limited to the skin and muscle. Neutrophil function is impaired, and IgG and IgM levels tend to be diminished (238, 414). In some cases, circulating immune complexes are detected.

Treatment is supportive with long-term antibiotic use, but the prognosis must be considered guarded. Until more is known about the mode of inheritance, close relatives should be screened for neutrophil function and immunoglobulin levels before being considered for a breeding program. Affected animals should not be bred.

X-LINKED SEVERE COMBINED IMMUNODEFICIENCY

Severe combined immunodeficiency (SCID) is a group of disorders in which the end result is severely impaired cellular and humoral immune responses. The condition is transmitted as an X-linked recessive trait and has been reported in the basset hound (442, 856) and the Cardigan Welsh corgi (856).

Thymocyte development is impaired, and peripheral blood lymphocytes do not proliferate when stimulated. Recent genetic sequencing has determined that the defect is located in the gamma chain of the interleukin-2 receptor (IL-2R) (310, 442). In both humans and dogs, the disease results from mutations in the gamma c chain, which is a common component of the receptors for IL-2, IL-4, IL-7, IL-9, and IL-15 (990, 991). The actual mutation varies with breed. Basset hounds have a four-base deletion, and Cardigan Welsh corgis have a single base addition to the gamma chain gene of the IL-2R gene (856).

Clinically, affected dogs are often stunted, lymph nodes are difficult to palpate, and tonsils are absent or small. Because of their lack of adequate immune responsiveness, affected animals are prone to opportunistic infections, such as pyoderma, enteritis, cystitis, and pneumonia. Male siblings may have succumbed to “fading puppy syndrome” or other vague conditions.

Absolute diagnosis is difficult. Lymphocyte counts typically are within normal limits or only mildly depressed, but lymphocyte stimulation tests tend to be abnormal, as are immunoglobulin A and immunoglobulin G levels. T-cell binding of IL-2 is minimal, and this makes a useful diagnostic tool. Finally, if a genetics laboratory is available, the defect can be detected on the short arm of the X chromosome (Xq13) in the gene coding for the gamma chain of the interleukin-2 receptor. No commercial test is currently available. On postmortem examination, thymic dysplasia and lymphoid hypoplasia are characteristic findings (988).

No specific treatment is curative, and therapy is aimed at the secondary infections. Bone marrow transplantation of lymphoid stem cells remains an option (308). Once the owners are aware of the extent of the abnormality, many of these dogs are euthanized.

Affected dogs should not be used for breeding, and the dam of any affected dog should be removed from the breeding population. Prior to being used in a breeding program, all siblings of the affected dog and its dam should be screened for IL-2 binding.

CHAPTER 8

Metabolic Disorders

Metabolic disorders reflect conditions that may affect more than one body system. Although the lysosomal storage diseases are often included in the classification of neurologic disorders, they clearly can and do affect other body systems. Diagnostic tests are now available for many of these disorders. When gene therapies are utilized, they likely will be used first to treat metabolic disorders, especially if they are controlled by a single gene and involve a lone defective enzyme.

AMYLOIDOSIS

Amyloidosis is a group of diseases characterized by the accumulation of an abnormal protein (amyloid AA) in tissues (96) or by the distribution of the deposits. Localized syndromes usually affect one organ, while systemic syndromes affect more than one organ and include reactive, immunoglobulin-associated, and heredofamilial syndromes (256). An underlying inflammatory or cancerous disease process is found in about 50% of dogs with amyloidosis. In the remaining dogs, a genetic basis is suspected. Much preliminary evidence suggests an inherited or familial disorder in the Chinese shar pei (487). In fact, the early-onset development of AA amyloidosis in the Chinese shar pei is similar to familial Mediterranean fever in people, which is known to be transmitted as an autosomal recessive trait (258). The condition in dogs is often referred to as familial shar pei fever (FSF). Another human condition with much similarity has been referred to as TRAPS, for TNF receptor-associated periodic syndrome. The defects have been determined to be dominant mutations to the tumor necrosis factor receptor 1 (653).

In primary nodular cutaneous amyloidosis, amyloid is deposited in the skin without evidence of systemic disease. In most cases, it seems to result from an immunoglobulin-producing accumulation of plasma cells, or a plasma cell tumor. On the other hand, systemic amyloidosis with cutaneous involvement tends to accompany multiple myeloma or defects in immunoglobulin metabolism (488).

Most Chinese shar peis that succumb to amyloidosis seem to develop problems in young adulthood (usually 12 to 24 months of age). Breeders may refer to the condition as "familial shar pei fever" or "swollen hock syndrome." Affected dogs develop a fever and may have swelling of their hocks, loss of appetite, increased thirst, increased urination, and signs of internal illness such as vomiting, diarrhea, and weight loss. Affected shar peis have transient fevers, potentially well above 106°F.

In addition to the Chinese shar pei (258), familial renal amyloidosis has been described in the beagle (80, 259), English foxhound (642), and Walker hound (259). Females seem to be more predisposed than males (259). In beagles, the glomerular deposits of amyloid typically do not cause problems until the dogs are 5 years of age or older. In the Chinese shar pei, the diagnosis typically is made between 1 and 6 years of age. The most common clinical signs include anorexia, lethargy, vomiting, weight loss, diarrhea, and polydipsia/polyuria.

No reliable screening tests are available for amyloidosis. The diagnosis is usually confirmed by biopsies for histopathologic assessment. Most shar peis have deposits of AA amyloid in their kidneys, but deposition in the liver and other tissues (adrenal glands, pancreas, intestines) is also possible. Blood tests aren't definitive, and leukocytosis and elevated IgG and IgM levels are most commonly seen. High levels of interleukin-6 have been reported in affected dogs, but this is not a commonly available test. Serum amyloid A (SAA) levels are usually predictive in people but haven't been fully studied in the dog. The best result will be with a genetic marker for the disease and its carriers. Work toward this end is in progress.

Amyloidosis has no cure. Affected individuals usually die from kidney or liver failure. Dogs that have hyperthermia require specific treatment (e.g., dipyrone) to lower the body temperature. In mild elevations, the temperature typically returns to normal within 24 to 36 hours without therapy. Medical therapies using colchicine and dimethyl sulfoxide (DMSO) have been used experimentally. Until a screening test is available, it is best not to buy or breed animals with a family history of amyloidosis.

CEROID LIPOFUSCINOSIS

Ceroid lipofuscinosis, also known as Batten disease and amaurotic idiocy, is a member of the lipidosis subgroup of the lysosomal storage diseases. At least two different forms have been found in the dog (495). The most common form is a specific enzyme defect (palmitoyl-protein thioesterase) that leads to the accumulation of toxic metabolites (sphingolipid activator proteins A and D) in nerve cells, and eventual death (810). In the other form, subunit c of mitochondrial ATP synthase is stored in various multilamellar profiles. It has been proposed that abnormal mitochondria in the neurons of affected animals may play a role in the pathogenesis of this condition (634).

The disorder has been reported in many breeds, including the American cocker spaniel (187, 633), Australian cattle dog (187, 350, 633), blue heeler (746), border collie (187, 633), Chihuahua (746), Dalmatian (187, 633), English cocker spaniel (741, 350), English setter (187, 633), Japanese retriever (187), miniature schnauzer (496, 987), Polish Owczarek Nizinny dog (1146), poodle (148), saluki (187), Tibetan terrier (187, 633), wire-haired dachshund (187, 633), and Yugoslavian sheepdog (187). A condition similar to ceroid lipofuscinosis, but referred to as amblyopia and quadriplegia, has been reported in the Irish setter as a simple autosomal recessive trait, lethal in the homozygote (903). Affected dogs are blind without apparent cause (amblyopia) and become unable to stand and ambulate (809).

The condition seen in miniature schnauzers is similar to the infantile form of the human disease, whereas most other affected canine breeds—namely the English setter, border collie, and Tibetan terrier—store subunit c of mitochondrial ATP synthase rather than sphingolipid activator proteins (497, 810). Cocker spaniels have generalized accumulation of a lipofuscin-like pigment in the smooth muscle of the intestine and other organs, imparting a brown discoloration (494). Both forms are presumed to be transmitted as autosomal recessive traits, as is the case in people (187, 496). This has been documented in border collies, English setters, and Tibetan terriers (187). Several genetic markers linked to the disease gene in English setters have been identified (602).

Clinical signs, such as diminished eyesight, dementia, abnormal behavior, and depression may be evident by 14 to 18 months of age in miniature schnauzers, and most affected animals are dead by 2 to 3 years of age. Behavioral changes include loss of learned behavior, fearfulness, and aggression (495). Dalmatians may be affected as early as 6 months of age, and Tibetan terriers as late as 6 years of age (350). For most other breeds, the age of onset is about 2 years of age, with an acute onset of clinical signs. The clinical presentation has much variability. Cerebral signs, such as behavioral changes, dementia, cortical blindness, circling, and seizures, are more common in English setters, border collies, Dalmatians and cocker spaniels. Cerebellar signs, especially ataxia, are more common in Australian cattle dogs and wirehaired dachshunds (633). In the Tibetan terrier, retinal blindness is the primary sign.

In most cases, the diagnosis is confirmed after death, upon which either subunit c or ATP synthase or characteristic granular osmiophilic deposits (GROD) can be detected in tissue sections of brain and retina (911). Severe neuronal loss in the cerebral cortex and the cerebellum is a hallmark feature in most breeds. Extraneural storage occurs in retinal pigment epithelium of English setters and border collies, and in breeds in which visceral storage is found (Australian cattle dog, cocker spaniel, border collie, English setter), no evidence of organ failure exists (633). Plasma carnitine levels are reduced 67% in affected dogs and 50% in carrier dogs (506). No treatment is available.

The parents of affected animals should be considered as carriers and not used for future matings. Hopefully, a diagnostic test will soon be available to determine carriers and thus allow us to prevent this devastating disease from occurring.

CHOLESTEROL ESTER STORAGE DISEASE

Cholesterol ester storage disease, also known as Wolman disease, is a rare lysosomal storage disease associated with a deficiency of lysosomal acid lipase (497). The result is an accumulation of triglyceride and cholesterol esters within macrophages of the liver and spleen, with death occurring before 1 year of age. A condition similar to cholesterol ester storage disease has been reported in fox terriers (412). Most affected animals don't live long enough to be bred, but parents and siblings should be considered as potential carriers of the trait and used cautiously, or not at all, in breeding programs.

> **Fucosidosis**
>
> Fucosidosis is a significant concern in the English Springer spaniel. The molecular defect has been determined and DNA testing will allow accurate identification of affected, unaffected, and carrier individuals. The diagnosis is most often confirmed by measuring blood levels of α-L-fucosidase.

FUCOSIDOSIS

Fucosidosis is a devastating fatal disease in English springer spaniels, associated with an inherited deficiency of the enzyme α-L-fucosidase. The condition is transmitted as an autosomal recessive trait, meaning that both parents of affected dogs are carriers (30, 187). The condition is more common in dogs bred in the United Kingdom and Australia but has been reported in the United States and Canada as well (982). The molecular defect is a 14-base pair deletion at the end of exon 1, which creates a frameshift and 25 novel codons in exon 2, followed by two premature stop codons so that a functional enzyme is not created. The enzyme deficit results in the accumulation of oligosaccharides, glycosaminoglycans, and glycoproteins with terminal fucose residues within cells.

Dogs are normal at birth but begin to show effects between 4 and 24 months of age. Most of the signs (dullness, behavior changes) are neurological but also may include weight loss, dysphagia, and changes in coat condition (1024). Some affected pups have a longer, thicker coat than their normal littermates.

Basic laboratory tests are typically normal, although the astute technician may detect vacuoles in white blood cells, caused by the accumulation of abnormal sugars. Most affected dogs die or are euthanized by 4 years of age. Post-mortem examination may reveal visibly enlarged optic, trigeminal, glossopharyngeal, vagal, and hypoglossal nerves (633). The diagnosis is confirmed by measuring blood levels of the enzyme α-L-fucosidase, which are very low (typically less than 5% of normal levels) in affected dogs and intermediate in carriers.

In the near future, a DNA test should be available, as sequencing of canine α-L-fucosidase cDNA has identified the causative deletion (788, 966). Although a PCR-based test has been designed to identify the presence of the mutant allele, it is not yet commercially available.

Even though fucosidosis cannot be cured, the hope is that gene therapy and bone marrow transplants may become available (313). Screening is important because most veterinarians are not familiar with the disorder and may not identify the problem in pups before they are bred. This is because the disorder is rare, the clinical signs can be vague, and the condition is seen only in Springer spaniels, not other breeds.

All English Springer spaniels intended for breeding should have blood samples tested for α-L-fucosidase levels. Affected animals often have blood levels 1/20th of normal, whereas most carriers have about 50% of the enzyme content of normal dogs. There is some variability in levels and, therefore, some overlap between carrier and normal animals is possible (30). It is hoped that a DNA test for fucosidosis will soon become available to give completely unequivocal results. The molecular defect has already been determined in Springer spaniels (and humans).

GALACTOSIALIDOSIS

Galactosialidosis is an extremely rare form of sphingolipidosis characterized by a combined deficiency of α-galactosidase and β-neuramidase enzyme activity caused by a peptide mutation (497). Only a single case has been reported, in a 5-year-old schipperke (534).

GLOBOID CELL LEUKODYSTROPHY (GCL)

Globoid cell leukodystrophy, also known as galactocerebrosidosis or Krabbe disease, is a lysosomal storage disease that is reported most commonly in the West Highland white terrier (633, 1080) and the Cairn terrier (633, 1080) but has also been seen in the bassett hound, beagle, Bluetick hound, Dalmatian, miniature poodle, and Pomeranian (187, 430, 497, 633, 728, 746). It is a neurological disease associated with an inherited (autosomal recessive in West Highland white terriers and Cairn terriers) lack of the critical enzyme galactocerebromide-β-galactosidase (galactosylceramidase) (430).

As part of their research on the human condition, researchers at the Jefferson Medical College, Division of Medical Genetics, have determined the gene mutation responsible. The mutation is an A to C transversion at cDNA position 473 for galactocerebriosidase (GALC), which results in an amino acid substitution in the peptide (1080). The amino acid sequence is 90% identical to that seen in the human condition.

Affected animals appear normal at birth but fail to develop normally with their littermates. The enzyme defect results in alterations in the cerebrum and cerebellum, and problems are usually evident by 11 to 30 weeks of age in West Highland white terriers and Cairn terriers (1080). In basset hounds, the age of onset is 1.5 to 4 years of age (633).

> **Globoid Cell Leukodystrophy**
>
> To test for GCL, collect a blood sample in a heparinized tube and send it to the GLC researchers at the Jefferson Medical College, 1100 Walnut Street, Room 410, Philadelphia, PA. A commercial test is not yet available from veterinary laboratories.

Animals tend to develop tremors, stilted gait, muscle weakness, and even behavioral changes. Most breeds have an ascending ataxia and paraparesis starting with the pelvic limbs. In other breeds, cerebellar signs accompany the pelvic limb ataxia (633). Magnetic resonance imaging reveals diffuse symmetrical white matter disease and can be used to monitor progression of the disease (212). The course is progressive and invariably fatal. In West Highland white terriers and Cairn terriers, however, the condition is rapidly progressive in pups older than 2 to 3 months (845), and in miniature poodles the condition is slowly progressive over 2 to 4 years (633).

Affected animals should not be bred. Both parents should be presumed to be carriers and not used in further breedings. The carrier state can be detected by appropriate blood tests.

> **Glycogen Storage Disease Type 1a**
>
> Blood samples for animals suspected of being affected or carriers for glycogen storage disease type Ia can be evaluated by the Department of Pediatrics, Division of Medical Genetics, Bell Building, Room 237, Duke University Medical Center, Durham, NC 27710.

If breeders believe that a carrier dog has other exceptional attributes and wants to breed, it is important to select a mate that is a non-carrier, and then to test all offspring and select only the dogs that are clear for perpetuating the line. The Institute for Genetic Disease Control in Animals (GDC) maintains an open registry for globoid cell leukodystrophy (GCL) in the Cairn terrier and West Highland white terrier.

GLUCOCEREBROSIDOSIS (GAUCHER'S DISEASE)

Glucocerebrosidosis is a rare lysosomal storage disease caused by a deficiency of the enzyme beta-glucosidase (glucocerebrosidase) (430). The condition is characterized by Wallerian degeneration of cerebral, cerebellar, and spinal cord white matter. Clinical signs, seen at 4 to 8 months of age, include ataxia, wide-based stance, tremors, hyperactivity, and a stilted gait. The condition has been reported in the Australian silky terrier (430, 633), in which it is suspected to have an autosomal recessive mode of inheritance (187).

The diagnosis can be confirmed by evaluating enzyme levels, and these also can be used to select appropriate breeding pairs in families afflicted with the disorder (301). In affected dogs, Gaucher cells, which are fixed macrophages containing glucocerebroside, can be found in the liver and kidney. Affected animals should not be bred, and parents and siblings should be considered as potential carriers of the trait.

GLYCOGEN STORAGE DISEASE TYPE IA

Glycogen storage disease type Ia, also known as von Gierke disease, reflects a glucose-6-phosphatase deficiency resulting from a transversion at position 450 of the coding sequence of the gene for glucose-6-phosphatase and an amino acid substitution in the peptide (528). Glucose-6-phosphatase helps to maintain a normal blood glucose during fasting. In this condition, both glycogenolysis and gluconeogenesis occur normally in response to hypoglycemia, but since glucose is not released from glucose-6-phosphate, blood glucose levels decline (819). The disorder is inherited as an autosomal recessive trait in the Maltese, in which a mutation in a single base pair results in a change in a crucial amino acid.

The diagnosis is often suspected in a young dog, typically a Maltese, with persistent hypoglycemia, even when fasted for as little as 2–4 hours. The diagnosis is confirmed by evaluating blood samples for glucose-6-phosphatase. In postmortem cases, biochemical analysis for glucose-6-phosphatase can be conducted on liver and kidney samples and compared to normal controls. Affected animals develop hypoglycemia, slow growth, an enlarged liver, distended abdomen, and failure to thrive (108). Although the disease has no treatment, some animals can be managed on a high-starch diet fed several times throughout the day. Raw cornstarch, rice cereal, grain products, and starchy vegetables are staples for managing the condition in people (819). Small amounts of protein provide needed amino acids and scant amounts of fat provide essential fatty acids and calories, but neither protein nor fat nor fruit sugars (fructose, galactose) contribute to the prevention of hypoglycemia and therefore should not form a significant portion of the diet. Affected animals and their parents should not be bred, and siblings should be considered as potential carriers.

GLYCOGEN STORAGE DISEASE TYPE II

Glycogenosis type II, or Pompe's disease, is a rare familial disorder (believed to be autosomal recessive) caused by an acid α-glucosidase deficiency. It has been reported in Swedish Lapland dogs (82, 1093). The enzyme alpha-glucosidase (acid maltase) is responsible for breaking down glycogen into its constituent sugar molecules, so an enzyme deficiency results in an accumulation of glycogen in tissues.

Clinically, affected dogs display progressive muscle weakness, frequent vomiting, and cardiac abnormalities by 6 months of age, and are dead by 24 months of age (1093). In people, different forms have been recognized, based on age of onset and severity of symptoms. The diagnosis is suspected based on electromyographic studies, electrocardiograms, echocardiograms, and biopsies in which there is massive glycogen accumulation in most organs. The diagnosis. however, can be confirmed only by evaluating specific serum enzyme levels (870). No treatment has been successful. Heterozygous carriers of the trait can usually be detected by their partial deficiency of acid α-glucosidase. Even though affected animals usually don't live long enough to breed, their parents should be considered obligate carriers of the trait and siblings as suspect carriers.

GLYCOGEN STORAGE DISEASE TYPE III

Glycogenosis type III, or Cori's disease, is a lysosomal storage disease inherited as an autosomal recessive trait in Akitas and German shepherd dogs (82). It refers to an enzyme deficit (amylo-1-6-glucosidase) that allows toxic substances to build up in cells (430). The result is catastrophic. By 6 to 12 weeks of age, affected pups have recurrent episodes of hypoglycemia, muscle tremors, incoordination, and seizures. By 8 months of age, affected animals will be dead. In humans, increasing dietary protein may be beneficial in providing amino acids for gluconeogenesis, muscle protein synthesis, and possibly as an alternate fuel for muscle metabolism (819). It is unknown whether this approach offers real hope for affected dogs.

The important news about this glycogen storage disease is that it can be prevented entirely by running screening tests, which will detect carriers are well as affected individuals. This is important in a breeding program, because carriers can look entirely normal and still contribute the trait to future generations. Accordingly, we can now completely eliminate this lysosomal storage disease from the Akita and German shepherd dog populations by using sensible screening and breeding strategies. Even though affected animals don't typically live long enough to be bred, parents should be considered as obligate carriers of the trait and siblings are suspect carriers.

GM-1 GANGLIOSIDOSIS

GM-1 gangliosidosis type 1 (Norman-Landing disease) belongs to the sphingolipidosis subgroup of the lysosomal storage diseases. This confusing disorder is inherited as an autosomal recessive trait and refers to an enzyme deficit (β-galactosidase) that allows toxic substances (GM-1 ganglioside) to build up in nerve cells (430, 509). The result is catastrophic. By 2 to 4 months of age, affected pups will have visual problems, have difficulty walking, and may appear depressed or lethargic. This progresses to ataxia and evidence of cerebellar involvement. By 8 months of age, affected animals will be dead.

The three breeds in which GM-1 gangliosidosis has been reported are the Portuguese water dog, beagle, and English springer spaniel (187, 497, 633, 746, 956). The condition in the Portuguese water dog and the English springer spaniel are similar biochemically, although they appear to represent different mutations of the beta-galactosidase gene (17). Portuguese water dogs tend to display a rapid progression of clinical signs, including ataxia, nystagmus, hypermetria, and intention tremors of the head (910). In springer spaniels, the condition is often accompanied by skeletal changes (dysostosis multiplex, dwarfism), coarse facial features, and hepatosplenomegaly (16, 17).

The important news about GM-1 gangliosidosis is that it can be entirely prevented by running screening tests, which will often detect carriers as well as affected individuals. Affected animals have low beta-galactosidase activity in the liver and marked elevation of GM1 ganglioside in the brain. This is important in a breeding program, because carriers can look entirely normal but contribute the trait to future generations. Accordingly, we now can completely eliminate this lysosomal storage disease from the purebred Portuguese water dog and English springer spaniel populations by sensible screening and breeding strategies. Affected animals should not be bred. Parents are carriers of the trait, and siblings are suspect carriers.

GM-2 GANGLIOSIDOSIS

GM-2 gangliosidosis belongs to the sphingolipidosis subgroup of the lysosomal storage diseases. This confusing disorder is inherited as an autosomal recessive trait and refers to an enzyme or activator deficit (β-hexosaminidases) that allows toxic substances to build up in nerve cells (430). The three subgroups of GM-2 gangliosidosis are:

1. Tay Sachs disease (Type B), characterized by deficient activity of hexosaminidase A
2. Sandhoff's disease (Type O), characterized by deficient activity of both hexosaminidase A and B
3. AB-variant (Bernheimer-Seitelberger disease), caused by an absence of an activator protein.

GM-2 gangliosidosis is reported primarily in German shorthaired pointers (Type B). Type AB cases also have been seen in a Japanese spaniel and in a mixed-breed dog (187, 219, 497, 633).

By 6 to 9 months of age, affected German shorthaired pointer pups will show both cerebral and cerebellar signs. The condition has been referred to as familial amaurotic idiocy (910), although this term has been applied to other conditions as well. In the other cases reported, the disorder wasn't recognized until approximately 18 months of age.

GM-2 gangliosidosis can be prevented entirely by running screening tests, which will detect carriers are well as affected individuals (964). This is important in a breeding program, because carriers can look entirely normal but contribute the trait to future generations. Accordingly, we now can completely eliminate this lysosomal storage disease from affected families through sensible screening and breeding strategies. Affected animals should not be bred. The parents should be considered as obligate carriers of the trait and siblings as suspect carriers.

HYPERLIPIDEMIA

Hyperlipidemia refers to serum elevations of cholesterol or triglycerides. Although this is common in people, hyperlipidemia is relatively rare in dogs. Familial hypertriglyceridemia, however, is believed to be heritable in miniature schnauzers (36, 41, 327), beagles (41, 1090), and briards (1097).

The diagnosis is confirmed by finding fasting plasma triglyceride concentrations above 500 mg/dl (55 mmol/L) on two consecutive occasions. The condition does not seem to predispose animals to heart disease, but the dog is treated to decrease the risk of pancreatitis.

Treatment is initiated with a reduced-fat diet. Because chylomicrons are exclusively of dietary origin, restriction of dietary fat is the most important part of treatment (326). Medium-chain triglycerides, marine oil, niacin, and gemfibrizal are reserved for patients that don't respond to dietary intervention alone. Animals with familial hyperlipidemia should not be used in breeding programs.

HYPERPHOSPHATEMIA

Benign familial hyperphosphatemia is seen in Siberian huskies, in which it bears significant resemblance to benign persistent familial hyperphosphatemia in humans (568). The mode of inheritance is not known precisely but is autosomal and likely recessive.

The condition is difficult to describe because it has few, if any, clinical manifestations. The problem is diagnosed when routine blood testing reveals marked elevations in the enzyme serum alkaline phosphatase. This can be apparent even in young pups. In this syndrome, the source of the enzyme activity appears to be a bone isoenzyme (568). Other blood tests and radiographs do not reveal any abnormalities.

The primary importance of this disorder is that owners (and veterinarians) of Siberian huskies should be aware of potential elevation of serum alkaline phosphatase levels as a familial trait in the breed and not necessarily as an indicator of internal disease. This is important because, without knowing of this breed peculiarity, veterinarians may continue to search for the source of these abnormal enzyme levels in an otherwise healthy dog. Whether affected animals should or should not be bred remains a breeder option.

LAFORA-BODY DISEASE

Lafora-body disease, also known as glycoproteinosis and α-glucosidase deficiency, is a rare neurodegenerative disease known to be autosomal recessive in the beagle, suspected autosomal recessive in the basset hound, and of unknown inheritance in the poodle (187, 233, 481). The genetic defect results in the accumulation of Lafora bodies in cells within the brain, skin, liver, and skeletal and cardiac muscles (233, 437, 481). The result is monoclonic and tonic-clonic seizures and progressive neurologic dysfunction.

The diagnosis can be confirmed by finding the classic Lafora bodies, which are PAS-positive inclusions consisting of polyglucosans with small phosphate and sulfate groups. Treatment consists of managing the seizures. Affected animals and their parents should not be used for breeding, and siblings should be considered as suspect carriers.

MALIGNANT HYPERTHERMIA

Malignant hyperthermia is a metabolic disorder of skeletal muscle, characterized by hypercatabolism and muscle contracture. An episode can be triggered by halothane anesthesia and occasionally other drugs such as succinylcholine and lidocaine. The condition has been determined to be an autosomal dominant trait in a strain of black Labrador retrievers, and suspected to be caused by a skeletal muscle ryanodine receptor mutation (RYR1) similar to that found in pigs and some humans with the condition (123, 1014). It has also been reported in various breeds of dogs, including the border collie, cocker spaniel, Doberman pinscher, greyhound, pointer, and St. Bernard (84).

Clinically, the onset of signs is insidious and might include increased heart and breathing rates, or fever. A more fulminant presentation is characterized by severe muscle rigidity, organ failure (heart, kidneys), and disseminated intravascular coagulation.

Diagnosis is suspected, based on characteristic clinical signs, typically after an animal has been anesthetized. *In vitro* tests have been used experimentally to determine genotype based on functional characterization of the calcium release channel of muscle homogenates. With pigs as the model, muscle activities are 50% greater in heterozygotes and 100% in homozygotes (781). Histopathologic examination of muscle fibers helps confirm the diagnosis. An *in vitro* muscle contracture test can be done to screen for animals suspected to be susceptible. When malignant hyperthermia is suspected, susceptible animals can safely undergo anesthesia if triggering agents are avoided (82).

Treatment is symptomatic and involves removing the triggering event (e.g., halothane anesthesia), lowering the body temperature with ice packs and chilled IV fluids, treating acidosis, and administering muscle relaxants such as dantrolene. Affected animals should not be bred. and closely related animals with breeding potential should be screened for susceptibility.

MUCOPOLYSACCHARIDOSIS I

Mucopolysaccharidosis I, also known as Hurler's syndrome and Scheie syndrome, is a rare connective tissue disease that has been reported as an autosomal recessive trait in Plott hounds (187), because of a deficiency of lysosomal alpha-L-iduronidase (633). The gene involved has been identified (668, 1009). Undegraded glycoproteins and glycolipids accumulate in a variety of tissues, including cartilage, bone marrow, skin, liver, and brain, as well as urine. Affected dogs can develop musculoskeletal anomalies and heart disease associated with thickened cardiac valves. Unlike most of the lysosomal storage diseases, affected animals can survive into adulthood and can be included inadvertently in breeding programs.

The diagnosis can be confirmed by measuring levels of alpha-L-iduronidase. Treatment with gene therapy has been attempted but has had limited success because of a humoral response to the alpha-l-iduronidase (959). Enzyme replacement has been used to successfully manage a dog for more than one year (501). Affected animals should not be bred intentionally. Because the condition is believed to be transmitted as an autosomal recessive trait, both parents of affected animals should be considered as obligate carriers of the trait. Siblings are suspect carriers.

MUCOPOLYSACCHARIDOSIS II

Mucopolysaccharidosis II, also known as Hunter syndrome, is a rare disease associated with a deficiency of iduronate sulfatase (430). The condition has been reported in the Labrador retriever (851). The diagnosis is suggested by the finding of glycosaminoglycans on metabolic urine screens. The diagnosis is confirmed by documenting the specific enzyme deficiency. There are no reports of successful treatment.

Affected animals should not be bred, and parents should be considered as obligate carriers of the trait. Siblings are considered to be suspect carriers.

MUCOPOLYSACCHARIDOSIS IIIA

Mucopolysaccharidosis IIIA, also known as Sanfilippo A syndrome, is a rare disease associated with a deficiency of heparan N-sulfatase. The condition has been reported in the wirehaired dachshund (317). Although many body systems can be affected, neurological dysfunction is most pronounced.

Unlike most other lysosomal storage diseases, clinical signs may not be apparent until affected animals reach adulthood (430). The diagnosis is suggested by the finding of glycosaminoglycans on metabolic urine screens. The diagnosis is confirmed by documenting the specific enzyme deficiency. There are no reports of successful treatment.

Affected animals should not be bred, and parents should be considered obligate carriers of the trait. Siblings are considered suspect carriers.

MUCOPOLYSACCHARIDOSIS VI

Mucopolysaccharidosis VI, also known as Maroteaux-Lamy disease, is a rare disease of connective tissue that is inherited in the miniature pinscher as an autosomal recessive trait (187, 430, 762). It also has been reported in the miniature schnauzer and the Welsh corgi (430). This disorder is characterized by a specific enzyme deficit (arylsulfatase B) that results in the accumulation of dermatan sulfate within cells, and eventual cellular dysfunction (432).

Clinically, mucopolysaccharidosis VI is characterized by severe bone disease (dysostosis multiplex), stunted growth, degenerative joint disease, clouding of the cornea, large tongue, and potential heart disease from thickening of the heart valves. The corneal clouding is typically evident to an astute examiner from about 8 weeks of age, and most clinical signs are apparent by 4 months of age. The musculoskeletal abnormalities become progressively more debilitating and, if left untreated, most dogs do not survive beyond 3 years of age.

The diagnosis can be difficult to confirm, as corneal clouding may be confused with corneal dystrophy, the latter of which is actually more common in the miniature pinscher. With routine hematologic assessment, granules may be seen within neutrophils and lymphocytes. Although these granules also may be seen with other lysosomal storage diseases, they may be the first clue that the problem is a metabolic disorder. Radiographs may reveal low bone density with thin cortices, which is quite characteristic. On urine screens, undegraded glycosaminoglycans are strongly indicative. Finally, confirmation is made by measuring lysosomal enzyme activity in serum or white blood cell pellets.

The therapeutic options for mucopolysaccharidosis VI are worth mentioning, because this is one of the few lysosomal storage diseases for which there is a treatment. Although it is expensive and experimental, bone marrow transplantation is a viable option. The donor white blood cells provide the body with the missing enzyme. If this is done in the young pup, before physical maturity, the animal has a possibility of leading a near-normal life. A normal littermate is needed to be the donor. Affected animals should not be used for breeding, and the parents should both be considered as carriers of the trait.

MUCOPOLYSACCHARIDOSIS VII

Mucopolysaccharidosis VII, also known as Sly syndrome, is a rare lysosomal storage disease characterized by accumulation of glycosaminoglycans within cells because of a deficiency of the enzyme beta-glucuronidase (431). Undegraded glycoproteins and glycolipids accumulate in a variety of tissues, including cartilage, bone marrow, skin, liver, and brain, as well as urine. Affected dogs can develop musculoskeletal anomalies and heart disease associated with thickened cardiac valves.

The diagnosis can be confirmed by measuring levels of beta-glucuronidase. Diagnostic tests using the canine beta-glucuronidase gene (exon 3) can be used to distinguish phenotypically between normal-appearing carriers and homozygous normal dogs (862). The condition is inherited as an autosomal recessive trait in people, and the same is believed to be true in the dog (432). The condition is rare enough that there are no clear-cut breed predispositions. Because the condition is believed to be transmitted as an autosomal recessive trait, both parents of affected animals should be considered as obligate carriers of the trait.

PHOSPHOFRUCTOKINASE DEFICIENCY

Phosphofructokinase (PFK) deficiency, also known as Tauri disease and glycogen storage disease VII, is a genetic disease that interferes with the metabolism of glucose in the body. It results in exercise intolerance, anemia, fever, and muscle disease. PFK deficiency is inherited as an autosomal recessive trait in the English springer spaniel and American cocker spaniel (358, 361, 426). The gene frequency is estimated to be about 10% of the springer spaniel population. Carriers show no signs of the disease but pass it along to the pups. When pups are affected, both parents must be carriers for the abnormal PFK gene. The molecular defect has been determined (975), and the gene sequence shares 90% homology with the human M-PFK gene (974).

An inherited metabolic defect, PFK deficiency is often first manifested by 2 to 3 months of age, but the changes are often not recognizable until at least 1 year of age. In fact, in some animals the condition may go unrecognized for years.

Phosphofructokinase-deficient muscle has limited oxidative capacity and a tendency to fatigue quickly, because of an inability to properly utilize glycogen and/or glucose (97). Muscle weakness, inability to properly exercise, and cramping are sufficiently nonspecific so that diagnosis is delayed until more characteristic changes are apparent. Owners may not always observe fever and pigment loss in the urine. PFK deficiency most often presents as a recurring mild hemolytic anemia. The anemia is attributable to a breakdown of red blood cells, and attempts are made to compensate, evidenced by increased reticulocyte counts, resulting in a macrocytic hypochromic compensated hemolytic anemia. When dogs experience an acute hemolytic crisis, they may hyperventilate. Affected dogs should not be allowed to overexert themselves.

The diagnosis can be confirmed in animals older than 3 months by measuring PFK activity in blood cells. A newly developed DNA test is even more specific. Nonspecific findings include leukocytosis, higher serum iron and ferritin, and lower serum haptoglobin (429).

No effective treatment for PFK deficiency has been found, but symptomatic therapy with L-carnitine, riboflavin, and coenzyme Q may improve the situation somewhat. Intravenous therapy, and antipyretic therapy with aspirin or dipyrone are needed during acute hemolytic crises, but blood transfusions are rarely needed.

Fortunately, PFK deficiency can be effectively prevented. Based on research conducted at the University of Pennsylvania, an extremely accurate DNA test (VetGen & GeneSearch) is available to identify affected, nonaffected, and carrier animals. With regard to English springer spaniels and American cocker spaniels, all breeding animals ideally should be clear, and can be registered with the Orthopedic Foundation for Animals (OFA). Mating a carrier to a clear animal is permissible if the carrier has obvious superior qualities in other areas.

NIEMANN-PICK DISEASES (SPHINGOMYELINOSIS)

The Niemann-Pick diseases are characterized by accumulation of sphingomyelin and cholesterol in tissues. Niemann-Pick disease type A exhibits a sphingomyelinase deficiency. Niemann-Pick type C is characterized by a cholesterol transport defect. These conditions are rare in dogs. Niemann-Pick type A (NPA) has been reported in a poodle (131), and Niemann-Pick type C (NPC) has been reported in a boxer (497).

The age of onset for NPC is about 2 months, and the clinical presentation includes ataxia, nystagmus, conscious proprioceptive deficits, paresis, and stupor (633). The age of onset for NPA is 5 months. The clinical presentation includes ataxia, head shaking, hypermetria, dysequilibrium, and hepatomegaly (633). Thus, the clinical signs are similar to the gangliosidoses.

NPA can be diagnosed with sphongomyelinase assays that will identify animals that are clear, carriers, and affected. NPC diagnosis requires a fibroblast culture assay system. The gene mutation for NPC has been determined in people (195), so testing methods will likely be refined in the near future. These diseases are rare, but can be eliminated from a purebred population by appropriate screening and breeding protocols.

SELECTIVE MALABSORPTION OF VITAMIN B12

Selective malabsorption of vitamin B12 has been reported as an autosomal recessive trait in giant schnauzers (303, 338) and border collies (1128). In giant schnauzers, a defect has been demonstrated in transport of intrinsic factor/cobalamin complex receptor to the ileal brush border membrane and is caused by defective glycosylation during synthesis of the receptor (332, 1128). It is characterized clinically by post-weaning onset of failure to thrive, hematological abnormalities, methylmalonic aciduria, and low serum vitamin B12 concentrations. The condition has some similarity to the inherited selective ileal malabsorption of vitamin B12 in people, where it is known as Imerslund-Grasbeck syndrome. In border collies, an autosomal recessive mode of inheritance is suspected (1128).

The diagnosis may be suspected in a breed at risk with proteinuria and a nonregenerative anemia with poikilocytosis and anisocytosis. Dogs do not have the classic macrocytic anemia associated with vitamin B12 deficiency in people. Evaluation for urinary amino acids typically reveals methylmalonic aciduria. Tests for malabsorption indicate a disorder limited to vitamin B12 absorption. Other tests of absorptive functions are expected to be normal.

Treatment involves parenteral administration of vitamin B12. Oral supplementation is not successful. Affected dogs should not be bred, and both parents should be considered obligate carriers of the trait. Siblings should be considered suspect carriers.

TYROSINEMIA

Tyrosinemia II is a rare metabolic condition associated with a deficiency of hepatic tyrosine aminotransferase. It has been reported in the German shepherd dog (555). Manifestations in the dog mimic tyrosinemia II in people, which is transmitted as an autosomal recessive trait. A similar condition in mink, sometimes called pseudodistemper, is also transmitted as an autosomal recessive trait

(372). The mode of inheritance has not been determined in dogs.

Clinically, the condition presents as erosions and ulcerations of the footpads and nose, as well as exudative ophthalmic lesions. Tyrosine crystals forming in the eye possibily initiate the exudative, inflammatory process.

The diagnosis is suspected based on elevated serum and urine levels of tyrosine. It can be confirmed by liver biopsy and assessment of hepatic tyrosine aminotransferase activity. Treatment is supportive and includes a low-phenylalanine, low-tyrosine diet (622). Affected animals should not be bred.

CHAPTER 9

Musculoskeletal Disorders

Musculoskeletal disorders include some of the most intensively studied conditions in veterinary medicine. In addition, registries have been in place for decades for conditions such as hip dysplasia. This has allowed opportunities for studies on heritability, the effects of selection pressure, and determining the best techniques to use, not only to diagnose the condition but also to predict future debility. Even though documenting the genetic basis for hip dysplasia and osteochondritic conditions has been problematic, major strides have been made in some of the rarer entities, such as muscular dystrophy.

ABDOMINAL HERNIAS

Abdominal hernias refer to defects in the external wall of the abdomen that may allow the protrusion of abdominal contents. This discussion will focus on "true" hernias in which there is a well-defined hernial ring and the contents remain surrounded by peritoneum, specifically umbilical hernias and inguinal hernias.

Congenital umbilical hernias are the most common abdominal hernias in dogs. They result from failure or delayed fusion of the lateral folds of the umbilicus from the umbilical cord (972). They are believed to be inherited in most cases, and both recessive (834) and polygenic threshold events (883, 972) have been postulated. In most breeds, the mode of inheritance remains unknown. Umbilical hernias are more commonly reported in females and the following breeds appear to be predisposed: Airedale, Basenji, Pekingese, pointer, and Weimaraner (328, 428, 461, 1134). However, umbilical hernias have been anecdotally reported in almost all breeds of dog.

Most umbilical hernias only trap fat in the umbilical ring and are of little clinical significance. Small hernias should be treated conservatively, since spontaneous closure can occur up to six months of age (883). Larger hernias, or those that trap abdominal viscera, require surgical correction. While it is often recommended that dogs with large umbilical hernias not be bred, the lack of specific knowledge regarding mode of inheritance suggests that this decision should remain a breeder option.

Inguinal hernias may arise as a result of congenital inguinal ring anomalies or following trauma. Whether they are heritable in most breeds is unknown (328). A breed predisposition is often cited for the Basenji, Basset hound, Cairn terrier, Pekingese, and West Highland white terrier, and males are more commonly affected (428, 435, 461, 1095, 1134).

Affected animals are most commonly presented with a painless inguinal mass of doughy consistency. The diagnosis can be confirmed via reduction of the hernia and palpation of the inguinal canal, although plain and/or contrast radiography is occasional required. Surgical correction is warranted. There is insufficient information on which to base breeding recommendations.

BOUVIER DES FLANDRES MYOPATHY

Bouvier des Flandres myopathy is a rare degenerative myopathy, with many features shared with the familial form of dysphagia and megaesophagus seen in the breed. Clinical signs in affected young adults include regurgitation, exercise intolerance, generalized muscle atrophy, and a peculiar gait. Megaesophagus is a common feature. Most dogs have elevated creatine kinase (CK) levels, and electromyographic studies demonstrate bizarre, high-frequency discharges in skeletal muscles.

Although the condition appears to be familial, a mode of inheritance has not yet been determined. Until the genetics of the condition are better understood, it still makes sense to recommend that affected animals not be used for breeding.

CRANIAL CRUCIATE LIGAMENT RUPTURE

Rupture of the cranial cruciate ligament in the knee is a common orthopedic problem in dogs. Two different etiologies have been identified, one a result of acute trauma and the other, ligament degeneration (279, 726). An isolated tear in the ligament can occur as a traumatic injury in any dog. Factors responsible for ligament degeneration are numerous and include obesity, osteoarthritis, cellular changes within the ligament, and genetics.

Breeds at increased risk for rupture of the cranial cruciate ligament include the Newfoundland, rottweiler, and Staffordshire terrier (727, 1101, 1118). Breeders report the condition with some consistency in the Kuvasz, mastiff, and bullmastiff as well. In smaller dogs (those less than 15-22 kg) degeneration of the cranial cruciate ligament is less severe and occurs later in life, compared to large dogs. Peak prevalence is in dogs 7 to 10 years of age (1118).

Clinically, cranial cruciate ligament rupture presents as acute hindleg lameness. If it is not treated, after a few weeks the inflammation in the joint decreases on its own and the stifle becomes stabilized by the thickening of periarticular tissues (727). The diagnosis can be confirmed by eliciting a cranial drawer motion of the tibia relative to the femur with the stifle joint extended, flexed, and/or in a neutral position. Anesthesia or sedation is warranted in animals with acute injury and inflammation. An alternative is stress radiographs taken with tibial compression, which is both a highly sensitive and a specific indicator of cruciate rupture (254).

Many surgical approaches have been described to remedy the situation (279, 727). To give informed opinions regarding breeding dogs with cranial cruciate ligament rupture is difficult, as a familial tendency has not been documented. Until more is known about the heritability of the condition, however, not breeding affected individuals, or at least making it a breeder option, is safest.

CRANIOMANDIBULAR OSTEOPATHY

Craniomandibular osteopathy is a bizarre proliferative bone disease that typically affects the lower jawbone (mandible), the tympanic bullae, and, occasionally, other bones of the head. Although the cause is unknown, the condition clearly is not cancerous or inflammatory—though it certainly appears that way. The condition is believed to be transmitted as a simple autosomal recessive trait in West Highland white terriers (1096), and affects Scottish, West Highland white, and Cairn terriers (804) predominantly. It has also been reported in the Boston terrier (181), boxer (1096), bullmastiff (1096), bull terrier (1096), Catahoula leopard dog (1096), Doberman pinscher (1096), English bulldog (1096), fox terrier (1096), German wirehaired pointer (1096), golden retriever (1096), Great Dane (1096), Great Pyrenees (330), Irish setter (1096), Kerry blue terrier (1096), Labrador retriever (281), Skye terrier (1096), Staffordshire terrier (1096), and Weimaraner (1096). Affected animals are typically younger than 1 year of age. Breeders may refer to the condition as scottie jaw, lion's jaw, or westie jaw.

The condition does not cause clinical problems in all cases. Affected animals, however, often have difficulty chewing and swallowing and may have some pain when opening the mouth.

The diagnosis is usually suspected when a young dog of a breed at risk experiences the clinical signs described. The diagnosis is confirmed by radiography in which selected bones of the head show thickening associated with proliferation of bone. Radiographs should be repeated every 3 months to monitor progression or regression of the condition. Blood profiles of affected dogs may show increased serum calcium levels and increases in some enzymes such as serum alkaline phosphatase. Work is under way to develop a DNA test for this disorder that will unequivocally identify animals that are affected, carrier, and unaffected.

No effective therapies are available, but luckily the condition is often self-limiting. The abnormal bone growth slows, often stops, and may even recede by about a year of age. In the interim, symptomatic therapy consists of anti-inflammatory therapy (e.g., aspirin), feeding soft foods, and perhaps tube feeding if opening the mouth is painful. If an animal cannot eat or is in uncontrollable pain, euthanasia may be necessary.

Affected animals should not be used for breeding, even if they recover completely. The parents should be considered as carriers, and siblings as suspect carriers. The Institute for Genetic Disease Control in Animals (GDC) maintains an open registry for craniomandibular osteopathy in all terrier breeds and a registry also exists with the Orthopedic Foundation for Animals (OFA). When a DNA test becomes available, selecting appropriate individuals for breeding will be an easy matter.

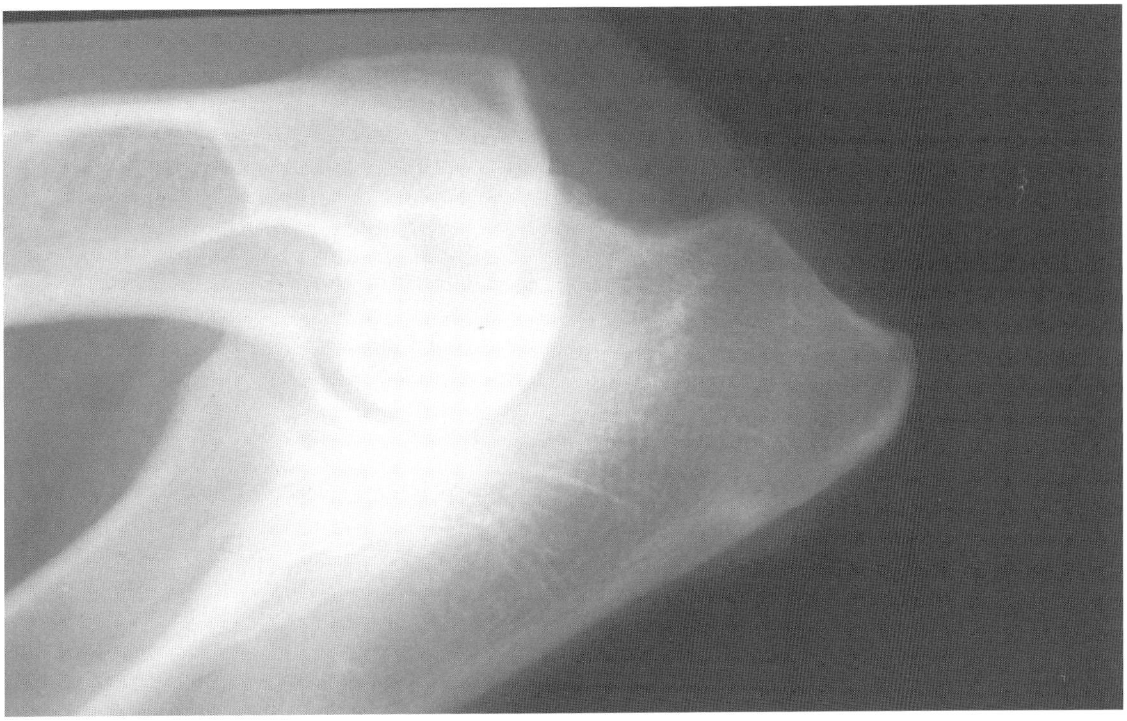

Figure 9-1 Elbow dysplasia
Courtesy of Jonathan T. Shiroma, Veterinary Radiologist, MedVet, Columbus, Ohio

ELBOW DYSPLASIA

Elbow dysplasia does not refer to just one disease but, rather, to an entire complex of disorders that affect the elbow joint (Figure 9-1). Several different processes might be involved, including ununited anconeal process (UAP), fragmented medial coronoid process (FCP), osteochondrosis of the medial humeral condyle, asynchronous growth of any of the bones that make up the elbow joint, or incomplete ossification of the humeral condyle. These topics are covered individually within this chapter. Following is a general description of elbow dysplasia.

Strong evidence supports the contention that osteochondritis dissecans (OCD) of the elbow is an inherited disease, likely controlled by many genes. Preliminary research (in Labrador retrievers) also suggests that the different forms of elbow dysplasia are inherited independently (805). Therefore, breeding stock should be selected from animals without a history of osteochondrosis, preferably for several generations. Unaffected dogs producing offspring with OCD, FCP, or both should not be bred again, and unaffected first-degree relatives (e.g., siblings) should not be used for breeding either.

The elbow registry of the Orthopedic Foundation for Animals (OFA) provides a standardized evaluation of the elbow joints for canine elbow dysplasia, regardless of specific cause. Radiographs are taken of the elbow joints and submitted to a registry for evaluation. Radiologists grade abnormal elbows from I to III, depending on the extent of joint damage, with Grade III being the worst. Normal elbows on individuals 24 months or older are assigned a breed registry number and are periodically reported to parent breed clubs.

The Institute for Genetic Disease Control in Animals (GDC) provides evaluation of elbows for degrees of arthrosis as recommended by the International Elbow Working Group, and also for joint incongruity, ununited anconeal process, fragmented medial coronoid process, and evidence of osteochondrosis. Swiss studies of elbow dysplasia in Bernese mountain dogs suggests that the incidence of elbow dysplasia should be based on primary lesions (ED score) in addition to arthrosis (ARTH) scores to improve specificity (565). In screening and control programs based on an open registry with access to family records, decreasing prevalence of elbow dysplasia can be expected, and related to selection of breeding stock (1017). Dogs with elbow dysplasia should not be bred, nor should any dog that produces a litter demonstrating elbow dysplasia. Ideally, first-degree relatives of dogs afflicted with elbow dysplasia should not be bred (805).

Elbow Dysplasia—Fragmented Coronoid Process (FCP)

The most common form of elbow dysplasia is fragmented coronoid process (FCP), in which part of the elbow joint breaks away from its bony anchor. It occurs in large breeds, especially Bernese mountain dogs, chow chows, German shepherd dogs, golden retrievers, Labrador retrievers, Newfoundlands, and rottweilers (74, 588). A genetic trend is thought to be important, but this has been truly documented only in rottweilers. Male dogs are affected more frequently than females (957). About 60% of cases also have a problem with OCD of the medial humeral condyle. At least in the Labrador retriever, fragmented coronoid process is thought to be inherited as a polygenic trait, independent of OCD of the humeral head (805). Apparently, not all cases of FCP are attributable to osteochondrosis; some are a result of mechanical stress (74).

Clinically, FCP is characterized by stiffness, stilted gait, or lameness. Most affected dogs show signs by 4 to 7 months of age. Pain can typically be elicited by flexion or extension of the elbow, but this is not specific for FCP. Special radiographic views and techniques are necessary to evaluate the coronoid processes (74). The craniolateral-caudomedial oblique (Cr15L-CdMO) projection provides the highest sensitivity for definitively identifying FCP (1143). It is difficult to actually see a fragmented coronoid process on radiographs because this area is often obstructed by other bones. Nevertheless, some telltale signs, such as bony deposits (osteophytes) found on the rim of the anconeal process, accompany the condition.

The coronoid process can be visualized with sophisticated linear tomography, but relatively few referral centers have this technology available. When dogs younger than 7 months of age have lameness suggestive of FCP but no radiographic changes, they should be reevaluated in 4 to 6 weeks to see if evidence of degenerative changes supports the diagnosis. If available, magnetic resonance imaging is extremely accurate and especially useful when radiographic findings are inconclusive (986). Arthroscopy through the cranial portal of the elbow allows access for both diagnosis and treatment (28). Sometimes, however, open surgery is necessary to confirm, as well as treat, the condition.

Conservative therapy should begin as soon as the diagnosis is made. This includes weight reduction, caloric restriction, use of chondroprotective agents, limited restricted exercise, and pain medication as needed. Anti-inflammatory agents must be used cautiously, because they decrease pain and encourage dogs to use the leg—not desirable for this condition, as it puts further stress on the joint. Several different surgical techniques are described for managing this condition (29, 770), although surgical intervention does not appear at present to improve the prognosis for dogs with FCP.

Dogs with elbow dysplasia should not be bred, nor should any dog that produces a litter evidencing elbow dysplasia. Ideally, first-degree relatives of dogs afflicted with elbow dysplasia also should not be bred (805).

Elbow Dysplasia—Incomplete Ossification of Humeral Condyle

Over the past decade, fractures of the humeral condyles of the elbow joint have been recognized to occur disproportionately in spaniels, especially cocker spaniels. In one published study of 28 affected dogs, 24 were cocker spaniels, 3 were Brittany spaniels and the last was a cocker spaniel-standard poodle cross (632). The condition also has been strongly suspected to occur in Cavalier King Charles spaniels, Boykin spaniels, and Clumber spaniels (632) and has been reported in the rottweiler (902). The cause is unknown, but a genetic basis is suspected.

Typically, the cartilage in this area turns to bone (ossifies) by 8 to 12 weeks of age. Ossification fails to occur completely in affected spaniels, and this causes the bone to become weak, and affected dogs may suffer from spontaneous fractures following even minor trauma. Most are adults (2 to 12 years of age; average 6 years of age) when they experience problems, and the majority so far have been males. Because these dogs are older, most veterinarians in clinical practice haven't considered a hereditary nature. Given the facts to date, however, incomplete ossification of the humeral condyle should be considered in any adult spaniel experiencing lameness of the front leg.

Diagnosis of the condylar fracture is not difficult with radiographs, but identifying affected individuals before the fracture occurs is more difficult. High-resolution radiographs may identify a fault in the condyles (always evaluate both front legs!), but this is determined more accurately by computed tomography (CAT scan), which is impractical for routine screening.

The fractures themselves require surgical correction. Transcondylar bone screws are recommended because of the weakness of the condyles for regular fixation methods. Because of the likely genetic nature of this problem, affected animals, their parents, and siblings should only cautiously be used for breeding.

Elbow Dysplasia—Osteochondrosis of the Medial Condyle

In some studies, osteochondrosis of the medial humeral condyle (elbow) is the most common form of osteochondrosis reported. In other studies, fragmented coronoid process is reported to occur 10 times as often as osteochondrosis of the medial humeral condyle (393). Accordingly, breed predispositions previously listed for this condition are unreliable. This discrepancy results, in part, from semantics. In many reports, elbow dysplasia and osteochondrosis of the elbow joint have been used synonymously. In others, osteochondrosis of the elbow joint and fragmented coronoid process have been used interchangeably. Statistics relayed by the orthopedic registries, the Orthopedic Foundation for Animals (OFA), and the Institute for Genetic Disease Control in Animals (GDC) refer only to elbow dysplasia.

This area is anatomically complex because it involves the intimate association of the bones of the forearm (radius and ulna) with the humerus. The medial aspect of the lower humerus (condyle) retains thicker cartilage longer than the lateral aspect, and, therefore, this site is more prone to osteochondrosis. When cracks and fissures form in the cartilage, it is prone to the classic changes of OCD (852). OCD of the medial humeral condyle is similar to the disorder seen in the shoulder. It just involves the lower end of the humerus rather than the upper part.

For OCD of the elbow, surgery is generally needed as soon as the condition is diagnosed. Treatment consists of surgical excision of the loose cartilage flap. Good clinical results can be achieved if surgery is performed before significant degenerative joint disease has developed. Degenerative joint disease usually continues, but at a much slower rate. Affected animals should not be bred.

Elbow Dysplasia—Ununited Anconeal Process (UAP)

Ununited anconeal process (UAP) occurs when the bone-growth center in the anconeal process of the elbow fails to unite with the ulna of the foreleg. This union normally occurs in medium- and large-breed dogs at 4 or 5 months of age. If it has not fused by 5 months of age, joint instability and the pain and inflammation associated with osteoarthrosis will result. There is a breed predisposition for the bloodhound, bullmastiff, German shepherd dog, Great Dane, Great Pyrenees, Irish wolfhound, Labrador retriever, Newfoundland, pointer, St. Bernard, and Weimaraner, as well as the chondrodystrophoid breeds such as the basset hound, French bulldog, and dachshund (461, 673, 960). Males are affected about twice as frequently as females, and the condition is bilateral in about 30% of cases (587).

The cause is still a matter of dispute, and genetics is but one of many putative etiologies. Incongruous growth of the radius and ulna has been proposed as the fundamental cause of UAP (960).

Foreleg lameness is the principal sign, typically when pups are between 5 and 12 months of age. The pathologic changes result from loss of the stabilizing effect of the anconeal process and from inflammation within the joint. The diagnosis is confirmed by a flexed lateral radiograph of the elbow, but this should not be attempted before the dog is 20 weeks old or interpretation will be difficult. In dogs with ununited anconeal process, a radiolucent line is seen between the anconeal and olecranon processes (215).

Surgical intervention seems to be warranted in cases of UAP. Whereas some surgeons prefer to remove the process and others choose to reattach it, the most successful approach seems to be ulnar osteotomy in which pressure is relieved on the anconeal process and it is allowed to reunite on its own (960). Affected animals should not be bred.

GRACILIS or SEMITENDINOSIS MYOPATHY

Myopathy of the gracilis or semitendinosis muscles is a rare and poorly understood entity. It is reported most commonly in the German shepherd dog and Belgian shepherd, and males are affected more than females (589). Affected dogs are typically adults, and they develop a characteristic hindlimb lameness with shortened stride and leg rotation. The diagnosis is confirmed by muscle biopsy demonstrating a scarring myopathy.

Neither medical nor surgical therapies seem to correct the problem consistently. A genetic trend, other than the breed predisposition, has not been documented for this disorder. It has some similarities to congenital torticollis in humans. Although affected animals should not be bred, information on which to base breeding recommendations is insufficient.

HEREDITARY MYOPATHY

Hereditary myopathy, also known as type II muscle fiber deficiency, is a rare, autosomal recessive

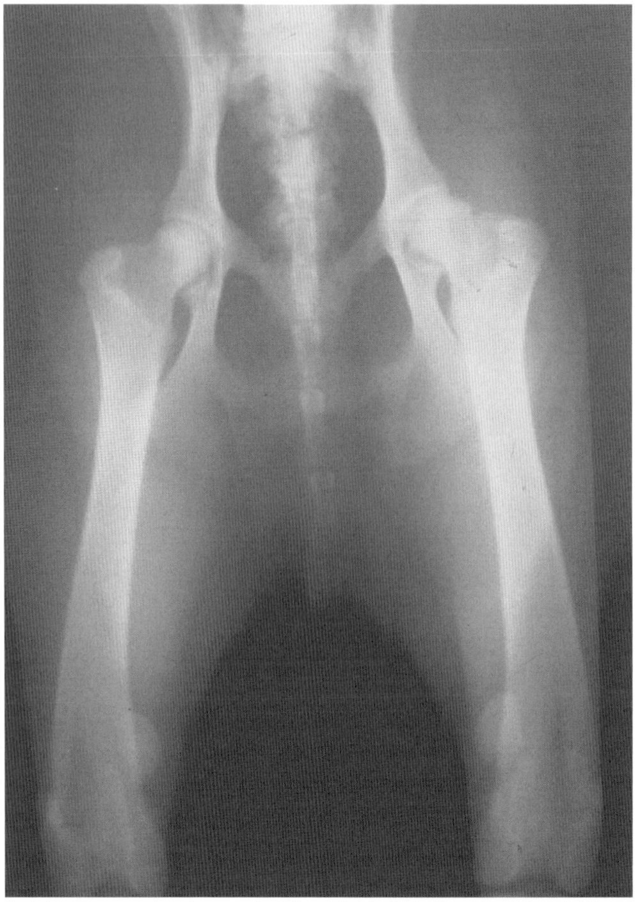

Figure 9-2 Hip dysplasia
Case supervised by Dr. Jeff Meinen, Mesa Veterinary Hospital, Mesa, Arizona

myopathy reported in the Labrador retriever (86, 459). It is characterized by a predominance of type I muscle fibers and a relative deficiency of type II fibers, particularly in older dogs and in certain muscle groups (18). The condition becomes obvious by 5 months of age, at which time a gait abnormality progresses to generalized weakness, exercise intolerance, and stunted growth (656). As the condition progresses, generalized atrophy of skeletal muscles develops (82). Despite their muscular changes, most animals remain bright and alert. In fact, most reach a clinical plateau, and some even show gradual but incomplete recovery (657).

The diagnosis is suspected with a profound creatinuria (up to 30 times normal) and abnormal electromyography (fibrillation potentials, positive sharp waves, and bizarre high-frequency discharges) and is confirmed by histochemical evaluation of muscle biopsies (662, 663, 729). Diazepam can alleviate some of the signs but, although animals are capable of living a normal life span, their prognosis for a normal life remains poor. Most are eventually euthanized.

Even if they are not incapacitated by the disorder, affected animals should not be bred. Both parents should be considered carriers of the trait and removed from breeding programs. Normal-appearing siblings should be considered as potential carriers. At this time, there is no way to detect heterozygous carriers.

HIP DYSPLASIA

Hip dysplasia is defined as an abnormal development of the hip (coxofemoral) joint and is actually a genetically transmitted tendency to develop laxity of the hip joints (618, 718) (Figure 9-2). The mode of inheritance is described as "polygenic"—meaning that the trait is influenced by several different genes (195). It also means that predicting with accuracy how pups will be affected when dysplastic parents are mated is not a simple task. In general, however, pups born to parents with normal joints are more likely to have normal hips themselves. Pups born to parents with hip dysplasia are at higher risk for developing hip dysplasia (618).

Understanding the different phenotypic expressions of hip dysplasia is not so difficult if one views the trait controlled by a set number of different, yet interrelated, genes. For example, if hip dysplasia were the product of three genes, there would be 8 possible combinations of genes in the gametes (e.g., XYZ, XYz, XyZ, Xyz xYZ, xYz, xyZ, xyz,), but 64 potential genotypes among the offspring. Considering both parents as heterozygous for all three gene pairs (XxYyZz) will illustrate the concept further. Phenotypically, the parents are likely going to be radiographically considered "good" or "fair" with respect to hip dysplasia. In the offspring of such a mating, the one genotype in which all three gene pairs are homozygous dominant (XXYYZZ) will have excellent hip conformation and will not transmit recessive hip dysplasia alleles to its offspring. However, of the 64 possible outcomes, this only involves one dog. Similarly, there is one outcome expected in which an offspring has all recessive alleles (xxyyzz). It is presumed that this dog will be severely dysplastic, despite the fact that both parents had decent hip conformation. Since we expect that most dogs are heterozygous for hip dysplasia genes, it should be expected that an entire spectrum of hip dysplasia traits may be seen in the offspring and this is exactly what is observed.

The heritability of the condition is typically cited as 0.2–0.6, with most near 0.25. Clearly, nongenetic factors play a role in expression as well (578, 790, 1003, 1044, 1045). It has been speculated that the heritability index of hip dysplasia may be as high as 0.9 if passive joint laxity is the criterion used for diagnosis (1045)

Although dogs may be born with a susceptibility or tendency to develop hip dysplasia, it is not a foregone conclusion that all susceptible dogs will eventually develop hip dysplasia. All dysplastic dogs are born with normal hips, and the dysplastic changes begin within the first 24 months of life, although they are usually evident within the first few months (195, 1044, 1045). The best evidence available suggests a genetic predisposition to hip dysplasia, with the involvement of multiple genes (11, 578).

It is now known that several factors combine to determine whether a susceptible dog will ever develop hip dysplasia. These include body size, conformation, growth patterns, pelvic muscle mass, caloric load, and electrolyte balance in the dog food (149, 618, 871). Hip dysplasia is especially devastating because if the joint laxity and femoral head subluxation progress, bone deformity and degenerative joint disease are the invariable results (335).

Clinically, the presentation of hip dysplasia can be quite diverse. Younger animals may have acute episodes of hindleg lameness that worsens with vigorous exercise or minor trauma. Eventually these dogs may have difficulty rising, walking, climbing, and running, with associated soreness. A period of accommodation may follow before the onset of degenerative joint disease and more consistent lameness. Affected dogs may try to shift their weight to the front legs and avoid putting pressure on their inflamed hip joints.

Interestingly, there does not seem to be a correlation between hip joint morphology and clinical signs (336). Some dogs with profound hip dysplasia display little discomfort, and others are in intense pain with only moderate joint changes.

When animals grow too quickly, it is more difficult for them to keep the hip joints stabilized. Susceptible dogs that are fed high-calorie diets have an increased risk of becoming dysplastic. Giving calcium or vitamin D supplements to susceptible dogs is not wise because these, too, can interfere with proper development of bones and joints (871).

Finally, some research suggests that the dietary electrolyte balance or "anion gap" of a dog food may affect the expression of hip dysplasia.

Hip Dysplasia

The Hip Dysplasia Registry is operated by the Orthopedic Foundation for Animals (OFA). Hip joint conformation is classified as excellent, good, fair, borderline, mildly dysplastic, moderately dysplastic, or severely dysplastic. Classifications of excellent, good, and fair are considered within normal limits, and if the dog is 2 years of age or older, a breed registry number is assigned. OFA concedes that preliminary evaluations done earlier than 2 years of age are reliable but that questionable cases should be reevaluated at 2 years of age (C041). OFA recommends that bitches not be radiographed for 3 to 4 weeks before or after a heat cycle or whelping, because they contend that hormonal changes can influence the radiographic appearance of subluxation. The ultimate purpose of OFA certification is to provide information to dog owners to assist in the selection of good breeding animals. Therefore, attempts to get a dysplastic dog certified will only hurt the breed by perpetuating the disease. The OFA maintains a database of hip evaluations for approximately half a million dogs (660).

PennHip Technique

A relatively new stress-radiographic technique, known as PennHip, involves direct measurement of joint laxity and is based on the supposition that joint laxity portends degenerative joint disease (979). Standard radiographs as well as additional radiographs are taken with the femoral heads in a compression view and a distraction view. To achieve the distraction view, a device is placed between the legs that acts as a fulcrum to displace the femoral head maximally. The relative degree of femoral head displacement from the acetabulum is quantified by calculating a distraction index (DI) that ranges from 0 to 1, with 0 representing full hip congruency and 1 representing complete subluxation.

Preliminary research showed that foods with a lower anion gap (difference between positively charged and negatively charged elements) led to a lower incidence of hip dysplasia in susceptible dogs (511). Although some breeders have favored vitamin C supplementation to help prevent hip dysplasia, this has absolutely no rational basis and no evidence that it does any good (with some evidence that it might do harm) (490).

Hip dysplasia is diagnosed by considering the history, clinical signs, and radiographic changes that are evident. It is rare for all but the most severely dysplastic dogs to have radiographic changes by 4 weeks of age. The earliest reliable test can be done at 16 weeks of age. This distraction test appears to be the best test available for predicting which dogs will eventually develop degenerative joint disease as a consequence of their hip dysplasia.

Also, two registries keep statistics on hip dysplasia. Dogs with no evidence of hip dysplasia can receive a registry number with the Institute for Genetic Disease Control (GDC) by 12 months of age, and from the Orthopedic Foundation for Animals (OFA) by 24 months of age.

Dogs diagnosed with hip dysplasia do have options. Some dogs with severe dysplasia experience little pain, and others that have minor changes may be extremely sore. The main problem is that hip dysplasia promotes degenerative joint disease (osteoarthritis or osteoarthrosis), which can eventually incapacitate the joint.

Medical management is indicated for young dogs with joint pain and for older dogs suffering from the pain and disability of degenerative joint disease (632). Aspirin and other anti-inflammatory agents, such as carprofen (Rimadyl) or etodolac (EtoGesic™), are suitable in the early stages. Surgery is needed when animals are in great pain, when drug therapy doesn't work adequately, or when movement is severely compromised. A variety of surgical techniques have been described, including total hip replacement (1046), triple pelvic osteotomy (661), and excision arthroplasty (659). Recent evaluation of the shelf arthroplasty has suggested that the procedure does not alter the progression of hip dysplasia in affected dogs (779). The same seems to be true for intertrochanteric osteotomy (294). Nutraceuticals, including polysulfated glycosaminoglycan, hyaluronic acid, glucosamine, and chondroitin, may also be of benefit, especially early on in the disorder (244, 660, 1042).

Preventing hip dysplasia in future generations has been an elusive ideal. There are many reasons for this expectation. Because hip dysplasia is a polygenic trait with a heritability of about 0.25, even intensive selection pressure merely shifts the mean toward the more desirable range. Hip joint morphology will still follow a normal distribution in the pups. The pups should not necessarily be expected to have the same preferred hip morphology as their parents. Although this can be frustrating for both owner and veterinarian, it is to be anticipated. Ridding a line of hip dysplasia is a slow process, involving many generations. See the discussion on heritability in the Introduction.

To minimize the risk of producing a dysplastic dog, it is best to start off with good stock. Ideally, clear hips will be a trait common for several generations in the animal's pedigree. Suitable animals can be selected from either a closed (OFA) or open (GDC) registry. These registries grade radiographs submitted by veterinarians for subjective morphologic criteria and maintain a database of animals evaluated. Some foreign registries also attempt to provide scores for hip joint morphology rather than just subjective descriptions (354, 1133). The statistics generated by these voluntary databases, however, are not entirely reliable because there is no requirement that a breeder submit radiographs from obviously dysplastic dogs. Sometimes breeders have a tendency to submit only radiographs that stand a fair-to-good chance of passing and gaining certification.

GDC Hip Registry

The Institute for Genetic Disease Control in Animals (GDC) recognizes that, with the USA as the exception, the world standard for screening for normal certification of hips is 12 to 18 months of age. Through the use of an open registry in Sweden and the evaluation at 1 year of age, the incidence of hip dysplasia has been reduced from 46% to 28% in 5 years in that country. To compensate for potential observer variations, the GDC requests reevaluation of any borderline cases at 2 years of age and withholds certification until that time.

Probably the best advice at this point is to evaluate potential breeding animals using a stress-radiographic technique (PennHip), which can estimate the susceptibility to hip dysplasia and degenerative joint disease in pups as young as 16 weeks of age. By calculating a distraction index for potential breeding stock, it is possible to make the selection process more standardized and somewhat more objective (850). PennHip also requires that *all* radiographs be submitted from each evaluation; owners are not allowed to pick and choose which results get submitted and which do not (at least in theory). Because the results of PennHip evaluations are not maintained by breed registries, such as the American Kennel Club (AKC), it is still advantageous to have breeding animals certified by one of the orthopedic registries—the OFA or GDC.

A dog with a distraction index (DI) of 0.4 has twice the passive laxity of a dog with a DI of 0.2. Also, a dog with a DI of 0.4 can be considered to be 40% luxated from the acetabulum. The closer the number is to 0, the "tighter" the hips; the closer to 1, the more lax the hip joint and greater the risk of hip dysplasia. The DI measurement is less influenced than other techniques by errors in positioning (978). Breed-specific differences in passive laxity continue to be identified in the PennHip database. For example, in German shepherd dogs, each 0.1 increase in DI is associated with a fourfold increase in risk of developing DJD; and in rottweilers, each 0.1 increase in DI is associated with a threefold increase in risk of developing DJD (846). A DI of 0.3 is believed to represent a biological threshold separating normal hip joints from joints susceptible to DJD (9, 978). Synovial fluid cavitation is relatively rare with distraction radiography but seems to be most common in Irish wolfhounds, Irish setters, Rhodesian ridgebacks, and Weimaraners (563).

As described, stress radiography (i.e., PennHip technique) allows the diagnosis of joint laxity in pups as young as 4 months of age. Because the technique is unreliable at younger ages, at least for German shepherd dogs, tests should be repeated at maturity for breeding dogs (980). A modification, in which dynamic ultrasonography is utilized to estimate passive hip laxity, has much clinical potential and has been used to estimate hip laxity in 6- to 8-week-old puppies (786).

If breeders start with pups that have less risk of hip dysplasia, the risk can be reduced further by controlling the dog's environment. For example, the food should contain a moderate amount of protein and super high premium and high-calorie diets should be avoided. Also, pups should be fed several times a day for defined periods (e.g., 15 minutes) rather than leaving the food down all day. Limiting food consumption has been shown to decrease the incidence of hip dysplasia in susceptible animals (510, 512). All nutritional supplements should be avoided, especially those that include calcium, phosphorus, or vitamin D. The pup should be engaged in controlled exercise rather than allowed to run loose. Unrestricted exercise in the pup can stress the joints, which are still developing. This won't affect the dog's genotype and its inherent risk for developing hip dysplasia, but it does have an impact on phenotype.

The best way to prevent hip dysplasia in future generations is to sanction the breeding only of dogs that have disease-free joints based on appropriate radiographic evaluation and that come from families with a history of disease-free joints. The distraction index is statistically the most predictive method for degenerative joint disease in pups (9). Heritability of DI is higher than that of hip scores and, thus, breeding pairs selected based on DI should result in faster genetic changes (578, 978, 981). This will lower the incidence of hip dysplasia but not remove it entirely. The incidence can be reduced further by selecting dogs for breeding based on family performance and progeny testing (578). Ideally, there should be no history of hip dysplasia for three generations back in any dog or bitch intended for breeding. It is also important to select animals with good hips from families in which the siblings also have good hips. In screening and control programs based on an open registry with access to family records, decreasing prevalence of hip dysplasia can be expected, and related to selection of breeding stock (1023).

Following is a list of breeding criteria that have been demonstrated to reduce the frequency of hip dysplasia in a population of dogs more rapidly (205, 1044, 1045):

1. Only normal dogs should be bred.
2. The normal dogs should come from normal parents and grandparents.
3. The normal dogs should have greater than 75% normal littermates.
4. The sire should have a record of producing normal pups that exceed the breed average.
5. Replacement dogs and bitches should have better hip conformation than their parents and grandparents.

This can be difficult in breeds with a high incidence of hip dysplasia. For example, the frequency of hip dysplasia in the fila Brasiliero is 58% (23) and many generations of selective breeding will be necessary to lower the prevalence of the disorder to an acceptable level. Much progress has been made in preventing hip dysplasia, and over the past 20 years an improvement has been noted in the hip joint phenotype of dogs in the United States, particularly male dogs (503). Nevertheless, the progress has not been fast enough for most veterinarians and breeders. It is hoped that in the next several years, DNA tests will become available to unequivocally identify hip joint genotype and take the guesswork out of our genetic selection.

HYPERTROPHIC OSTEODYSTROPHY

Hypertrophic osteodystrophy, also known as Moeller-Barlow disease, is a developmental condition affecting primarily young, rapidly growing large-breed dogs. It is reported most commonly in the boxer, Doberman pinscher, German shepherd dog, Great Dane, Irish setter, Labrador retriever, rottweiler, and Weimaraner (743, 924, 1101, 1102). The condition is thought to be familial, but a mode of inheritance has not been determined (1140). Males are affected more often than females (748). The condition has some similarity to Paget's disease in humans, and a viral infection is thought to possibly precipitate the condition in dogs (743). This condition can affect the metaphysis of any long bone but is most often recognized in the distal radius, ulna, and tibia (587, 743).

Clinical signs may develop between 2 months of age and the time the growth plate closes, typically 5 to 8 months of age. There is variable lameness and pain on palpation, and some dogs experience fever, anorexia, and depression. Most dogs recover spontaneously in a few weeks, but relapses can occur (743).

The diagnosis is confirmed radiographically by finding metaphyseal sclerosis and linear radiolucency parallel and subjacent to the physis. Treatment is usually attempted with analgesics, nonsteroidal anti-inflammatory agents, and sometimes fluids and enteral nutrition. Because the genetics of the condition have not been determined, the only reasonable advice at this time is not to breed affected individuals.

IDIOPATHIC MULTIFOCAL OSTEOPATHY

Idiopathic multifocal osteopathy is a poorly documented condition seen in Scottish terriers. It is characterized by multifocal absence of bone in the skull, cervical spine, and proximal extremities (434). Some of the characteristics are shared with human osteolysis syndromes, particularly Winchester syndrome and vanishing bone disease. Affected dogs are reluctant to move, and when they do, they walk with a stiff, stilted gait. Carpal valgus, ligamentous laxity, and dysphagia are also reported. The heritability of the condition has not been determined. Based on a very limited number of reported cases, diagnosis should be based on survey radiographs and histopathologic assessment. The prognosis is considered guarded, and affected dogs should probably not be bred.

LEGG-CALVÉ-PERTHES DISEASE

Legg-Calvé-Perthes disease, also known as Legg-Perthes disease and aseptic necrosis of the femoral head, is a disorder of the hip joint seen in young, small-breed dogs, such as the affenpinscher (802), Bichon frisé (802), Border terrier (802), Cairn terrier (153), Lakeland terrier (153), Manchester terrier (153), miniature pinscher (153), miniature poodle (924), silky terrier (181), West Highland white terrier (153), and Yorkshire terrier (892). Males and females are affected with equal frequency (587). Typically the disease is seen in dogs between 4 and 12 months of age, and in most cases (85%) only one leg is affected (587). A genetic trend has been suspected, involving an autosomal recessive trait with incomplete penetrance (885, 1074).

Affected dogs are typically lame on one leg and in great pain. The affected area may show substantial atrophy of muscle. The diagnosis can be suspected on the basis of radiographs, but surgical biopsies are needed for confirmation. If an early diagnosis is made, before significant bony changes occur, placing the affected leg in a non-weight-bearing sling may allow the femoral head to revascularize and correct the situation. Otherwise, treatment involves surgically removing the damaged femoral head. Because most cases are found in small dogs that aren't bearing a lot of weight on the hip joint, further reconstructive surgery is not usually necessary.

The Institute for Genetic Disease Control in Animals (GDC) maintains an open registry for Legg-Perthes disease in terriers and miniature and toy poodles. It should thus be possible to select animals with no family history of Legg-Calvé-Perthes disease and, hopefully, eliminate the trait from the gene pool. Affected animals should not be bred, and parents should be considered carriers. Siblings are suspect carriers.

MASTICATORY MYOSITIS

Masticatory myositis, also known as eosinophilic myositis, is an immune-mediated disease in which antibodies are directed against type II M fibers in masticatory muscles (20). It is most commonly reported in the German shepherd dog (84). Masticatory muscles contain a unique myosin isoform, unique myosin light chains, and unique myosin heavy chains. Studies have suggested that transforming growth factor-beta (TFG-beta), and latent transforming growth factor-beta binding protein (LTBP), a modulating protein, may play a role in muscle tissue repair, inflammation, and fibrogenesis in this condition (1083).

Clinical signs result when the masticatory muscles become painful and swollen. The diagnosis is made on the basis of consistent clinical signs, histopathology, and immunopathology. Serologic testing may reveal elevated creatine phosphokinase (CPK), significant ANA titers, and positive titers to type II M myosin antibodies (20). The condition does tend to respond well to immunosuppressive therapy and may enter a period of permanent or semi-permanent remission. Affected animals should not be bred, but information is not sufficient to make more specific breeding recommendations.

MITOCHONDRIAL MYOPATHY

Mitochondrial myopathy is a rare metabolic disorder reported in young Clumber and Sussex spaniels. Similar disorders have been described in the Old English sheepdog (82, 100) and Jack Russell terrier (791). Although the cause is still a matter of some debate, inheritance is believed to play at least some role, and the condition is thought to be associated with abnormal mitochondrial function. Because mitochondrial DNA is inherited exclusively from the cytoplasm of the mother's egg, the disorder should pass only from the maternal line to both sexes.

The condition usually becomes evident by 3 months of age. Affected pups tire easily and may collapse in sternal recumbency when pressure is applied while the dog is walking on a leash. Afflicted dogs develop excessive panting and tachycardia because of metabolic acidosis. The disorder is suspected when mild exertion results in metabolic acidosis with elevated lactate and pyruvate concentrations. Electromyographic studies reveal increased insertional activity and complex repetitive discharges (82). Ultrastructural evaluation of muscle biopsies reveals subsarcolemmal accumulation of mitochondria (791).

There is no treatment, and the prognosis should be considered poor. Supplementation with ascorbic acid may be beneficial, although results have not been impressive to date. Even though the genetics of this disorder have not been conclusively determined, it would seem appropriate that the dam be considered a carrier of the trait and not used for future matings. If inheritance is indeed cytoplasmic, affected males should not transmit the disorder to their offspring, but females can.

MUSCULAR DYSTROPHY

Alaskan malamutes, golden retrievers, Groenendaeler (Belgian) shepherds, Irish terriers, miniature schnauzers, rottweilers, and Samoyeds are susceptible to an X-linked myopathy, similar to Duchenne-type muscular dystrophy in humans (82, 459, 543, 544, 778, 940, 952, 1060, 1068, 1136). A similar dystrophin deficiency has been reported in German shorthaired pointers (917). A colony of Pembroke Welsh corgis with a form of x-linked muscular dystrophy has been established from a single proband (1142). The underlying defect in these disorders is believed to be an inability to produce dystrophin, a protein in muscle fibers, and dystrophin is lacking in the skeletal and cardiac muscles of affected dogs (82). It is now apparent that not all cases have a complete absence of dystrophin. In golden retriever muscular dystrophy, a truncated dystrophin protein of 390 kD has been detected that is only 5% of the size of normal dystrophin. It results from a frameshift mutation in exon 7 that predicts a stop codon early in exon 8 (1142). A muscular dystrophy associated with myofiber atrophy, mild myonecrosis, and decreased muscle carnitine levels has been demonstrated in rottweilers (415). This distal muscular dystrophy does not seem to be related to major dystrophin abnormalities. Rottweiler muscular dystrophy is caused by a point mutation in exon 58 of the dystrophin gene, which results in a truncated dystrophin protein (1136). There is a high rate of dystrophin mutations in humans, and the same appears to be true in dogs.

Being a sex-linked trait, X-linked muscular dystrophy is carried by females and manifested in males. Problems start in 6- to 8-week-old pups and progress rapidly. The neck becomes rigid and the gait stiff, but the first sign is usually difficulty in swallowing. Most muscles wither, but the tongue and hamstring muscles become variably more developed. Clinical signs progress slowly during the first 6 months of life and then tend to stabilize (82).

The diagnosis is suspected based on elevated muscle enzymes (e.g. creatine kinase, aldolase, lactate dehydrogenase), and confirmed by muscle biopsy, electromyography, and neurological examinations (543, 1059). A DNA test has been designed to detect affected, carrier, and clear golden retrievers (39), but it is not yet commercially available. There is no treatment, and animals get progressively worse. Potential strategies for gene therapy are being pursued in people as well as dogs (462). The dam should be considered an obligate carrier and removed from breeding programs. Affected animals should not be bred.

MYOCLONUS

Familial myoclonus is a rare condition of muscular hypertonicity that has been reported in Labrador retrievers (546). When stimulated, affected dogs fall to their sides and exhibit extensor rigidity and opisthotonos. This is usually evident even in young pups. A mode of inheritance has not been determined. Some improvement is noted with drugs such as diazepam and clorazepate. Affected animals should not be bred.

MYOSITIS OSSIFICANS

Myositis ossificans is a rare muscle disorder characterized by bone formation within muscles (607). The cause is not known with any certainty, but the condition in people is believed to be congenital or hereditary. Clinical signs include progressive weakness, swollen muscles, muscle pain, stiffness, and bony deposits within muscles (88). The diagnosis is confirmed by histopathologic assessment of affected tissue. The prognosis is guarded in generalized cases, but in focal mineralization, surgical excision may be successful. Affected animals should not be bred.

MYOTONIA

Myotonia is a disorder of skeletal muscle characterized by delayed relaxation of the muscle fiber in response to voluntary, mechanical, or electrical stimulation. The pathophysiology of congenital myotonia remains controversial. A mutation in a gene controlling or regulating ionic transport in muscle membranes may be responsible for the condition in people, in which both dominant and recessive variants are recognized. Congenital myotonia in the dog closely resembles nonprogressive myotonia congenita in people.

The condition is seen most often in chow chows, in which it is believed to have an autosomal recessive inheritance (302, 459, 547, 958). Isolated cases have also been described in the American cocker spaniel, Great Dane, Labrador retriever, miniature schnauzer, Rhodesian ridgeback, Staffordshire bull terrier, and West Highland white terrier (82, 450, 547, 957, 1086). A deficiency in type I fibers has been reported in the Staffordshire terrier (82), in which there seems to be a familial trend (547).

The diagnosis is rendered following electromyography (repetitive discharges that wax and wane in frequency) and histopathological and histochemical evaluation of muscle biopsies. Procainamide, quinidine, and phenytoin have been used to halt the progression of clinical signs, but they do not correct the underlying problem. Until more is known about the genetics of myotonia in the dog, affected animals should probably not be bred. In the chow chow, in which autosomal recessive inheritance is suspected, both parents of affected dogs should be considered as carriers of the trait.

OSTEOCHONDROSIS

Osteochondrosis is a disorder of growth cartilage that occurs in specific locations and is prevalent in specific breeds. The term osteochondrosis itself is a matter of controversy, as the initial process does not involve bone. Other terms for the disorder include osteochondritis dissecans, osteochondrosis dissecans, and dyschondroplasia. Focal failure of endochondral ossification leads to retention of cartilage, rather than conversion to bone (286). The etiology is complex, with trauma, genetics, growth rates, nutrition, and ischemia all having a role. Genetic factors clearly do have a role, and breed predispositions have been recognized (286).

In time, when osteochondrosis causes flaps of cartilage to be exposed in the joint, inflammation results. At this time, it is referred to as osteochondritis dissecans (OCD), describing the inflammatory component and the fact that cartilage has become "dissected" and exposed. If the flap becomes dislodged, it may be referred to as a "joint mouse." In dogs, the condition affects the front legs preferentially (shoulder, elbow) but also can affect the back legs (hip, stifle) and even the vertebrae in the neck (refer also to the earlier discussion on elbow dysplasia).

The factors that cause osteochondrosis are many, and trauma, poor nutrition, and hereditary abnormalities have all been explored. The most likely associations made to date suggest that feeding diets high in calories and calcium promote the development of osteochondrosis in susceptible dogs (969). Dietary protein content does not seem to play a significant role in the disturbed regulation of endochondral ossification (755). Also, animals that are allowed to exercise in an unregulated fashion are at increased risk, as they are more likely to sustain cartilage injuries (969). The fact that OCD occurs mainly in large-breed dogs suggests that the increased weight-bearing needs of the cartilage may make it prone to damage. Some evidence also shows that a variety of hormones (such as calcitonin, somatotropin, thyrotropin, and sex hormones) may influence the development of osteochondrosis.

Osteochondrosis is a disorder of young dogs. Problems usually start between 4 and 7 months of age. Large-breed dogs are most likely to be affected, but there is great breed variability depending on the exact regional type of osteochondrosis encountered.

In the early stages of osteochondrosis, usually no clinical signs are apparent. Only when a cleft forms in the cartilage and inflammation ensues is the condition clinically evident. The usual manifestation is a sudden onset of lameness. In time, the continued inflammation results in arthritis in those affected joints.

The diagnosis of OCD is often strongly suspected when a young dog of a breed at risk suddenly becomes painfully lame. This lameness may worsen in wet or cold weather or when the leg is extended. Careful manipulation can usually pinpoint the site of the problem. The manipulation must be exact so as not to confuse elbow problems with those in the shoulder, or hip problems with those in the stifle. The opposite limb also should be carefully evaluated, even if no problems are clinically evident.

Radiographic studies of the joints are useful for establishing a diagnosis. Unfortunately, cartilage does not show up well on radiographs. Heavy sedation or anesthesia is usually necessary so that the painful limb can be stretched and properly positioned. If finances allow, taking radiographs of both limbs is worthwhile for comparison purposes. Radiographs also should be taken of other joints on the same limb (e.g., elbow and shoulder) to evaluate for other potential sites of involvement. Early cases may show a minimal decrease in bone density; moderate cases may have a flattened contour; and advanced cases are often associated with a concave defect and considerable arthritis.

The management of dogs with OCD is a matter of much debate and controversy. Some recommend surgery to remove the damaged cartilage before joint damage is permanent. Others recommend conservative therapy of rest and analgesics. Each side has proponents. The most common drugs used are aspirin and polysulfated glycosaminoglycans. Most veterinarians agree that the use of corticosteroids creates more problems than it solves in treating this condition. What seems clear is that some dogs respond to conservative therapies and others need surgery.

The conservative approach utilizes nonsteroidal anti-inflammatory drugs such as aspirin and polysulfated glycosaminoglycans. Aspirin reduces pain and lameness but doesn't promote healing. Complex sugars, such as hyaluronate, glucosamine, pentosan polysulfate, and PSGAGs (chondroitin sulfate), also known as chondroprotective agents, may help protect joint tissues and be a useful adjunct in OCD. They seem to inhibit enzyme-mediated degradation of articular cartilage in osteoarthritis.

Surgery is often helpful if it is performed before joint damage is significant. With a bone curette or scalpel, the edges of the cartilage defect are trimmed back to healthy bone. The central portion of the defect is completely removed. The defect then fills with fibrous cartilage. The results vary from fair to excellent, depending upon which joint is affected and whether the surgery was performed before arthritis set in. Dogs that have recurring problems after surgery likely have progression of degenerative joint disease within the affected joint.

Preventing osteochondrosis involves not breeding dogs with a family history of OCD and controlling as many environmental issues as possible. The Institute for Genetic Disease Control in Animals (GDC) maintains open orthopedic registries to help in the selection process of breeding animals.

High energy intake, either from feeding high-calorie diets or ad libitum feedings, affects the speed of cartilaginous and bone growth, as well as affecting endocrine regulatory mechanisms (872). Strategies to help minimize the risk of developing OCD include feeding a measured amount of food given the pup's energy requirement, keeping the energy density of the food below 4 kcal/g, maintaining the calcium level at 1% of a DM basis, not giving any vitamin or mineral supplements, and keeping the dog slim by monitoring weight, height and body condition and making any management changes necessary (872).

OSTEOCHONDROSIS OF THE SHOULDER

Osteochondritis dissecans of the humeral head is a common cause of foreleg lameness, and arguably the most prevalent form of osteochondrosis in the dog. Trauma within the shoulder joint is believed to damage the articular cartilage and form a cartilage flap in the caudal-central region of the humeral head (491). Although large breeds such as the golden retriever, Labrador retriever, Newfoundland, and rottweiler are commonly predisposed, smaller breeds such as the Chihuahua, greyhound, miniature poodle, and whippet can also be affected. Breeders report the condition frequently in the Kuvasz, but the true incidence in the breed has not been determined. Males are affected approximately twice as frequently as females (491).

Most cases are seen in pups younger than 7 months of age, but one-third of cases are not detected until 1 year of age. The classic picture is one of lameness, and usually only one leg is involved initially. This lameness tends to worsen following exercise and improves after a period of rest. Affected dogs can't support their weight on the leg, so they walk with a shortened stride, often raising their heads as they place the weight on the bad leg. In about 50% of cases, both front legs eventually become involved. In time, if the problem is not addressed, the joint eventually becomes incapacitated with arthritis.

The diagnosis is suspected when the animal has pain following flexion or extension of the shoulder joint, and is confirmed by radiography of the shoulder joint. Sedation is required to allow proper positioning and to minimize pain. The dog is positioned in lateral recumbency with the affected limb down, the head and neck extended, and traction applied to the affected limb to avoid superimposition of the shoulder on the thorax and neck (491). Because the condition can be bilateral, radiographs should be taken of both limbs. Arthrography and arthrotomy are useful for identifying joint "mice" within the bicipital tendon sheath (491).

Although there is some debate regarding the merits of conservative versus surgical therapy, dogs with clinical signs and radiographic evidence of shoulder lesions are best managed surgically. The recovery period following surgery is much shorter than with conservative therapy, and with a much higher success rate (491). Several different surgical approaches have been documented, and arthroscopic surgery is also an option. The prognosis for full recovery is good unless degenerative changes are already present within the joint. Affected animals, and those with a family history of shoulder OCD, should not be used in breeding programs.

The best form of prevention is to breed only individuals without a family history of osteochondrosis. The Institute for Genetic Disease Control in Animals (GDC) maintains open orthopedic registries to help in the selection process of breeding animals.

OSTEOCHONDROSIS OF THE HINDLEGS

Osteochondrosis of the hindlegs is much less common than OCD of the shoulder or elbow. In addition, some cases heal spontaneously, which may explain in part why it is reported more rarely. Affected dogs have lameness of one or both hindlegs and a shortened stride on the affected leg. Also, the joint capsule may be swollen on the affected leg. Osteochondrosis of the femur is a developmental disorder affecting cellular differentiation of cartilage cells in this region. Even though osteochondrosis of the stifle, hock, and the femoral head have all been reported, too few cases involving the femoral head have been documented to allow any meaningful interpretation. This discussion, thus, will deal only with problems in the knee and hock joints.

Breeds at risk for osteochondrosis of the stifle (knee) joint include the German shepherd dog, Great Dane, golden retriever, Labrador retriever, Newfoundland, and rottweiler (417, 924, 1101), although the condition has also been documented in the Akita, border collie, boxer, bull terrier, chow chow, collie, Doberman pinscher, greyhound, Irish wolfhound, mastiff, Samoyed, schnauzer, standard poodle, and Staffordshire bull terrier (720). The most common presentation is hindleg lameness

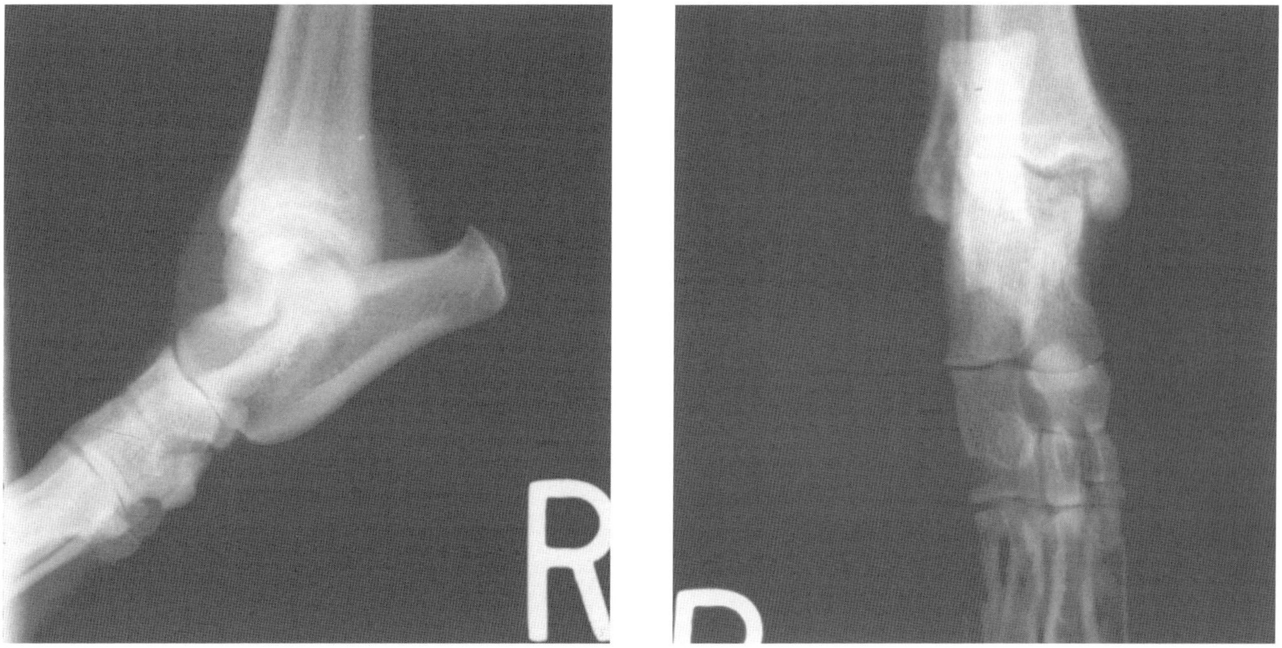

Figure 9-3 Osteochondrosis of the tarsus
Courtesy of Dr. Jeff Meinen, Mesa Veterinary Hospital, Mesa, Arizona

that becomes worse following exercise. Most affected dogs develop problems by 5 to 7 months of age. Of the cases reported, approximately three-quarters are males (587). Osteochondrosis of the physis between the apophysis and the cranioproximal tibial diaphysis has been suggested as a cause of avulsion of the tibial tuberosity in Doberman pinschers (1048), greyhounds (967), and rottweilers (1048).

Osteochondrosis of the tibiotarsal (hock) joint is a rare form of osteochondrosis, most commonly reported in the Australian cattle dog, bull terrier, bullmastiff, Labrador retriever, and rottweiler (318, 587, 1101). More than 70% of all cases have occurred in the rottweiler and Labrador retriever (719). Unlike most other forms of OCD, males don't seem to be overrepresented in this entity. Most dogs are 6 to 12 months of age when they are first affected, developing progressive hindleg lameness. Both legs are affected in approximately 40% of cases (719). Most cases of tarsal OCD involve the medial trochlear ridge, except the rottweiler, in which the lateral trochlea is most commonly affected (318, 1063).

The diagnosis is confirmed through use of radiography, and circular radiolucent condylar defects, joint effusion, and joint "mice" may be evident (417). The lesion may cause a flattened or irregular contour of the affected condyle (720). Excellent radiographic technique and multiple positions may be necessary to document OCD of the tibiotarsal joint, as standard radiographic techniques usually fail to allow complete visualization of both medial and lateral trochlear ridges because other anatomic structures are usually in the way. Confirmation of the diagnosis is necessary, as other conditions can mimic OCD clinically. For example, rottweilers are also prone to fragmentation of the medial malleolus, which can present similarly. OCD flaps in this joint often contain bone, in contrast to OCD flaps in other joints, which usually contain cartilage.

Other changes in and around the joint may provide important clues to diagnosis. OCD of the stifle results in flattened and irregular contours and loss of bone density. In the greyhound condition, radiography revealed partial or complete avulsion of the tibial tuberosities (967). If facilities allow, arthroscopic surgery can be used to diagnose and treat OCD of the hindlegs. Although medical therapy may be suitable for mildly affected individuals, surgery is recommended for progressively lame patients with large osteochondral defects or intracapsular joint "mice."

Most clinicians report increased success for surgically removing the OCD flap using minimally invasive procedures (318), preferably before 12 months of age, when permanent changes may have already compromised the joint. Although dogs improve clinically after surgery, they still may develop lameness after heavy exercise or in cold weather (1101). Conservative therapy does not seem to be as successful in managing this condition.

The best form of prevention is to breed only individuals without a family history of osteochondrosis. The Institute for Genetic Disease Control in Animals (GDC) maintains open orthopedic registries to aid in the selection process of breeding animals.

OSTEOCHONDRODYSPLASIA

The term osteochondrodysplasia refers to a developmental abnormality of cartilage and bone resulting from delayed endochondral ossification (formation of bone from cartilage) (Figure 9-3). The condition is seen primarily in the Alaskan malamute (1013), German shepherd dog (1108), Great Pyrenees (55), Irish setter (416), Labrador retriever (154), Norwegian elkhound (56), Samoyed (680), Scottish deerhound (102), and Shetland sheepdog (461).

The defect in Alaskan malamutes in often termed nonselected chondrodysplasia, but some breeders simply refer to it as "dwarfism," which is an imprecise term. The mode of inheritance for nonselected chondrodysplasia in the Alaskan malamute has been determined to be autosomal recessive (1013). In many cases, multiple littermates are affected. The condition affects primarily the M'Loot malamute line.

The condition in the Samoyed is also inherited as an autosomal recessive trait. Affected animals have chondrodysplastic bone changes and ocular anomalies such as cataracts and retinal degeneration (680). In Labrador retrievers, the condition of osteochondrodysplasia together with cataracts and retinal degeneration is also apparent but occurs with great variability (154, 855). Studies in the Labrador retriever and Samoyed suggest that the syndrome is caused by one abnormal gene, which has recessive effects on the skeleton and incompletely dominant effects on the eye (155, 350, 855).

In the Scottish deerhound, osteochondrodysplasia is inherited as an autosomal recessive trait (102). Stunted growth is evident by 4 to 5 weeks of age and is accompanied by short, bowed limbs and exercise intolerance. Skeletal deformities worsen progressively with age.

Chondrodysplasia has been reported in the Great Pyrenees (55), but a mode of inheritance has not been determined. Hypochondroplastic dwarfism has been verified as an autosomal recessive trait in the Irish setter (416).

The picture of the chondrodysplastic Alaskan malamute is one of short, bowed legs and thickened joint capsules. Although most dogs are not crippled by the disorder, affected animals have a higher incidence of arthritis and joint pain. In addition, a mild regenerative anemia (hereditary stomatocytosis) occurs with chondrodysplasia but typically does not require treatment.

Diagnosis is not difficult but can be confirmed with radiographs if necessary. Similarly, animals can be "screened" for chondrodysplasia between 3 and 13 weeks of age using radiography. Most affected dogs also have increased urinary excretion of glycosaminoglycans, particularly chondroitin sulfate (680).

Surgery is of little benefit in "fixing" a chondrodysplastic dog, but corrective osteotomy is sometimes attempted to more properly align limbs. Periodic use of analgesics and anti-inflammatory agents (e.g., aspirin) are sometimes necessary for animals that have joint pain.

To prevent chondrodysplasia, breeding animals should have a clear ancestry going back at least five generations. The condition is autosomal recessive in most breeds studied, so affected animals should not be bred and parents should be considered obligate carriers of the trait. In the Alaskan malamute, breeders often voluntarily limit themselves to mating animals with a chondrodysplasia rating of not more than 6.25%, corresponding to the animal having one carrier as a great-great-great grandparent. Siblings of affected animals are suspect carriers. The Institute for Genetic Disease Control in Animals (GDC) maintains an open research database for chondrodysplasia in the Great Pyrenees. It is hoped that in the near future a DNA test will be available for chondrodysplasia, allowing the identification of animals that are clear, affected, or carriers.

OSTEOGENESIS IMPERFECTA

Osteogenesis imperfecta is a rare heritable condition associated with bone brittleness. It has been reported in the Bedlington terrier, Norwegian elkhound, and poodle (461, 673). A mode of inheritance has not been determined. Affected dogs have structural abnormalities in type I collagen (145). Diagnosis can be suspected when there are multiple fractures with no evidence of trauma or metabolic disease. Confirmation requires culturing fibroblasts (e.g., from a skin biopsy) to demonstrate the collagen abnormality (145). Affected dogs and their parents should not be used for breeding.

PANOSTEITIS

Panosteitis ("pano" to many breeders) is an inflammatory condition that affects the leg bones. The

Orthopedic Foundation for Animals (OFA) Classification of Patellar Luxation

Grade	Features
1	Intermittent patellar luxation causing the limb to be carried occasionally. The patella easily luxates manually at full extension of the stifle joint but returns to the trochlea when released. No crepitation is apparent. The medial or, occasionally, lateral deviation of the tibial crest (with lateral luxation of the patella) is minimal, and there is very slight rotation of the tibia. Flexion and extension of the stifle is in a straight line with no abduction of the hock.
2	There is frequent patellar luxation, which, in some cases, becomes more or less permanent. The limb is sometimes carried, although weight bearing routinely occurs with the stifle remaining slightly flexed. Under anesthesia, it is often possible to luxate the patella by turning the tibia, but the patella reluxates when the manipulation ceases. After many years, the constant luxation may cause erosion of the articulating surface of the patella and the trochlea. This results in crepitation becoming apparent when the patella is luxated manually.
3	The patella is permanently luxated with torsion of the tibia and deviation of the tibial crest of between 30 and 50 degrees from the cranial/caudal plane. Flexion and extension of the joint causes abduction and adduction of the hock. The trochlea is very shallow or even flattened.
4	The tibia is twisted and the tibial crest may show further deviation with the result that it lists 50 to 90 degrees from the cranial/caudal plane. The patella is permanently luxated, and a space can be palpated between the patellar ligament and the distal end of the femur. The trochlea is absent or even convex.

basset hound (461), Doberman pinscher (924), German shepherd dog (461, 924), Labrador retriever (924), and rottweiler (1101, 1102) are the breeds most commonly affected. The condition affects males more frequently than females and often is recurrent or periodic in nature. It is characterized by excessive bone remodeling (742). Most dogs are younger than a year of age, but occasionally as old as 6 years of age, when they are first affected.

Affected animals typically show lameness in one or more legs, which may appear to "migrate" between legs. Pain is severe in some dogs and mild in others. Associated problems are lack of appetite, weight loss, and muscle wasting. The diagnosis can usually be confirmed by radiography in which there is an increased radiolucency of the medullary cavity in the region of the nutrient foramen, followed by a granular increased radiopacity (587).

No specific treatment is available for panosteitis, but the condition usually responds to enforced rest and mild anti-inflammatory agents (e.g., aspirin). Many breeders recommend the use of diets with lower protein and fat content, although a dietary role for the condition has not been established. Others have used dietary supplements combining immune enhancers (e.g., dimethylglycine) with nutritional joint protectors (e.g., chondroitin sulfate, glycosaminoglycans). Affected dogs should not be used for breeding, but not enough is known about the heritability of the condition to make breeding recommendations for parents, siblings, or other close relatives.

PATELLAR LUXATION

Patellar luxation refers to the condition in which the kneecap slips out of its usual resting place and lodges on the medial aspect or lateral aspect of the knee. This is a congenital problem of dogs, but the degree of patellar displacement may increase with time as the tissues stretch and the bones continue to deform (312). Medial patellar luxation is seen primarily in small and toy breeds of dogs, including the affenpinscher, Boston terrier, Cairn terrier, Chihuahua, cocker spaniel, papillon, Pekingese, Pomeranian, toy and miniature poodle, silky terrier, Yorkshire terrier, and the chondrodystrophoid breeds (181, 924, 936). Lateral patellar luxation, also referred to as genu valgum, is most commonly reported in the

Great Dane, Irish wolfhound, rottweiler, and St. Bernard (1101).

Medial patellar luxation is evident in young dogs and is considered a heritable trait. Lateral patellar luxation in large breeds is usually apparent by 5 to 6 months of age, but not until 5 to 8 years of age in toy and miniature breeds. A heritable nature has not been proven for lateral patellar luxation.

Medial patellar luxation may be graded as to the extent of laxity in the patella. The condition can be diagnosed by manipulating the knee joint to see if the kneecap luxates toward the inner (medial) or outer (lateral) aspect of the leg. Usually, little or no pain is associated with this process. No laxity is preferred, and affected individuals may have Grade 1 (mild) through Grade 4 (severe) luxations.

1. Grade 1 luxation may not even be noticed by owners but can be manually moved over the bony ridge, although it spontaneously returns to normal position once released.
2. Grade 2 luxation is characterized by a patella that may skip off its bony ridge occasionally, resulting in lameness. It does eventually return to its normal position.
3. Grade 3 luxation varies from occasional lameness to a more persistent weight-bearing lameness. The kneecap tends to spontaneously luxate out of its normal position when the leg is manipulated.
4. Grade 4 luxation is characterized by persistent lameness, and the patellae no longer remain in their normal positions.

Radiography can be used to document persistent luxation and to evaluate for other abnormalities such as arthritic changes.

Older dogs and those that are mildly affected may respond to conservative therapy, but surgery is often recommended for young dogs before arthritic changes become evident. Several surgical techniques have been used successfully. After surgery, dogs should have enforced rest for 6 weeks while healing, and leash activity only during that time. The results are excellent in most cases.

The best form of prevention for this disease is to purchase only those animals that have no family history of patellar luxation. Registries are maintained by the Orthopedic Foundation for Animals (OFA) for all breeds, and specific open-breed registries exist at the Institute for Genetic Disease Control in Animals (GDC) for miniature and toy poodles, terriers, Great Pyrenees, Chinooks, and Belgian sheepdogs.

CHAPTER 10

Nervous System Disorders

Many neurological disorders have been extensively studied, which has produced an impressive body of information on genetic transmission of many traits. Within this chapter are topics with some crossover to other disciplines, especially the musculoskeletal disorders. Glycogen storage diseases, which are often grouped with the neurological diseases, can be found in Chapter 8, dealing with metabolic disorders.

AGGRESSION

Aggression is a behavior intended to threaten or injure another animal or person. However, it is not a single entity. Aggression can result as a manifestation of dominance, fear, territoriality, or predation. Animals that are in pain or have medical disorders can also display aggression. It is important to realize that there is a significant difference between a fearful Pomeranian in a veterinary office, a Great Dane that protects it food bowl from children and other dogs, and a terrier that pounces on a wayward gerbil. There is little doubt that genetics plays an important role in behavior, but it is also clear that it is dangerous to make generalizations about the heritability of aggression.

While aggression cannot entirely be controlled through genetics, heritability calculated for behavioral traits can be used as a selection tool (840, 1135). In one British study, owners of aggressive English cocker spaniels were more likely to be tense, emotionally unstable, shy, and undisciplined, than were owners of dogs that weren't aggressive (839). While no studies have been definitive, the heritability of fearfulness and aggression are believed to be 50% or greater (1134). While many reports cite specific breeds as being "aggressive," most are not controlled studies and are of dubious value. In fact, the dogs implicated most often for biting people are mixed breeds (1144). Because of the danger to the public, it is safe to recommend that no dog that demonstrates unprovoked aggression towards people be bred, regardless of other redeeming qualities.

CEREBELLAR ABIOTROPHY

Cerebellar abiotrophy results from selective cell death of Purkinje and/or granule cells. It is an inherited trait in many breeds. Purkinje cells complete their migration and differentiation during gestation, whereas granule cell migration and maturation is not complete until approximately 10 weeks postnatally (633). Neonatal cerebellar abiotrophy has been reported in beagles and Samoyeds (1148).

Although the mode of inheritance is not known, it is thought to be familial (187). Postnatal cerebellar abiotrophy has been reported in Airedales, Australian kelpies, Bern running dogs, Bernese mountain dogs, border collies, Brittany spaniels, bullmastiffs, bull terriers, English springer spaniels, Finnish harriers, German shepherd dogs, Gordon setters, Irish setters, Kerry blue terriers, Labrador retrievers, miniature poodles, and rough-coated collies (187).

The mode of inheritance has been determined for some breeds, namely Australian kelpies, bullmastiffs, and Gordon setters, and has been found to be autosomal recessive (187, 995). A familial trend has been recognized in Airedales, Bernese mountain dogs, Finnish harriers, Labrador retrievers, and miniature poodles (187).

Even though signs of progressive cerebellar abiotrophy are seen in all breeds, the age of onset and rate of progression differ significantly between breeds. For example, Labrador retrievers, collies, border collies, and Australian kelpies are affected at an early age (6 to 12 weeks) and progression is rapid.

In Gordon setters, age of onset is 6 to 36 months, and progression is slow. Bullmastiffs show signs between 1 and 7 months of age. Brittany spaniels have a late onset (10 years) and slow progression (449). For breeds in which an autosomal recessive mode of inheritance has been documented, affected animals should not be bred. Parents are obligate carriers, and siblings are suspect carriers. Until more information is available on a mode of inheritance of other forms, breeders should be cautious when selecting breeding animals from a family with a history of cerebellar abiotrophy.

Another form of cerebellar abiotrophy has been reported in Kerry blue terriers (245) and rough-coated collies; it occurs as an autosomal recessive trait (187, 633). This form differs from the one just discussed in that extrapyramidal and other motor systems degenerate as well. The condition affects young pups, and progression of clinical signs is much more rapid in rough-coated collies than in Kerry blue terriers. Affected animals should not be bred, and parents are considered obligate carriers. Siblings are suspect carriers.

CEREBELLAR ATAXIA

Cerebellar ataxia has been documented as an X-linked recessive trait (XCA) in English pointer dogs (782). Clinical signs begin at about 12 weeks of age and progress from an awkward gait with disorientation and nystagmus to marked ataxia by 16 months of age. The diagnosis can be confirmed on post-mortem examination, which shows a striking reduction in the number of Purkinje cells throughout the cerebellar cortex.

The dams of affected males should be considered as obligate carriers and removed from breeding programs. An androgen receptor marker does appear to be linked to the disease gene and can be used to identify affected males at birth, as well as carrier females (483)

CEREBELLAR HYPOPLASIA

Cerebellar hypoplasia refers to a collection of disorders in which the cerebellum does not develop normally because of an absence of cells. Although secondary forms exist, a genetic malformation is presumed in the wire fox terrier, Irish setter and chow chow (746). A subtype is cerebellar vermian hypoplasia, seen in Boston terriers and bull terriers, which is similar to Dandy-Walker syndrome in humans (546). Clinical signs, noted at about 2 weeks of age, include ataxia, dysmetria, intention tremors, and, in some dogs, vestibular signs (545).

A definite pattern of inheritance has not been established. Dogs with cerebellar hypoplasia have an early onset of hypermetria, ataxia, and intention tremor. The diagnosis is suspected based on clinical signs and can be confirmed only on necropsy. Although no treatment is available, affected animals may make acceptable pets because the condition tends not to be progressive. They should not be bred, though.

CERVICAL VERTEBRAL INSTABILITY

Cervical vertebral instability, also known as cervical vertebral malformation/articulation, cervical spondylomyelopathy, and Wobbler syndrome, is caused by an instability in the intervertebral disks in the neck area. Vertebral canal stenosis results from malformed vertebral laminae or hypertrophy of the ligamentum flavum, articular facet enlargement, or pariarticular tissue hypertrophy (596). About 75% to 80% of Wobbler cases have spinal cord compression associated with hypertrophy of the dorsal annulus fibrosis (1067).

Doberman pinschers and Great Danes represent about 80% of the cases presented (942). The condition also has been reported in the basset hound, beagle, boxer, borzoi, bullmastiff, chow chow, fox terrier, German shepherd dog, golden retriever, Great Pyrenees, Irish setter, Irish wolfhound, Labrador retriever, Old English sheepdog, Rhodesian ridgeback, and rottweiler (187, 474, 546). The mode of inheritance is unknown for all breeds but has been suggested to be autosomal recessive in the Great Dane, Doberman pinscher, and borzoi, and familial in basset hounds and bullmastiffs (474, 546). Males are more commonly affected than females (1028, 1065), except in borzois, in which females seem to have a predilection.

When the disk destabilizes and puts pressure on the spinal cord, the result is severe neck pain. Unlike most other affected breeds, Dobermans may also develop rigid front legs (132). Affected Great Danes start with problems between 3 and 18 months of age; Dobermans usually develop clinical signs later, between 4 and 10 years of age. Affected dogs develop clinical signs associated with narrowing of the spinal canal and compression of the spinal cord. Preliminary research suggests that excess dietary calcium, genetic factors, and overfeeding may all be involved.

The diagnosis is confirmed by taking radiographs, and contrast studies are often used to help outline the defect (Figure 10-1). Computed tomography provides additional information that is not obtained by conventional myelography (951).

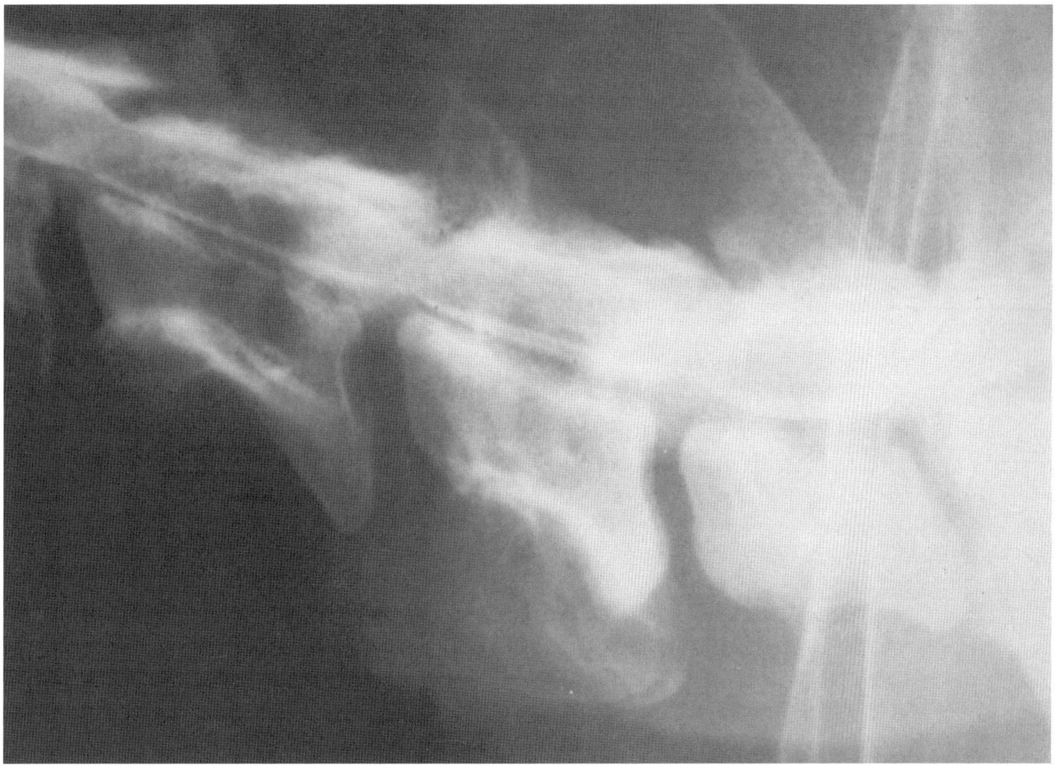

Figure 10-1 **Caudal cervical spine/myelogram of Doberman with Wobbler's syndrome**
Courtesy of Renee Leveille, Assistant Professor, The Ohio State University, Columbus, Ohio

Doberman pinschers often suffer from Hansen's type II disk protrusion, and the disk failure is typically noted at C5-C6 or C6-C7. When both disk unions are affected, this is often accompanied by significant vascular compromise and onset of neurologic signs (596).

Initial treatment consists of strict rest and antinflammatory therapy (usually with corticosteroids) to quickly reduce the amount of inflammation in the spinal canal. This conservative therapy often improves the clinical signs but cannot be expected to correct the underlying spinal defect. Although some dogs can be maintained on long-term corticosteroid therapy with adequate control, most others eventually develop progressive problems. If permanent damage is not evident, surgical decompression and stabilization is the treatment of choice.

The best way to prevent Wobbler syndrome is to avoid calcium supplementation, feed several small meals daily (rather than one large meal), or *ad libitum* feedings, and not purchase a pup with a family history of vertebral instability. Because this condition isn't usually evident before a first breeding, however, breeders may not be aware of the condition when breeding young dogs. Several generations of affected animals could actually be produced before anyone recognizes a problem. Accordingly, animals with a family history of Wobbler syndrome should be cautiously selected to participate in a breeding program. It is probably best not to breed affected animals and to consider parents and siblings as potential carriers of the trait.

COMPULSIVE BEHAVIORS

Compulsive behaviors refer to behaviors that are usually brought on by conflict, but that are subsequently shown outside of the original context (612). On the other hand, stereotypies are generally defined as unvarying repetitive or constant behavior patterns that have no obvious goal or apparent function (564). Stereotypies can be performed as components of displacement behaviors or compulsive disorders. In veterinary medicine, most of these conditions are recognized as bizarre behaviors with striking breed predispositions. Acral lick dermatitis is discussed separately in the chapter on dermatologic conditions.

Tail chasing is not an unusual pursuit in dogs, but compulsive tail chasing behavior has been variously described as a subepileptic episodic behavior, a neuropathological disorder, a psychosis, an opioid-mediated compulsive disorder, and a displacement behavior (266, 564). An intense spinning and whirling disorder has been described in terriers, especially bull terriers, but occasionally American Staffordshire terriers, miniature bull terriers, and Jack Russell terriers (721). Most cases are first noticed at 3 to 12 months of age.

The diagnosis is suspected when tail chasing behavior and spinning is seen in a breed at risk with no evidence of medical problems. An abnormal electroencephalogram is noted in many affected dogs (266). Management is based on treating the underlying cause and contributing factors. Combining behavior modification with drugs used to manage obsessive-compulsive disorders, seizure disorders, or narcotic antagonists is the most successful option. Clomipramine appears to be the treatment of choice for dogs suspected of exhibiting compulsive behavior (447, 721), and anticonvulsants are most useful for those suspected of having complex partial seizures (266). Affected dogs should not be bred.

Flank sucking represents a poorly understood condition in which a dog nurses a patch of skin on its flank. The Doberman pinscher is the breed most commonly affected, and the trait has been followed through certain bloodlines, suggesting a hereditary component (564). Flank sucking becomes the operative diagnosis when no physiological reasons can be found for the behavior. In many cases, no treatment is necessary, since the damage is localized and the behavior often appears to calm the animal. Behavior modification and medical intervention is used when the physical damage is considerable or the compulsion contributes to other behavior problems. Affected animals are best not bred, but this is considered a breeder option.

CONGENITAL PERIPHERAL VESTIBULAR DISEASE

Congenital vestibular disease is presumed to be inherited in the Akita, beagle, Doberman pinscher, English cocker spaniel, German shepherd dog, Shetland sheepdog, and Tibetan terrier (85, 546, 746). Although some of these conditions may indeed be inherited, a familial trend has not been determined. Clinical presentation includes head tilt, ataxia, circling, and deafness without nystagmus, seen in pups younger than 4 months of age. No treatment is available, but vestibular dysfunction improves in some dogs, although deafness is permanent. Affected animals probably should not be bred, although evidence is lacking that this is a heritable trait.

DEAFNESS

Deafness is a loss of hearing, which can be complete or partial. Inherited deafness is a sensorineural deafness resulting from degeneration of inner ear structures and neurons of the spiral ganglion, with clinical signs apparent from a few weeks to a few months of age (619). Predominantly white, merle (e.g., American foxhound, collie, dappled dachshund, harlequin Great Dane, Norwegian dunkerhound, Old English sheepdog, Shetland sheepdog), or piebald (beagle, bulldog, bull terrier, Dalmatian, English setter, Great Pyrenees, greyhound, Samoyed, Sealyham terrier) coat coloring predisposes dogs to inherited deafness.

Interestingly, deaf dogs are not born that way; they lose their hearing between 3 and 4 weeks after birth (1011). The mode of inheritance is predominantly autosomal dominant (619). Recessive inheritance, however, has been described in the bull terrier (1012), Doberman pinscher (85), pointer (1004), and rottweiler (83). In the Dalmatian, deafness is attributable to an autosomal recessive multifactorial gene with incomplete penetrance (386). The condition in Dalmatians seems to be slightly more prevalent in females (1138).

Deafness is most commonly reported in Dalmatians, English setters, Australian shepherds, border collies, and Shetland sheepdogs (619) but has also been reported in many other breeds (85, 461, 533, 1011, 1012). Breeds affected by congenital deafness are as follows, with the breeds having the highest incidence in italic type:

Akita
American cocker spaniel
American Staffordshire terrier
Australian blue heelers
Australian cattle dog
Australian shepherd
Beagle
Border collie
Boston terrier
Boxer
Bull terrier
Catahoula leopard dog
Collie
Dappled dachshund
Dalmatian
Doberman pinscher
Dogo Argentino
English bulldog
English setter
English springer spaniel

Foxhound
Fox terrier
German shepherd dog
Great Dane
Great Pyrenees
Greyhound
Ibizan hound
Jack Russell terrier
Kuvasz
Maltese
Miniature pinscher
Miniature poodle
Norwegian dunkerhound
Old English sheepdog
Papillon
Pointer
Rhodesian ridgeback
Rottweiler
St. Bernard
Schnauzer
Scottish terrier
Sealyham terrier
Shetland sheepdog
Shropshire terrier
Siberian husky
Toy poodle
Walker American foxhound
West Highland white terrier
Whippet

Prevalence is highest in the Dalmatian, in which 8% are bilaterally deaf and approximately 22% are unilaterally deaf (454). In a British study, 5.3% were bilaterally deaf and 13.1% were unilaterally deaf (1139). The heritability of deafness in Dalmatians has been calculated as 0.21 (298). The prevalence is as high as 75% in all-white Norwegian dunkerhounds; and in dappled dachshunds, 18% are bilaterally deaf and 36%, unilaterally deaf (1011). The prevalence of deafness in the bull terrier, English setter, English cocker spaniel, and Australian cattle dog is one-half to one-third that of the Dalmatian. (1011).

The merle gene (M) is dominant, so heterozygous dogs (Mm) still retain the pattern. Breeding two merles (Mm), however, may produce genotypic homozygotes (MM) that may be white in coloration and have an increased incidence of deafness, blindness, and sterility. The chances of deafness increase with the amount of white in the coat (1011). The piebald (sp) and extreme piebald (sw) genes affect the amount and location of white coloration. The inheritance of this form of deafness does not seem to be dominant and likely involves more than one recessive gene pair, or incomplete penetrance (1011). In the Doberman pinscher, neither the merle nor the piebald gene is involved and deafness in the breed is inherited as an autosomal recessive trait (1125).

Because deaf dogs don't usually make good pets (and definitely shouldn't be used for breeding), all breeding animals of breeds at risk should have hearing tests and pups should be tested when they are weaned at 6 to 8 weeks of age and before they are sold. Whereas dogs that are deaf in one ear can still make good pets, they should be neutered so they will not contribute genetically to future generations. Dogs that are deaf in both ears make poor pets because they are difficult to teach and because they are easily startled.

You can tell subjectively if a dog can hear by shaking keys, clapping your hands, or otherwise trying to attract the dog's attention while out of sight. The definitive way to test, however, is known as BAER (Brainstem Auditory-Evoked Response) testing, which is completely painless and can detect any loss of hearing in one or both ears. This testing is available from veterinary schools and referral centers. Ideally, every dog of a susceptible breed and color pattern should be BAER-tested before breeding, and all breed-susceptible pups should be BAER-tested before being sold.

Studies have shown that prevalence is strongly associated with parental hearing status (1139), so breeding stock should be selected from families in which deafness is not a problem. Because the defective gene for type I Wardenburg syndrome in humans has been identified, it is hoped that a DNA test for inherited deafness will eventually become available for dogs, too. The Institute for Genetic Disease Control in Animals (GDC) maintains an open registry for deafness in all breeds.

DEGENERATIVE MYELOPATHY

Degenerative myelopathy is a neurodegenerative disease of the spinal cord, characterized by widespread loss of myelin and axons beginning in the thoracolumbar area (183). Deposition of immunoglobulin and complement in spinal cord lesions suggest that an immune-mediated destruction of nerve tissue is involved in the pathogenesis (27). This condition is seen primarily in the German shepherd dog, and the age of onset for clinical signs is typically 5 to 9 years of age (183, 1043). In the Siberian husky, it may not be apparent until 10 to 12 years of age (995). It has also been reported in other breeds, including the Belgian shepherd, boxer, Chesapeake Bay retriever, Dutch Kooiker dog, golden retriever, Irish setter, Irish terrier, Kerry blue terrier, Labrador retriever, Old English sheepdog, Pembroke Welsh corgi, pug, Rhodesian ridgeback, rough-coated collie, and Weimaraner (184, 187, 311, 629, 1028). A familial predisposition is suggested in the German shepherd dog (1043). The hereditary necrotizing myelopathy described in Dutch Kooiker dogs has an autosomal recessive mode of inheritance (629). See also the leukodystrophies and peripheral neuropathies, later in this chapter, for related conditions.

Affected dogs develop proprioceptive loss, followed by progressive posterior ataxia. Dogs may first knuckle their hind toes when walking. Their movements become progressively more awkward. By the time that upper motor neuron dysfunction is evident (e.g., hyperactive tendon reflexes, crossed extensor reflexes), the chances of successful treatment are greatly diminished. Dogs that develop lower motor neuron dysfunction have an even worse prognosis. The condition progresses to involve the front legs and eventually the brainstem.

The diagnosis is rendered in a breed at risk, with characteristic neurologic signs supported by consistent laboratory and radiographic findings. Routine and contrast radiographs are normal with uncomplicated degenerative myelopathy. Protein may be elevated mildly in the cerebrospinal fluid (CSF), but this is nonspecific. Tests of immune dysfunction offer the most promise. There is depressed cell-mediated immune responsiveness, as determined by lymphocyte stimulation assays. Also, circulating immune complexes may be detected (184). A serum marker will likely be determined eventually, to help confirm the diagnosis.

Treatment involves exercising the dog to preserve muscle tone, and treating with nutritional supplements and, potentially, immunosuppressive therapies. Corticosteroids are typically tried first, as the condition is presumed to be immune-mediated. Nutritional supplementation with vitamin E, vitamin B12, and aminocaproic acid is sometimes initiated in treatment protocols. Although aminocaproic acid seems to be the most effective of the supplements, other nutraceuticals may be used concurrently (183).

Because the genetics of degenerative myelopathy are not yet understood in most breeds, designing a preventive breeding program is difficult. Until more is known about the disorder, it is best to avoid breeding dogs from families in which degenerative myelopathy has been recognized. In Dutch Kooiker dogs, in which an autosomal recessive mode of inheritance has been determined, affected dogs should not be bred and parents should be considered carriers of the trait. Siblings are suspect carriers.

DYSMYELINOGENESIS

Dysmyelinogenesis refers to abnormal myelination, and hypomyelinogenesis implies a lack of myelin in the nervous system. An X-linked genetic basis has been proven for the congenital form in Welsh springer spaniels (187, 390) in which there is a point mutation in exon 2 of the proteolipid protein gene; non-X-linked dysmyelinogenesis has been reported in Bernese mountain dogs, chow chows, a Dalmatian, Lurchers, Samoyeds, and Weimaraners, (271, 471, 604, 746, 995, 1091). A familial trend has been suggested in the chow chow, Samoyed, and Weimaraner, and an autosomal recessive mode of inheritance is presumed in the Bernese mountain dog (187, 471). The condition in the chow chow and Weimaraner is also believed to be autosomal recessive in nature (608).

In the chow chow, Lurcher hound, Samoyed, and Weimaraner, the process is generalized in the central nervous system (CNS). The condition presents as tremor in puppies, often accompanied by ataxia and hypermetria, without weakness. In the chow chow, the process begins at 2 weeks of age with bunny hopping, rocking horse motions, hypermetria, and intention tremors. Signs peak at 6 to 8 months of age, and by 12 months, affected animals are clinically normal (271). In springer spaniels, affected male dogs develop a gross tremor of the head, body, limbs, and extraocular muscles at 10 to 12 days of age (471). If females are affected, as heterozygotes, the changes are typically subtle, and most recover by 1 month of age. In affected males, the clinical signs are less severe when the animals are sleeping, but otherwise they are progressive and unrelenting. Additional signs include inability to stand or walk, inability to eat, and consequent weight loss. Affected animals rarely survive past 3 to 4 months of age unless owners make an extraordinary effort.

In Weimaraners, tremors of variable severity begin at 1 to 3 weeks of age, but animals typically recover and are clinically normal by 1 year of age. In Lurcher pups, clinical signs begin at about 2 weeks of age and include fine tremors of the head and limbs that improve during rest or sleep. Some affected animals can be expected to return to clinical normalcy. Fewer cases have been reported in Samoyeds, but they also show clinical symptoms by about 3 weeks of age, developing tremors of the head and body, no menace response, and hypermetria.

The diagnosis may be suspected based on magnetic resonance imaging (MRI) but can be confirmed only on necropsy. Although no treatment exists, affected chow chows, Weimaraners, and Bernese mountain dogs typically improve to virtual normalcy

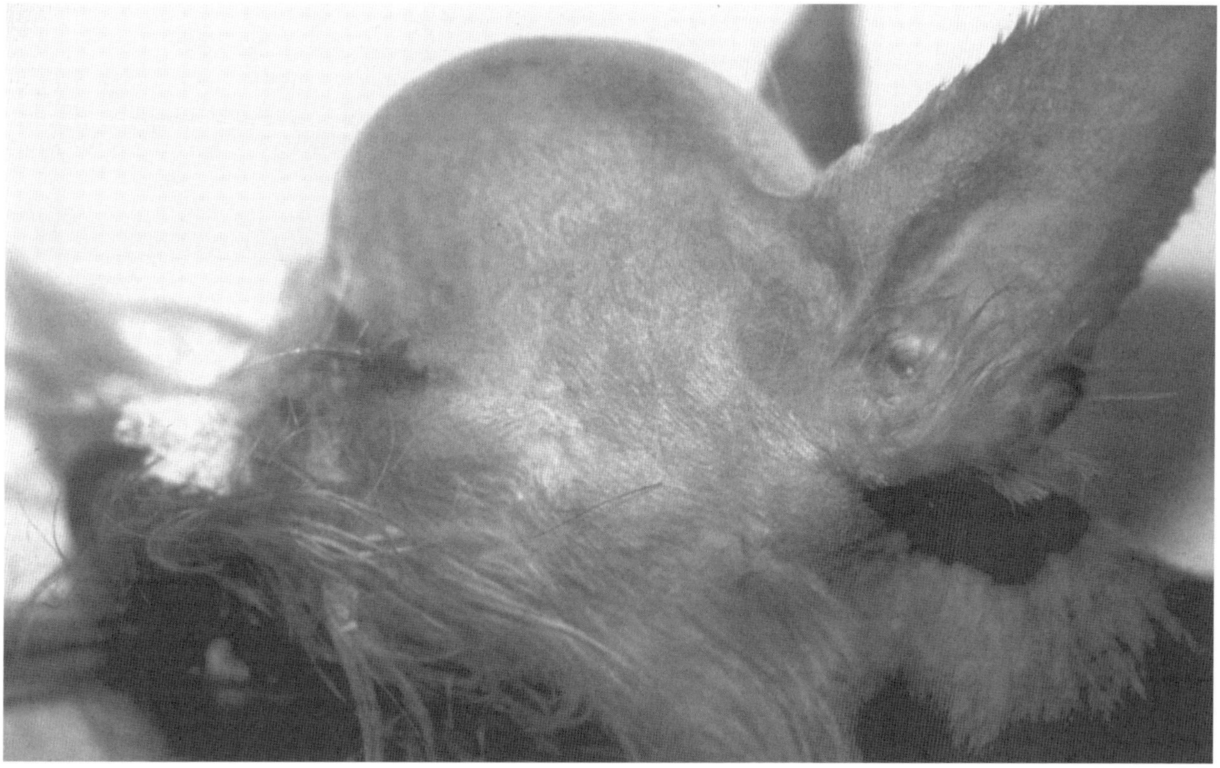

Figure 10-2 Young dog with hydrocephalus displaying skull expansion
Courtesy of Dr. Don Levesque, Veterinary Neurological Center, Phoenix, Arizona

by 1 year of age (271, 746). Affected male Welsh springer spaniels do not seem to improve over time and rarely survive until adulthood. Whether they do or do not recover, affected animals should not be used for breeding. The dam of affected Welsh springer spaniel males should be considered as an obligate carrier. Normal-appearing female littermates are suspect carriers. In the Bernese mountain dog, both parents should be considered as obligate carriers and all siblings as suspect carriers.

HEMIVERTEBRA

Hemivertebra results when the vertebra does not develop properly, typically because of persistence of the notochord or lack of ossification. Hemivertebra is seen most frequently in the screw-tailed breeds—the Boston terrier, bulldog, French bulldog, and pug (26). The kinked tail is attributable to hemivertebrae in the caudal vertebrae. In the German shepherd dog and German shorthaired pointer, hemivertebra occurs as an autosomal recessive disorder (187, 550). The condition is also considered inherited in the English bulldog and Yorkshire terrier (1028) and has been reported in the Doberman pinscher and rottweiler (187).

Affected animals may appear clinically normal or may display signs of myelopathy consistent with the region of the spinal cord affected. The diagnosis typically is made with radiographs, but myelograms of the entire spine are indicated to determine the impact of the defect and to look for evidence of other congenital disorders that may occur concurrently. In uncomplicated cases, surgical decompression and stabilization are usually satisfactory to resolve the clinical situation.

The condition can be prevented by intelligent breeding practices. Affected animals should not be bred. In the German shorthaired pointer and German shepherd dog, both parents should be considered to be carriers of the trait and should be removed from breeding programs. Siblings should be considered as potential carriers of the trait. In other breeds, it is best not to breed animals from families known to be affected with the trait.

HYDROCEPHALUS

Hydrocephalus is a condition in which the brain swells from the accumulation of cerebrospinal fluid (CSF) (Figure 10-2). The cause can be either congenital or secondary to some obstructive process to the outflow of CSF (423). Congenital hydrocephalus is thought to possibly result from infections, toxins, or nutritional disorders while pups are still in the womb.

Although the mode of inheritance for hydrocephalus has been determined in cats, only a familial trend in brachycephalic and small dogs has been documented. Breeds predisposed to hydrocephalus include the Boston terrier, Cairn terrier, Chihuahua, English bulldog, Lhasa apso, Maltese, Manchester terrier, Pekingese, Pomeranian, pug, shih tzu, toy poodle, and Yorkshire terrier (187, 423, 546, 962). In young bullmastiffs, hydrocephalus has been described in association with cerebellar ataxia (150).

Primary hydrocephalus causes seizures, problems with vision, and behavioral abnormalities. In young dogs, the skull may expand as the cerebrospinal fluid accumulates and forces the skull outward. Even with treatment, affected animals may have permanent learning deficits.

Confirmation of the diagnosis often requires specialized tests such as electroencephalography (EEG), ultrasonography through fontanels, or computed tomography (CT scans). Neurological examinations, radiographs of the skull, and pressure measurements of the cerebrospinal fluid are often highly suggestive but not confirmatory in all cases.

Treatment for hydrocephalus is directed at lowering the volume of cerebrospinal fluid and encouraging proper drainage. Corticosteroids such as prednisone are thought to decease the production of CSF, but long-term use is dangerous. Diuretics such as furosemide may also be helpful in this regard.

For animals with severe disease, surgical drainage may be contemplated. This is a sophisticated procedure in which a permanent drainage tube (ventriculovenous shunt) is placed in the brain. When seizures result, they must be treated with appropriate medications, such as phenobarbital.

Until more is learned about the heritability of the condition, affected animals should not be used for breeding. Animals with a familial history of hydrocephalus should be used cautiously in breeding programs.

INTERVERTEBRAL DISK DISEASE (IVD)

Vertebrae are joined by two types of joints: the diarthrodial joints with their articular facets and the amphiarthrodial joint stabilized by the intervertebral disk (963). Intervertebral disks are located between all vertebrae except the atlantoaxial joint (C1-C2) and the sacrocaudal vertebrae. The disk itself consists of an inner gelatinous nucleus pulposus (NP) and an outer, fibrous annulus fibrosus (AF). The intervertebral disk is like a jelly donut with a tough, fibrous outer layer and a jelly-like inner layer. In some instances, the jelly-like inner layer protrudes, or herniates, through the fibrous layer and puts pressure on the spinal cord. This causes intense pain and limited use of the limbs supplied by those obstructed nerves.

The intervertebral disks in chondrodystrophoid breeds, such as the bassett hound, dachshund, French bulldog, Pekingese, and Welsh corgi, undergo chondroid metaplasia throughout life, in which the disk becomes more like cartilage than fibrous tissue (963). Scottish terriers and Alaskan malamute dwarfs are not included in this category. They are similar to the larger group of nonchondrodystrophoid breeds in which the disks slowly undergo fibroid metaplasia, characterized by slow fibrous change. Breeds with the highest incidence of IVD include basset hounds (187), beagles (187), cocker spaniels (95, 187), dachshunds (95, 187, 963), French bulldogs (187), Lhasa apsos (95, 187), poodles (95), Pomeranians (95), shih tzus (187), and Welsh corgis (187). Dachshunds account for 45% to 70% of all canine cases (95). A familial trend is suspected but unproven.

The distinction between breeds is important because it impacts on the risk of disk herniation and the age at which it occurs. For example, in the chondrodysplastic breeds, disk herniation occurs at a younger age, 75% between 3 and 6 years of age. In one study of dachshunds, almost 30% evidenced disk calcification by 1 year of age (1006). Although the overall incidence of intervertebral disk disease is about 2% of the canine population, 45% of dachshunds between 4 and 7 years of age are affected with clinical disk disease (963). In addition, in the nonchondrodystrophoid breeds, disk degeneration is typically confined to a single disk, whereas in chondrodystrophoid breeds, degeneration occurs simultaneously in many or all disks (95). The Doberman pinscher is the only large, nonchondrodystrophic breed commonly affected with cervical intervertebral disk disease (1047).

Approximately 85% of herniated disks occur in the lower back, and 15% in the neck region. In the dachshund, most involve the disks T10-11 to L7-S1, where the discs tend to be small, the dorsal zone of the annulus fibrosus is very narrow, and the nucleus pulposus is located far dorsally (923). The cardinal sign of IVD disease is intense pain. When a disk ruptures in the lower back (thoracolumbar disk disease) the hindlegs become paralyzed and the herniated material applies pressure onto the disk. Dogs with thoracolumbar disk disease that have back pain without neurologic deficits may still have substantial compression of the spinal cord (1016). In a short time, the pain subsides as the spinal cord damage interferes with the ability to recognize pain. These cases are surgical emergencies. Dogs with cervical intervertebral disk disease experience neck pain, a stiff gait, and spasms of the neck and shoulder muscles; pain in the front legs is seen in 50% of cases, but paralysis is relatively uncommon (1047).

Two types of intervertebral disk prolapse are described that have breed applicability. Type I prolapses are associated with considerable damage and hemorrhage and are seen in the chondrodystrophoid breeds. Type II prolapses can be seen in geriatric animals of any breed and are slowly progressive and not nearly as debilitating.

When IVD syndrome is suspected, radiographs are usually taken of both the neck and the thoracolumbar areas, even when the clinical picture suggests where the problem is likely to be. This is because other areas of potential herniation will have to be evaluated. Occasionally, myelography has to be performed to identify the exact location of the problem.

Intervertebral disk disease can be managed medically or surgically. Definitive guidelines are available to suggest which is most appropriate. Medical therapy may be adequate when the dog has mild-to-moderate pain but no evidence of spinal cord damage (e.g., paralysis). For dogs with thoracolumbar disk disease, paralysis, and loss of deep pain sensation, surgery should be immediate. If the pressure on the spinal cord is not reduced within about 24 hours, permanent nerve damage is likely.

To offer meaningful guidelines regarding breeding programs is difficult because IVD is common in some breeds, yet a mode of inheritance has not been determined. Until more is known about the genetics of this condition, it is best not to breed affected animals, and close relatives should be carefully scrutinized before being included in breeding programs.

LEUKODYSTROPHIES

Leukodystrophies are so named because they primarily affect the white matter in the nervous system. Because the leukodystrophies differ so dramatically between breeds, they are discussed below as separate topics.

Rottweiler leukodystrophy, also known as leukoencephalomyelopathy of rottweilers, is a bilaterally symmetric demyelination of white matter in the spinal cord, cerebellum, trigeminal nerve, brainstem, and optic tracts (341). It is presumed to be an autosomal recessive trait (187, 633). Clinical signs include ataxia, and perhaps hypermetria and tetraparesis. Age of onset is 1.5 to 4 years, with rapid progression to recumbency in 6 to 12 months. The condition is progressive and can be confirmed only on necropsy (179, 746). Because some animals do not begin to show signs until 4 years of age, affected animals sometimes have been bred already. Affected animals should not be bred, and parents and siblings are considered suspect carriers until the mode of inheritance has been documented conclusively.

Dalmatian leukodystrophy has an onset of 3 to 6 months of age and is also believed to be an autosomal recessive trait (61, 187, 633, 995). Clinical signs include visual deficits, ataxia, and weakness, with demyelination occurring in cerebral white matter, optic nerves, and additional white matter tracts (61). Affected animals should not be bred, and parents should be considered carriers of the trait. Siblings are suspect carriers.

Miniature poodle leukodystrophy is a rapidly progressive demyelinating disorder of the cervical spinal cord and brainstem. Age of onset is 2 to 4 months of age (187). Clinical signs include upper motor neuron paraplegia that progresses to tetraplegia (633). The cranial nerves are unaffected, patellar reflexes remain intact, and cerebral activity seems basically normal (1062). Until more is known about the genetics of this disorder, affected animals should not be bred and close family members should be considered as suspect carriers.

Hereditary polioencephalomyelopathy produces a vacuolar degeneration affecting primarily the gray matter in the central nervous system of young Australian cattle dogs (101). Clinical signs include seizures followed by progressive spastic tetraparesis. Diagnosis can be confirmed by histopathologic assessment, which typically includes malacia in the cerebellum, brainstem, and spinal cord with vacuolation of glial cells and marked mitochondrial accumulation in astrocytes. An inherited biochemical defect, possibly mitochondrial, has been postulated (101). Affected animals should not be bred. The diagnosis is strongly supported by characteristic distribution of signal abnormalities with magnetic resonance imaging, but are not necessarily pathognomonic for hereditary polioencephalomyelopathy (101).

Hereditary ataxia, also known as *progressive ataxia*, is seen in smooth fox terriers and Jack Russell terriers. The condition has been documented to be autosomal recessive in smooth fox terriers (1028) and has been presumed to be autosomal recessive in Jack Russell terriers (187). Clinical signs are apparent by 2 to 6 months of age as a slowly progressive ataxia with intention tremor. The damage consists of axonal degeneration with

Wallerian-type demyelination. Most dogs are eventually euthanized; they rarely live more than 2 years. Occasionally the process stabilizes so animals experience minimal loss of function (995). If animals survive to breeding age, they definitely should not be bred and parents should be considered carriers of the trait. Normal-appearing siblings should be considered as suspect carriers.

Hound ataxia is a poorly documented disorder seen in beagles, foxhounds, and harrier hounds, characterized by demyelination of most spinal tracts (187). It affects dogs 2 to 7 years of age, and the signs progress for as long as 18 months (995). The hindlimbs become ataxic while forelimb function remains normal. At present, hound ataxia seems more likely attributable to environmental causes (perhaps nutritional) than to genetics (995). Until more is learned about the inheritance of this condition, however, affected animals should not be used in breeding programs.

Nervous system degeneration in Ibizan hounds is presumed to be an autosomal recessive cause of axonal degeneration with spheroid formation throughout the spinal cord (1028). Clinical signs, apparent by 4 to 6 weeks of age, include ataxia, hypermetria, and absent patellar reflexes. Seizures may also be a feature of this disorder. Although most owners would not consider breeding affected individuals, parents should be considered as potential carriers of the trait and normal-appearing siblings as suspect carriers.

Labrador retriever central axonopathy is presumed to be an autosomal recessive severe degeneration of axons and myelin in the spinal cord white matter (246, 1028). Clinical signs are apparent by 4 to 6 weeks of age and include ataxia, tetraparesis, and hypermetria. The animals become nonambulatory by 5 months of age. Clinical signs reflect spinal cord and cerebellar dysfunction, and necropsy findings include a diffuse symmetrical axonopathy and involvement of cerebellar Purkinje cells (246). Even though most breeders would not consider breeding affected individuals, parents should be considered as potential carriers of the trait and normal-appearing siblings, suspect carriers.

Hereditary myelopathy of Afghan hounds, also known as *Afghan myelomalacia*, is presumed to be an autosomal recessive severe myelinolytic disorder of white matter with cavitation and necrosis, resulting in rapidly progressive upper motor neuron (UMN) paraparesis (995, 1028). The mid-thoracic region is affected most profoundly. Clinical signs are apparent by 3 to 13 months of age and may progress to tetraparesis (187). The dog usually retains some motor function. Affected dogs may not be able to stabilize themselves while standing, and they fall to the side. Segmental spinal reflexes are preserved initially, but in chronic cases these reflexes may become abnormal (1062). Most breeders would not consider breeding affected individuals, but parents, too, should be considered as potential carriers of the trait and normal-appearing siblings as suspect carriers.

Spongiform leukodystrophy has been reported as a hereditary condition in Labrador retrievers, Samoyeds, and silky terriers, and also has been reported in association with toxicity reactions. Clinical signs include tremors, ataxia, and hypermetria, starting as early as 2 weeks of age (633, 783). Affected animals should not be bred unless the cause is documented to be nonhereditary.

Fibrinoid leukodystrophy, also known as *Alexander's disease*, is a rare disorder of demyelination that has been reported in Bernese mountain dogs (1104), Labrador retrievers (187, 995), miniature poodles (187), and Scottish terriers (210). The condition becomes clinically evident by 6 to 9 months of age. This is believed to be an inborn error of astrocyte metabolism (633). The diagnosis is confirmed by histopathologic evaluation in which large, eosinophilic Rosenthal fibers, presumably remnants of astrocytes, are found around blood vessels (995). Most breeders would not consider breeding affected individuals, but parents should be considered to be potential carriers of the trait and normal-appearing siblings to be suspect carriers.

LISSENCEPHALY

Lissencephaly is a congenital condition of the brain in which the normal convoluted appearance is absent and the brain surface is smooth. It is believed to be genetically transmitted in the Lhasa apso (546) and also has been reported in the wire fox terrier and Irish setter in association with cerebellar hypoplasia (187, 746). It is believed to be a developmental disorder of neuronal migration and proliferation. Behavioral abnormalities, seizures, and visual deficits are evident early in life. Electroencephalographic findings are characteristic, but confirmation requires MRI or necropsy examination. Although no specific treatment is available, prognosis is fair if seizure activity can be controlled. Affected animals should not be used for breeding.

MENINIGITIS

Most cases of meningitis and meningoencephalomyelitis occur as a result of infection. Some breed-specific forms, however, seem to have a heritable basis. Because they tend not to have many clinical features in common, they are discussed below as separate entities.

Beagle pain syndrome affects beagles from 5 to 10 months of age and results in fever, depression, reluctance to move, and intense cervical hyperesthesia (669). In all likelihood, it is a manifestation of juvenile polyarteritis syndrome (546), which is discussed more thoroughly in Chapter 6, covering hemolymphatic disorders, under the heading of "Vasculitis." Clinical signs may wax and wane over 2 to 4 weeks. Diagnosis is based on clinical presentation and laboratory abnormalities consisting of neutrophilia, nonregenerative anemia, and neutrophilic pleocytosis on CSF evaluation. No microbes are detectable. Most cases respond to corticosteroid therapy. Until more is learned about the genetics of the condition, affected animals should not be bred.

Bernese mountain dog aseptic meningitis is a severe necrotizing vasculitis that is not uncommon in the Bernese mountain dog population, although a mode of inheritance has not been determined (669). The age of onset is 3 to 12 months, with sudden onset of fever, cervical rigidity, spinal pain, and stilted gait (670). Clinical signs may wax and wane. Diagnosis is based on clinical presentation and laboratory abnormalities consisting of neutrophilia and neutrophilic pleocytosis with elevated protein levels on CSF evaluation. No microbes are detectable, and cases respond to immunosuppressive agents such as prednisone. An estimated 1% to 2% of the Bernese mountain dog population may be affected, and the condition is familial (669). Although most breeders would not consider breeding affected individuals, the parents should be considered as potential carriers of the trait and normal-appearing siblings as suspect carriers.

Necrotizing meningoencephalitis, also known as *pug encephalitis*, is a chronic progressive neurologic disorder. Although it is seen most commonly in pugs (201, 747), similar conditions have been reported in the Maltese (1003) and Yorkshire terrier (1039) breeds. Most dogs are in young adulthood when they are first affected. Although the cause of the disease is not known, genetic and viral etiologies have been suggested. It might represent a genetically programmed neurologic disorder or a genetically determined abnormality of the immune system, making affected dogs susceptible to an infectious agent (669).

The most common clinical presentation is seizures, but other manifestations include depression, circling, head pressing, and blindness (747). In the Yorkshire terrier, clinical signs are indicative of either cerebral or brainstem involvement (1039). Diagnostic testing usually reveals leukocytosis in the cerebrospinal fluid (CSF), consisting predominantly of lymphocytes, and elevations of CSF protein.

Most dogs die despite treatment, typically within 6 months of onset of clinical signs. The diagnosis is confirmed on post-mortem examination. The disease is characterized by nonsuppurative meningoencephalitis with extensive necrosis. The histopathological presentation is identical between the breeds mentioned, except that in the Yorkshire terrier the process is not necessarily limited to the cerebrum (500). Because almost nothing is known about the genetics of the disorder, individuals from affected families should not be used in breeding programs unless they have other genetic qualities that are clearly desirable.

MYASTHENIA GRAVIS (MG)

Myasthenia gravis (MG) is a disease affecting the interaction of nerves and muscles. Both congenital and acquired forms occur in the dog. Congenital MG results from an autosomal recessive defect in the nicotinic acetylcholine receptors, which causes a transmission error at the junction of nerve and muscle. This recessive trait has been documented in the English springer spaniel, Gammel Dansk honsehund, Jack Russell terrier, Samoyed, and smooth fox terrier (187, 467, 517, 593, 940). Although it is not discussed further here, acquired immune-mediated myasthenia gravis also has definite breed predilections but no defined mode of inheritance.

The clinical picture of myasthenia gravis is one of muscle weakness. In the congenital form, weakness is noted by 6 to 8 weeks of age when the pups are just learning to walk. When walking, the stride may be shorter than usual, but the pups typically recover after a short rest. With fatigue, the face may droop and animals may even have difficulty holding up the head. Chewing and swallowing may become difficult, and megaesophagus is seen occasionally, although more commonly with acquired MG and with the congenital form in the smooth fox terrier breed (688). This can result in pneumonia if ingested foods are retched up and then enter the respiratory passages (aspiration pneumonia). Owners may note that the animal is vomiting, but in most cases it is regurgitation—a passive process.

The most-used diagnostic test for MG is the Edrophonium chloride (Tensilon) response test, but it should be administered by experienced individuals, as side effects may be noted. Dogs with MG tend to improve within 30 seconds of the injection, then revert to fatigue within 5 minutes. A modification of this test can also be performed with neostigmine methylsulfate (Prostigmin). The diagnosis also can be made using nerve conduction studies. Immunologic studies demonstrating anti-acetylcholine receptor antibodies are not useful for diagnosing the congenital form of this disease.

Little can be done for pups with congenital myasthenia gravis. Pyridostigmine bromide (Mestinon) is currently considered the drug of choice for acquired MG in dogs. Although it does not repair the defect, it does delay the destruction of acetylcholine, giving it the maximum opportunity to interact with the nerve muscle junction. Neostigmine (Prostigmin) also has been used for this purpose. Whether these drugs have any real benefit when treating congenital MG is uncertain. When using these anticholinesterase agents, caution must be exercised in selecting any other drug to be used with the affected dog. That is because several other drugs, including some antibiotics, heart medications, and anticonvulsants, may interfere with, and actually may potentiate, the signs of myasthenia gravis.

> **Edrophonium Chloride Challenge for MG**
>
> Administer 0.2–5 mg Edrophonium chloride IV
>
> Results in temporary improvement in most cases

Some dogs with myasthenia gravis still can make acceptable pets. It is best to feed them on an elevated platform to reduce the risk of regurgitation and aspiration. A low-energy, low-stress existence will minimize the incidence of "attacks." Affected animals should not be bred, and their parents should be recognized as obligate carriers of the trait. Normal-appearing siblings are suspect carriers.

MYELODYSPLASIA

Myelodysplasia, also known as spinal dysraphism, refers to a variety of related malformations of the spinal cord. In Weimaraners, it is probably inherited as a co-dominant gene with variable penetrance that is lethal in homozygotes (546), and it is reported sporadically in the Alaskan malamute (874), Chihuahua (187), Dalmatian (995, 1028), English bulldog (546), Labrador retriever (187), rottweiler (1028), Samoyed (1028), and Siberian husky (187, 995). The result is a variety of anomalies of the spinal cord (e.g., myeloschisis, hydromyelia, syringomyelia) that cause nonprogressive neurologic dysfunction.

Mildly affected animals tend to bunny hop and have an awkward gait, but otherwise they are not in distress. The diagnosis is almost impossible to confirm in the living animal and is based on clinical signs and exclusion of other possibilities. No treatments are available. Affected animals should not be bred—especially Weimaraners, in which the mode of inheritance appears to be co-dominant.

NEUROAXONAL DYSTROPHIES

Neuroaxonal dystrophies are inherited errors of metabolism resulting in swellings (or spheroids) along a region of the axon. They may be primarily inherited or may occur secondarily to other disease processes. This discussion is confined to primary hereditary disorders, each of which is described separately.

Rottweiler neuroaxonal dystrophy is an autosomal recessive hereditary disorder in which spheroids appear throughout the brain and spinal cord (187, 995). The end result is an awkward gait in all four limbs and a progressive head tremor. The defect may not be noted until the dog is 12 to 24 months of age (179). Conscious proprioception, attitude, and strength are unaffected. These latter features distinguish this disorder clinically from rottweiler leukodystrophy. Patellar reflexes are hyperactive, with clonus, and laryngeal paralysis is sometimes present (47). The condition is slowly progressive and usually commences before 1 year of age. Head and neck incoordination and intention tremors are obvious by 5 to 6 years of age (179). The diagnosis is suspected on the basis of breed affected and clinical signs and is confirmed with histopathologic evaluation. Affected dogs should not be bred. Parents are considered obligate carriers, and normal-appearing siblings are suspect carriers.

Jack Russell terrier neuroaxonal dystrophy is similar in many ways to the disorder in rottweilers, but these terriers also show bilateral hydrocephalus, hypoplasia of the corpus callosum, and absence of the septum pellucidum (633). Histopathologically there is extensive axonal swelling, principally in the gray matter of the brainstem, and the presence of spheroids, suggesting similarities with human infantile neuroaxonal dystrophy (Seitelberger's disease) (908).

Other forms of neuroaxonal dystrophy also have been described. In the Chihuahua, the condition affects gray matter structures in the brainstem and spinal cord with spheroids in white matter tracts (633). In collies, a suspected autosomal recessive neuroaxonal dystrophy affects pups at 2 to 4 months of age, and spheroids are detected with mild Wallerian degeneration in cerebellar structures (187). An autosomal recessive disease of bullmastiffs results in neuroaxonal dystrophy, intramyelinic vacuolization, and hydrocephalus (150). In papillon pups, neuroaxonal dystrophy causes ataxia and hypermetria resulting from widespread changes in both white and gray matter, characterized by axonal swellings (331). A unique condition in young Labrador retrievers selectively affects cerebral white matter while sparing the brainstem and cerebellum (763).

PERIPHERAL NEUROPATHIES

Peripheral neuropathies represent a collection of neurological disorders affecting the peripheral nervous system (PNS), but not necessarily exclusively. Because these conditions are often quite distinct, each will be discussed separately.

Giant axonal neuropathy is considered to be an autosomal recessive trait in German shepherd dogs (83, 87, 187, 273, 467). Not strictly a peripheral neuropathy, the central nervous system can be involved as well. Affected dogs develop paraparesis at just over a year of age, with progression to the front legs, proprioceptive deficits, hypotonia, and muscle atrophy (87, 995). Megaesophagus and laryngeal paralysis also can be a feature of this disorder and can lead to aspiration pneumonia as an additional consequence. Electrophysiologic studies often reveal decreased amplitude of evoked compound muscle action potentials and denervation potentials (87). The prognosis is poor. Even though most breeders would not consider breeding affected individuals, parents should be considered as potential carriers of the trait and normal-appearing siblings as suspect carriers.

Hereditary polyneuropathy is believed to be an autosomal recessive trait seen in Alaskan malamutes (709). This results in paraparesis between 6 and 18 months of age, with gradual progression to the front limbs. As with giant axonal neuropathy, megaesophagus and marked atrophy of the laryngeal muscles can be features of this disorder. Pathologic findings include neurogenic muscle atrophy, loss of myelinated nerve fibers, myelinoaxonal necrosis, and variable demyelination or remyelination (92). Dogs sometimes recover sufficiently to become suitable house pets, but the paresis may recur after months or years. Affected animals and their parents should not be used for breeding, and normal-appearing siblings should be considered as suspect carriers.

Polyneuropathy is believed to be an autosomal recessive trait seen in rottweilers (467). The condition results in distal axonal degeneration in both motor and sensory fibers, with secondary demyelination. Paraparesis is seen in adult dogs, eventually progressing to tetraparesis. Pronounced neurogenic atrophy is present is skeletal muscle biopsies (94). Pathologic findings suggest that this is a dying-back distal sensorimotor polyneuropathy with some similarities to hereditary motor and sensory neuropathy (HMSN) type II in humans. Although most breeders would not consider breeding affected individuals, they should consider parents as potential carriers of the trait and normal-appearing siblings as suspect carriers.

Progressive axonopathy in boxers is believed to be an autosomal recessive disorder, with axonal swellings in spinal nerve roots and lateral and ventral funiculi of spinal cord (83, 272, 467). Because affected axons are swollen by accumulated membranes and organelles, this disorder most likely results from defective axoplasmic transport (995). Affected dogs develop pelvic limb ataxia as pups, and this progresses to the front limbs by 1 year of age (995). Proprioceptive deficits, hypotonia, patellar areflexia, and head bobbing are common manifestations (272). Conscious proprioception decreases only late in the disease, and pain sensation is unaffected (546). Muscle atrophy is not a feature of this disorder. The diagnosis is suspected on the basis of breed, age of onset, loss of patellar reflexes without muscle atrophy, slow progression of signs, and electrophysiologic evidence of reduced sensory potentials, decreased motor nerve conduction velocities, and spontaneous activity (87, 388, 389). Animals can function as acceptable pets for many months or years, but eventually they develop pronounced gait disability. Affected boxers should not be bred, and parents should be considered as obligate carriers of the trait. Normal-appearing siblings are considered to be suspect carriers. A similar condition is reported in the Great Pyrenees (187).

Hypomyelinating neuropathy is suspected to be a heritable neuropathy of golden retrievers, characterized by reduced myelination in peripheral nerves (467). Affected dogs have hindlimb ataxia by 2 months of age, but progression is minimal. They often maintain a crouched stance, hindlimb muscle atrophy, weakness, and possible bunny hop when attempting to run. Motor nerve conduction velocities are significantly reduced in sciatic-tibial and ulnar nerves, and electromyography reveals rare denervation potentials in a few muscle groups (91). Affected individuals should not be bred. Information on which to base other breeding recommendations is insufficient.

Hypertrophic neuropathy is likely an autosomal recessive disorder of recurrent demyelination and remyelination, seen in Tibetan mastiffs (187, 467). Affected dogs develop pelvic limb ataxia by 2 months of age, quickly progressing to tetraplegia. Although individuals seem to improve over 1 to 2 months, weakness often remains. Cerebrospinal fluid analysis may reveal elevated protein levels, and electrophysiologic studies may show deceased nerve conduction velocities and occasional denervation potentials (87). No treatment is available, and the prognosis is poor. Most breeders would not consider breeding affected individuals, but they should also consider parents as potential carriers of the trait and normal-appearing siblings as suspect carriers. The condition should be considered extremely rare, even in the Tibetan mastiff.

Sensory neuropathy is thought to be an autosomal recessive loss of axons in primary sensory nerves and has been reported in longhaired dachshunds (83, 187, 467). Affected animals develop ataxia by 2 months of age, with diminished pain perception. Although the condition is nonprogressive, urinary and fecal incontinence and genital self-mutilation can be extremely problematic. Electrodiagnostic studies show decreased velocity of sensory conduction but not motor nerve conduction (995). In contradistinction to sensory neuropathy in pointers with acral mutilation syndrome, this sensory neuropathy spares the spinal ganglia (272). The prognosis is poor. Even though most breeders would not consider breeding affected individuals, they should consider parents as potential carriers of the trait and normal-appearing siblings as suspect carriers.

Dancing Doberman disease is a progressive neuromuscular disease of unknown etiology, but genetics likely plays some role, as the condition is seen only in the Doberman pinscher (467). A mode of inheritance, however, has not been determined (995). It is not even known if this is, in fact, a peripheral neuropathy. Clinical signs are seen in young adult Dobermans, starting as persistent flexion of one hindleg, and the other hindleg becoming involved shortly thereafter, resulting in a shifting leg lameness. The presentation seems to be quite variable. Most dogs have exaggerated hindlimb reflexes, and some have conscious proprioceptive deficits and muscle atrophy. Electromyographic studies are often characteristic, but diagnosis is typically based on breed and clinical presentation alone. The condition is slowly progressive, but animals can remain functional for years. The mode of inheritance is not known for this disorder, but prudence would dictate that affected animals not be included in breeding programs.

Serotonin Antagonist Challenge for the Diagnosis of Scotty Cramp

- Give methysergide 0.3 mg/kg PO
- Exercise animal 2 hours later
- Potentiates cramping in mildly affected dogs

RAGE SYNDROME

Rage syndrome appears to be a form of dominance aggression. Seen in English springer spaniels, it seems to be familial and is extremely dangerous (564). Although the pathophysiology of this and other forms of dominance aggression is poorly understood, preliminary studies have found that the afflicted dogs may have identifiable neurochemical changes. These cases have been likened to episodic dyscontrol, a form of epilepsy. The affected dogs may respond to antiepileptic drugs such as phenobarbital or primidone. Until more is known about the pathophysiology and inheritance of this trait, affected animals should not be bred.

SACROCAUDAL DYSGENESIS

Sacrocaudal dysgenesis is a malformation of the sacrocaudal vertebrae and spinal cord segments. It is believed to be inherited in the English bulldog and also has been reported in the pug and Boston terrier (1028). Clinical signs are apparent by 4 to 6 weeks of age, with lower motor neuron signs such as incontinence, bunny hopping, ataxia, weak flexor reflexes, and muscle atrophy. Plain and contrast radiography can be used to confirm abnormalities of the sacral and caudal vertebrae. Meningoceles can be treated surgically, but, otherwise, management is symptomatic only. Affected animals should not be used for breeding.

SCOTTY CRAMP

Scotty cramp is a paroxysmal hyperkinetic disorder of Scottish terriers believed to be transmitted as an autosomal recessive trait (746, 995). The disease involves a functional defect in the neural pathways that control muscle contraction. Similar conditions have been reported in young Norwich terriers and Dalmatians (187). Clinical signs are evident by 1 to 18 months of age, appearing as a stiff gait, hypertension of the hindlimbs, and spasms of the cervical and facial muscles. Personality remains unaffected during episodes, and these episodes seem to be stimulated by exercise, excitement, or stress.

The diagnosis can be made on the basis of clinical signs or with a methysergide challenge that induces clinical signs. Symptomatic therapy consists of vitamin E, diazepam, or acepromazine. Affected animals and their parents should not be used for breeding, and normal-appearing siblings should be considered to be potential carriers of the trait.

SEIZURE DISORDERS

Although seizures certainly can be nonspecific, epileptic seizures imply that the seizures are neural in origin. Epileptic seizures have many classifications, the easiest, from a clinical perspective, of which is to differentiate partial from generalized seizures. Partial seizures are a manifestation of a focal epileptogenic event in the cerebral cortex, and generalized seizures erupt from both cerebral hemispheres (50, 841). Generalized seizures also can be subdivided into convulsive (grand mal) and nonconvulsive (petit mal) varieties. Convulsive, generalized seizures are the most commonly seen in dogs (841), reported in about 75% of epileptic dogs (473).

Although genetics seem to play an important role in transmission of at least some cases of canine epilepsy, the genetic mechanism by which this transmission occurs is not yet clear (220). A genetic basis for epilepsy has been established for the following breeds:

Beagle	(54, 220, 925)
Belgian Tervuren	(220, 297, 816, 925)
Dachshund	(220, 816)
German shepherd dog	(295, 816, 925)
Golden retriever	(475, 841, 925, 999)
Keeshond	(220, 410, 816, 925)
Labrador retriever	(187, 351, 423, 448 475, 816, 925)

Idiopathic epilepsy runs in families, and breeding studies have shown a genetic basis for the disorder in the families listed above. It is believed to be inherited in other breeds as well, such as the bichon frisé (181), border collie (816, 841), boxer (816), cocker spaniel (187, 816, 925), collie (816), Irish setter (816, 841, 925), poodle (187, 816, 925), St. Bernard (187, 816), Shetland sheepdog (816), Siberian husky (816), Springer spaniel (816), Welsh corgi (816), and wire fox terrier (187, 816). Most breeders acknowledge that the condition is prevalent in the Brittany, but the true incidence in this breed remains unknown. In the Belgian Tervuren, the heritability of the disorder has been estimated to be 0.77% (297), and as much as 17% of the breed may be affected (296).

Although the mode of inheritance is unknown, the condition is presumed to be familial. More important, it probably is different in each unrelated breed. As more research is done, it is expected that the epilepsy trait will be found to be genetically heterogeneous among breeds, but monogenic and likely recessive. Epilepsy is slightly more commonly reported in males (300), and some report a male-to-female sex ratio of as high as 6-to-1, depending on breed (46). It is believed that genetically determined "factors" may make the brain more susceptible to triggering or precipitating events (842).

If the condition in dogs is similar to that in humans, in any given animal the disease is likely attributable to a single gene defect. Unfortunately, that gene defect probably is different in each breed. Thus, there is some hope that some specific genetic defects will be detected that are breed-specific. This would make it possible to design breed-specific DNA tests to allow breeders to reduce the frequency of the disease by selective breeding.

Epilepsy is usually first seen in dogs between 1 and 3 years of age. The condition is similar to that reported in people, and the seizures follow the same pattern. The generalized seizure usually involves the following defined phases.

1. *Aura.* The animal may appear restless, fearful, abnormally affectionate, or show other behavioral changes.
2. *Ictus.* This is the actual seizure phase. The animal usually loses consciousness and the limbs become stiff. This is followed by paddling movements of the limbs. Crying, urination, defecation, and salivation may also occur. This phase may last from seconds to minutes.
3. *Post-ictus.* This phase takes from seconds to minutes, marked by confusion, circling, blindness, or sleepiness. It may last from several minutes to a few days. The post-ictus phase and the length or severity of the ictus phase apparently have no correlation.

The diagnosis is made by pairing a history of seizures with normal test results for other potential causes. In dogs younger than 1 year of age or older than 7 years of age when the seizures are first noted, a more thorough evaluation is strongly recommended to consider seizures as a secondary manifestation of an underlying disease. Otherwise, no specific laboratory tests are available to confirm epilepsy. If abnormalities are detected, electroencephalographic features are consistent and unique in dogs with idiopathic epilepsy (473). Low levels of gamma-aminobutyric acid (GABA) and high levels of glutamate (GLU) are typically found in the cerebrospinal fluid (CSF) of epileptic dogs. The GABA value tends to vary inversely with body weight (843).

The most common anti-seizure medication used in veterinary medicine is phenobarbital, which is highly effective in preventing seizures and has few side effects. While they are becoming accustomed to the drug, animals may have increased appetite and thirst and, occasionally, temporary weakness. The level of phenobarbital in the blood should be checked periodically. This is done by taking a blood sample immediately before giving the anticonvulsant medication so the concentration of drug is measured at its lowest. This blood level indicates if the amount of drug given should be increased, decreased, or remain the same. Potassium bromide is considered an option for animals that don't respond well to phenobarbital, or it can be used in combination with phenobarbital; therapeutic serum concentrations of both drugs should be monitored during therapy (1049). Partial seizures may be adequately treated with felbamate. Although these measures may not result in complete elimination of seizure activity, it is still important to reduce the seizures in both intensity and frequency as much as possible.

Affected animals should not be used for breeding. Selection studies in the Belgian Tervuren have shown that breeding only non-epileptic dogs produces offspring with a probability of 0.99 of never having a seizure (296). Thus, until more information is known about epilepsy in specific breeds, any animals with a history of primary epileptic seizures, and their parents, should not be bred (296). The Institute for Genetic Disease Control in Animals (GDC) maintains an open research database for idiopathic epilepsy in Labrador retrievers, Irish setters, and Bernese mountain dogs.

SHAKER SYNDROME

Shaker syndrome, also known as generalized tremor syndrome, little white shaker syndrome, and generalized sporadic acquired idiopathic tremors, is a poorly understood condition of young dogs that involves intention tremors of the head and limbs, hypermetria, and ataxia (1091). It is most commonly reported in Maltese and West Highland white terriers (817), which might explain why it was originally believed to be associated with white coat color. It has also been reported in the beagle, bichon frisé, Samoyed, spitz, and Yorkshire terrier (187).

The condition develops over 1 to 3 days and remains static until it is treated, although some cases improve spontaneously. The diagnosis is suspected with the clinical presentation and the fact that spinal and higher reflexes, cranial nerves, and personality remain unaffected. Treatment with corticosteroids and/or benzodiazepines typically results in prolonged remission (1091). Although the recommendation is not to use affected animals in breeding programs, evidence for heritability of the condition is lacking.

SLEEP DISORDERS

Narcolepsy and cataplexy are two sleep disorders recognized in dogs. Narcolepsy consists of a disturbed sleep pattern including excessive daytime sleepiness and uncontrollable sleeping episodes. Cataplexy refers to a sudden episode of muscle weakness without loss of consciousness. In the veterinary literature, most sleep disorders have been reported as narcolepsy. Although many breeds have been affected, the condition has been documented to be inherited as an autosomal recessive trait in the dachshund (842), Doberman pinscher (163, 686), Labrador retriever (505, 686), and miniature poodle (842). The allele is referred to as canarc-1 (686).

The condition is not completely recessive, and heterozygotes have increased susceptibility of manifesting cataplexy upon administration of certain drugs (687). Interestingly, litters of narcoleptic dogs are not at increased risk for mortality (163). Other breeds reported with narcolepsy/cataplexy include the Airedale, Afghan, Alaskan malamute, English springer spaniel, giant schnauzer, Irish setter, rottweiler, St. Bernard, and Welsh corgi (842).

Dogs with sleep disorders are typically diagnosed when they fall asleep while being challenged with interesting opportunities such as feeding and play. There is some variability as to when this is detectable. In dachshunds and Labrador retrievers,

Testing for Sleep Disorders

Food-Elicited Test

- Place 10 pieces of food in a row, 1 foot apart from each other.
- Record time to eat all food, and number of attacks.
- Positive = takes > 2 minutes and has 2 or more attacks.

Yohimbine Response Test

- Administer 50 mcg/kg yohimbine IV bolus.
- Wait 30 minutes, then challenge.
- Positive response = 75% reduction in attacks.

the condition is usually evident by 3 to 5 months of age. In the miniature poodle, it may not be detectable until as late as 18 months of age (187). The diagnosis can be made by a food-elicited test, yohimbine response test, physostigmine challenge, atropine response test, imipramine challenge, and electrophysiologic testing. Because linkage markers have been identified for the narcolepsy gene canarc-1, DNA tests will likely be available for some affected breeds. In addition, for breeds in which the condition is widespread, identifying heterozygotes by using drug challenge to initiate cataplexy may be possible (687).

Treatment can be initiated with yohimbine, methylphenidate, or imipramine. Recent studies suggest that thyrotropin-releasing hormone (TRH) and its analogs can significantly reduce cataplexy (777). Affected animals and their parents should not be used for breeding, and siblings should be considered to be potential carriers.

SPINA BIFIDA

Spina bifida, part of the spinal dysraphism group of neurological disorders, refers to a developmental failure in part of the vertebra. Sometimes, no clinical abnormalities are associated with the defect (spina bifida occulta), and other cases have an open communication from the spinal cord (spina bifida aperta). The condition is thought to be heritable and is reported most commonly in the English and French bulldog (26, 1028). Other breeds in which the condition is seen include the beagle, Boston terrier, Chihuahua, Dalmatian, pug, and Samoyed (187, 1028). Environmental factors have also been shown to produce the malformation.

Clinically, spina bifida aperta is evident at birth, with either a direct opening to the spinal cord or a protruding cystic structure. Milder forms of the disorder may present just a whorled pattern of hair on the midline, a draining tract, or a dimple at the site of malformation. In spina bifida occulta, no clinical lesions are evident.

Most defects are seen in the lower lumbar or sacral spine. Neurological signs may or may not be present, depending on the extent of the malformation. When neurological signs are evident, they typically pinpoint the site of the defect. The diagnosis can be confirmed with radiography, but the entire spinal cord should be radiographed to survey for other congenital defects that might appear concurrently.

Treatment is generally not attempted for severely affected individuals. Mildly affected animals may respond to reconstructive surgical procedures (26). Because the genetics of the condition are not entirely known, any animals with a family history of spina bifida should probably not be bred.

SPINAL MUSCULAR ATROPHY

The term spinal muscular atrophy is applied to most of the inherited motor neuron diseases in humans in which motor neurons are affected preferentially but not necessarily exclusively (203). This probably represents a spectrum disorder, from focal degeneration seen in German shepherds to the multisystemic disease seen in Cairn terriers. Because these disorders differ significantly from one another, they are best discussed separately. One disorder, Stockard's paralysis, will not be discussed in any detail because it has not been reported since 1936 (1062) and is only of historic interest. The paralysis occurred in the crossbreeding of St. Bernards or bloodhounds with Great Danes.

Focal spinal muscular atrophy in German shepherd dogs affects motor neurons in the cervical intumescence and causes asymmetric foreleg weakness (218), typically by 1 to 2 months of age (995). The disorder is presumed to be inherited (217). A genetic basis is also suspected for the motor neuron disease in Doberman pinscher pups, which develop a disorder characterized by forelimb extension and hindleg paresis (217). A similar condition has been reported in the Griffon Briquet Vendeen dog (628).

Hereditary progressive spinal muscular atrophy is presumed to be an autosomal recessive trait in pointers (83, 466, 467). Lipid accumulated in spinal motor neurons and brainstem neurons causes pelvic limb weakness by 6 months of age, progressing to tetraparesis, and progressive muscle atrophy. There is hyporeflexia, but the animal retains sensation (546). Electromyograms show fibrillation potentials and positive sharp waves in epaxial and appendicular muscles (87). Affected dogs show progressive involvement of lower motor neurons (466). The prognosis is poor.

Even though most breeders would not consider breeding affected individuals, they also should consider parents as potential carriers of the trait and normal-appearing siblings as suspect carriers.

More advanced yet is a familial motor neuron disease of female rottweiler pups associated with paraparesis and tetraparesis, the process affecting sensory as well as motor neurons (217). Pups develop paraparesis by 4 weeks of age, and some develop megaesophagus as well (83, 954). An intention tremor and loss of gag reflex also may be noted. The condition is characterized by swelling and central chromatolysis of the nerve cell body, neuronal necrosis, and some neurophagia in the large motor neurons (955). Wallerian degeneration may be seen in some of the myelinated fibers in the peroneal and sciatic nerves (955). Most breeders would not breed affected individuals, and they also should consider parents as potential carriers of the trait and normal-appearing siblings as suspect carriers.

Another form of spinal muscular atrophy, seen in Brittany spaniels, is believed to be an autosomal dominant trait with variable penetrance (83, 87, 467). It shares certain features with human amyotrophic lateral sclerosis (ALS), also known as Lou Gehrig's disease (838, 1052). Because of the variability in clinical presentation, at least three forms are recognized (202, 610):

1. Tetraparesis by 3 to 4 months of age in homozygotes
2. Tetraparesis by 2 to 3 years of age in heterozygotes
3. A more chronic form in heterozygotes that is slowly progressive over many years.

Clinical signs begin with weak limb and trunk muscles, hyporeflexia, waddling, and progressive atrophy of hindlimb and lumbar muscles (87). The most definitive diagnostic technique in dogs older than 6 months of age is muscle biopsy. Aspartate, glutamate, and N-acetylaspartate are reduced in the spinal cord of homozygotes (1052). The prognosis is poor. Although most breeders would not breed affected individuals, they should also consider parents as potential carriers of the trait and normal-appearing siblings as suspect carriers. In family lines that have a problem with this disorder, individuals should not be bred until they are at least 3 years of age to make detection of heterozygotes easier.

Neuronal abiotrophy is thought to be an autosomal recessive trait and has been described in Swedish Lapland dogs (467, 995). These dogs develop leg weakness at 5 to 7 weeks of age, which progresses quickly to tetraparesis. Spinal hyporeflexia and distal limb muscle atrophy are also present (546). Severe cases include limb deformity and arthrogryposis. Electromyographic findings consist of fibrillation potentials and positive sharp waves of the pelvic musculature and reduced conduction velocities in tibial and peroneal nerves (1062). Affected animals do not recover (87). Most breeders would not breed affected individuals, but they should consider parents as likely carriers of the trait and normal-appearing siblings as suspect carriers.

A neuronal degeneration in the brain without spinal cord lesions has been reported in cocker spaniels and is presumed to be autosomal recessive in nature (187). Affected animals usually are 10 to 14 months of age. Clinical signs include ataxia, hypermetria, seizures, abnormal behavior, absence of menace response, and depressed postural reactions (476). Laboratory profiles and cerebrospinal fluid analysis are usually unremarkable. The condition is progressive and does not respond to treatment. The diagnosis can be confirmed on necropsy by determining neuronal degeneration (gliosis, demyelination, diffuse nerve cell loss, and axonal degeneration) in the brain. Affected animals should not be bred, and parents should be considered as carriers of the trait; siblings should be considered as suspect carriers.

Finally, the most debilitating form is the multisystemic chromatolytic neuronal degeneration in Cairn terriers, associated with paraparesis, quadriparesis, ataxia, loss of spinal reflexes, and head tremor (217, 808). There is often an exercise-induced deterioration of clinical signs (1150). The condition is typically seen in animals 4 to 7 months of age and is considered familial, although an exact mode of inheritance has not been determined (187). Affected animals should not be bred and close relatives should be carefully evaluated before being considered for a breeding program.

VERTEBRAL STENOSIS

Vertebral stenosis is a rare narrowing of the spine present at birth. It can occur alone or in association with other congenital anomalies of the spinal cord. A strong association has been demonstrated between stenotic lumbosacral transitional vertebrae (L7-S1) and cauda equina syndrome in the German shepherd dog (733). A thoracic vertebral stenosis has been recognized in Doberman pinschers (26), which might be confused with vertebral instability. The defect, however, is typically in the T3–T6 region. The condition has also been reported in beagles, Lhasa apsos, and toy poodles (187), though it may not become clinically apparent until middle age (3 to 8 years of age).

Vertebral stenosis may be subclinical if it is mild, or clinical if it results in spinal cord compression. The diagnosis can be confirmed radiographically. Myelography is helpful, but the defect usually can be seen on plain radiographs if it is profound. Computed tomography and magnetic resonance imaging allow more accurate characterization of the bony changes. Mildly affected animals may be maintained with anti-inflammatory drug therapy and enforced rest. Decompression surgery is best if it is performed early, prior to significant spinal cord compression. Internal stabilization may also be necessary. Individuals from families known to be affected with vertebral stenosis should not be including in breeding programs.

CHAPTER 11

Ophthalmologic Disorders

Ophthalmic diseases in purebred dogs have received a great deal of scrutiny over the years. Much of this is a result of efforts of the Canine Eye Registration Foundation (CERF) (see Appendix). CERF maintains a purebred registry of dogs that have been examined and certified annually. The Institute for Genetic Disease Control in Animals (GDC) maintains all-breed registries for heritable eye diseases, as well as registries and databases of conditions in specific breeds (see Appendix). Although most eye diseases are diagnosed by clinical evaluation, some forms of progressive retinal atrophy can be confirmed by DNA testing.

CATARACTS

A cataract is an opacity of the lens of the eye. Although cataracts have many causes, most cataracts are inherited. Cataracts can be further subdivided by stage (incipient, immature, mature, hypermature), location (anterior or posterior capsule, anterior or posterior cortex, equator, nucleus), mode of inheritance, and age of onset (congenital/perinatal, juvenile, adult onset, or senile). Regarding age of onset, the designations are fairly arbitrary, with congenital/perinatal designating that the cataract was present when the eyes first opened, juvenile when recognized at less than 2 years of age, and adult-onset implying cataract detection at 2 to 6 years of age. Geriatric or senile cataracts are not believed to have a heritable basis.

Breeds may be susceptible to more than one form of cataract. German shepherd dogs, for example, are prone to congenital cataracts that are autosomal dominant and also juvenile cataracts that are transmitted as an autosomal recessive trait. Table 11-1 lists various cataract conditions by breed, time of onset, mode of inheritance, and form of the disease.

The diagnosis of heritable cataracts is best made on ophthalmic examination and by precluding other causes. Although no medical or nutritional therapies seem to be suitable for treating inherited cataracts, removal of the lens can be accomplished through several techniques (370, 1120, 1130). The prognosis is good to excellent, and most dogs do extremely well following cataract extraction. Sudden, large increases in intraocular pressure can occur following lens extraction and require monitoring to avoid complications (693, 983).

Heritable cataracts can be prevented by proper genetic counseling based on the specific breed involved, and the Canine Eye Registration Foundation (CERF) maintains a registry. The Institute for Genetic Disease Control in Animals (GDC) maintains an open registry of inherited eye diseases for all breeds.

COLLIE EYE ANOMALY

Collie eye anomaly (CEA), the incomplete development of the eye, is inherited as a simple recessive defect (in the collie), but a cluster of genes is believed to control the severity and susceptibility. That is how pups from the same litter can show such variability. Although it is called collie eye anomaly (CEA), the condition does affect other breeds, including the border collie, Shetland sheepdog, Australian shepherd, and Lancashire heeler terrier (34, 43, 1108). Choroidal hypoplasia may be seen as an inherited trait in Australian shepherds, border collies, and Shetland sheepdogs (350).

Most collies with CEA don't have vision problems, but some have serious hemorrhages within the eye, as well as severe defects of the optic nerve

Table 11-1 Cataract Conditions

Breed	Onset	Inheritance	Reference
Afghan	Juvenile	Autosomal recessive	345, 827, 1119
Affenpinscher	Juvenile	ND	903
Akita	Congenital	Autosomal recessive	293, 802
Alaskan malamute	Juvenile	Recessive?	293, 903, 1119
American cocker spaniel	Congenital, Juvenile, Adult	Suspected AR Autosomal recessive or polygenic	135, 293, 345, 350, 365, 827, 1147
American Staffordshire terrier	Juvenile	ND	1119
American water spaniel	Juvenile	ND	903
Australian shepherd	Congenital, Juvenile, Adult	ND	293, 903
Basenji	Congenital	ND	293
Beagle	Congenital	Dominant, incomplete penetrance	345, 827, 1119
Bearded collie	Juvenile–Adult	ND; males predominate	903, 1119
Bedlington terrier	Juvenile	Autosomal recessive	365, 903
Belgian Tervuren	Juvenile	ND	903
Bernese mountain dog	Juvenile	ND	903
Bichon frisé	Juvenile	ND	903
Border collie	Adult	Familial	903, 1119
Border terrier	Adult	ND	903
Borzoi	Juvenile–Adult	ND	903
Boston terrier	Congenital, Juvenile, Adult	Autosomal recessive	293, 345, 350, 903
Bouvier des Flandres	Congenital, Juvenile, Adult	ND	903, 1119
Boxer	Juvenile	ND	903
Brussels griffon	Adult	ND	903
Cairn terrier	Juvenile, Adult	ND	903
Cavalier King Charles spaniel	Congenital, Juvenile	ND	293, 350
Chesapeake Bay retriever	Juvenile or Adult	Incomplete dominance	345, 349, 350, 1119
Chow chow	Congenital	ND	293, 350
Collie	Congenital	ND	293, 903
Curly-coated retriever	Juvenile; Adult	ND	350, 903
Doberman pinscher	Congenital	Dominant, incomplete penetrance	293
English bulldog	Juvenile	ND	903
English cocker spaniel	Congenital	Autosomal recessive suspected	293, 1119
English cocker spaniel	Juvenile	Familial	903
English springer spaniel	Congenital, Juvenile, Adult	Familial	350, 903
English toy spaniel	Juvenile	ND	350, 903
Entlebucher mountain dog	Juvenile	Autosomal recessive	997
Field spaniel	Juvenile/Adult	ND	903

(continued on next page)

Table 11-1 Cataract Conditions (continued)

Breed	Onset	Inheritance	Reference
Flat-coated retriever	Juvenile or Adult	ND	293, 903
French bulldog	Juvenile	ND	365, 903
German shepherd dog	Congenital	Autosomal dominant	293, 345, 827
German shepherd dog	Juvenile	Autosomal recessive	33, 350
German shorthaired pointer	Juvenile	ND	365, 903
German wirehaired pointer	Juvenile	ND	903
Golden retriever	Juvenile or Adult	Incomplete dominance	223, 345, 827
Gordon setter	Juvenile or Adult	ND	903
Great Dane	Juvenile	ND	903
Ibizan hound	Juvenile, Adult	ND	903
Irish setter	Juvenile	ND	827
Irish water spaniel	Juvenile, Adult	ND	903
Irish wolfhound	Juvenile, Adult	ND	903
Italian greyhound	Juvenile or Adult	ND	350, 903
Keeshond	Juvenile, Adult	ND	365, 903
Kerry blue terrier	Juvenile	ND	903
Komondor	Juvenile–Adult	ND	903
Kuvasz	Juvenile	ND	903
Labrador retriever	Congenital	Incomplete dominance	223, 293
Labrador retriever	Juvenile or Adult	Incomplete dominance	345
Lakeland terrier	Juvenile	Autosomal recessive	903
Lhasa apso	Juvenile–Adult	ND	903
Manchester terrier	Adult	ND	903
Miniature pinscher	Juvenile	ND	903
Miniature schnauzer	Congenital	Autosomal recessive	293, 345, 827, 953
Miniature schnauzer	Juvenile	Autosomal recessive	31, 32, 1119
Miniature schnauzer	Adult	ND	903
Norfolk terrier	Adult	ND	903
Norwegian buhund	Congenital	Autosomal dominant	59
Norwegian elkhound	Juvenile	ND	903
Norwich terrier	Juvenile	Autosomal recessive	365, 903
Old English sheepdog	Congenital	Familial, Autosomal recessive?	345, 350, 536, 1119
Old English sheepdog	Juvenile–Adult	ND	903
Papillon	Juvenile–Adult	ND	903
Pembroke Welsh corgi	Congenital, Juvenile	ND	365, 903
Pointer	Juvenile	Dominant, incomplete penetrance?	903, 1119
Pomeranian	Adult	ND	903, 1119
Poodle, toy, miniature	Juvenile or Adult	Autosomal recessive	293, 827, 1119
Poodle, standard	Juvenile	Autosomal recessive	35, 345, 827, 1119
Pug	Juvenile–Adult	ND	903
Rhodesian ridgeback	Juvenile–Adult	ND	903
Rottweiler	Juvenile or Adult	Familial	350, 1119

(continued on next page)

Table 11-1 Cataract Conditions (continued)

Breed	Onset	Inheritance	Reference
Russian terrier	Congenital	ND, familial?	609
St. Bernard	Juvenile	ND	903
Samoyed	Congenital	Autosomal recessive	293
Samoyed	Juvenile–Adult	ND	903
Schipperke	Adult	ND	903
Schnauzer, standard	Congenital	Autosomal recessive	903
Schnauzer, standard	Juvenile	ND	350
Scottish terrier	Adult	ND	903
Sealyham terrier	ND	Recessive suspected	1119
Siberian husky	Juvenile	Autosomal recessive	345, 827
Silky terrier	Adult	ND	903
Staffordshire bull terrier	Congenital	Autosomal recessive	345, 350
	Juvenile	Autosomal recessive	903, 1119
Tibetan terrier	Juvenile	ND	903
Welsh springer spaniel	Congenital, Juvenile	Autosomal recessive	32, 293, 345
Welsh terrier	Juvenile	ND	365, 903
West Highland white terrier	Congenital	Autosomal recessive	293, 345, 756, 1119
	Juvenile	ND	
Whippet	Adult	Familial	903
Wire fox terrier	Juvenile	Autosomal recessive suspected	673, 1119
Yorkshire terrier	Juvenile	Autosomal recessive	903, 1119

ND = Not determined

(colobomas). The condition is not fatal but can result in blindness. An estimated 80%–90% of collies have some of these signs without apparent visual disturbance and, fortunately, the condition tends to be nonprogressive (724). The condition seen in Shetland sheepdogs, often referred to as Sheltie eye anomaly, rarely involves retinal detachment and intraocular hemorrhage, and the heritability has not been determined (724).

Because the condition is present at birth, pups can be checked as early as 5 to 6 weeks of age, although 6 to 10 weeks is preferred. Characteristic funduscopic changes include choroidal hypoplasia, coloboma, retinal detachment, retinal vascular tortuosity, and intraocular hemorrhage (1108). The biggest problem is that carriers can't be detected by any known diagnostic tests, including examination with an ophthalmoscope. This is significant because many collies are carriers for the trait. Diagnosis of the condition in merle-colored dogs can be difficult.

There is no treatment for collie eye anomaly. The best form of prevention is to register all pups with the Canine Eye Registration Foundation (CERF) and purchase pups from parents that have been registered and have not previously produced affected pups. Only normal-eyed Australian shepherds should be used for breeding. Mildly affected pups (grades 1 or 2) can still make acceptable pets, but their parents are definite carriers and should not be used for further breeding.

CORNEAL DYSTROPHY

Corneal dystrophy refers to corneal conditions that are bilateral, noninflammatory, and inherited; they involve the corneal epithelium, stroma, or endothelium (197). Corneal degeneration is a more appropriate term for nonhereditary conditions of the cornea. The age of onset is quite variable depending on the breed affected, with onset from 4 months in Airedale terriers to 13 years of age in Chihuahuas (363).

In most cases, the corneal dystrophy is epithelial and/or stromal and consists of an abnormal collection of lipids in the clear cornea of the eye, which results in a hazy or crystalline opacity. The majority of cases are attributable to lipid stromal opacities and are associated with hypercholesterolemia and hypertriglyceridemia (172). Most animals are older than 6 months of age when the opacity is first noticed. Ophthalmologists describe the location of the opacities as anterior, mid-, or deep stromal. The condition is usually slowly progressive or nonprogressive, and in most cases does not completely interfere with vision.

Calcium opacities also occur in dogs but are not believed to be heritable. In young Yorkshire terriers, a subepithelial geographic corneal dystrophy has been described, which slowly resolves by 4 months of age (903). Strict epithelial dystrophies include the chronic ulcerative keratitis of boxers (described below) and a poorly characterized disorder of multiple punctate corneal opacities seen in Shetland sheepdogs (749).

Endothelial dystrophy and endothelial degeneration refer to corneal dystrophies affecting Descemet's membrane or the corneal endothelium, and are usually seen in middle-aged and older animals. A hereditary form, similar to Fuch's corneal dystrophy in humans, is seen in the Boston terrier, Chihuahua, cocker spaniel, and dachshund, and is recognized in middle-aged and older animals (344, 527). In the American cocker spaniel, posterior polymorphous dystrophy is believed to be dominant or incompletely dominant, and endothelial dystrophy of the Boston terrier and Chihuahua has not be characterized genetically (527). The posterior polymorphous dystrophy of American cocker spaniels is seen in adult dogs as corneal opacities of the endothelium, without edematous changes (350).

The Siberian husky is prone to a stromal dystrophy of axial triglyceride deposits, and Airedales develop anterior stromal deposits of triglycerides (827). Deep opacities also occur with persistent pupillary membranes and with anterior chamber cleavage syndrome. This syndrome consists of microphthalmia, absence of the anterior chamber, lens abnormalities, and retinal dysplasia. It is seen in the Doberman pinscher and St. Bernard (527).

Corneal ulcers are commonly seen in older boxers and may result in visual impairment (350). Similar conditions are seen in the older Alaskan malamute, Boston terrier, Brussels griffon, Dandie Dinmont terrier, golden retriever, Japanese chin, Lhasa apso, Pekingese, pug, rottweiler, Samoyed, and shih tzu (903). A mode of inheritance has not been determined in any breed. This condition of refractory corneal epithelial ulcers may represent inadequate function of basement membrane complexes necessary for epithelial adhesion (761).

Proliferative episcleritis, also known as nodular fasciitis, nodular episcleritis, nodular granulomatous episclerokeratitis, and fibrous histiocytoma, is likely an immune-mediated inflammatory disease in which fleshy masses are seen on the cornea, sclera, nictitating membrane, lips, and conjunctivae. It is reported most commonly in the collie (270, 350), but similar granulomatous processes have been reported in the American cocker spaniel, border collie, golden retriever, miniature poodle, and Shetland sheepdog (255, 824). The condition responds to immunosuppressive therapy. The possible genetic nature of this disorder has not been determined.

Table 11-2 lists the various manifestations of corneal dystrophy by breed and any indication of heritability.

The diagnosis of corneal dystrophy is typically made by a veterinary ophthalmologist after thorough clinical evaluation and testing for underlying causes of cholesterol elevation, such as hypothyroidism. No effective therapies are available for corneal dystrophy, but most don't interfere with vision. In breeds in which the condition is clearly familial, affected animals should not be bred and parents should be considered potential carriers of the disorder. In other breeds, such as the Afghan hound, the hereditary link is more tenuous and the choice to breed or not to breed becomes a breeder option (350). The Institute for Genetic Disease Control in Animals (GDC) maintains an open registry of inherited eye diseases for all breeds.

DERMOID

Dermoids are congenital collections of cutaneous tissue (skin, hair follicles, sebaceous glands, fat) found on the conjunctiva or cornea. A mode of inheritance has not been determined, but there seems to be a breed predilection for the dachshund, Dalmatian, German shepherd dog, and St. Bernard, (365, 827, 903). It has been suggested that the condition is inherited as an autosomal recessive trait in the miniature longhaired dachshund (903). The condition is treated with surgical excision at 12 to 14 weeks of age. Incomplete excision may lead to recurrence. Until more is known about the heritability of the condition, affected animals should not be bred.

DISTICHIASIS

Distichiasis refers to eyelashes that may project toward the surface of the eye from abnormal locations, such as the openings of specialized (Meibomian) glands in the eyelids. Breeds with a high incidence of distichiasis include the

Table 11-2 Corneal Dystrophy

Breed	Infiltrate	Inheritance	Reference
Airedale terrier	Lipid	Sex-linked	344, 363, 527, 827
Afghan hound	Lipid	ND	344
Alaskan malamute	Lipid	ND	903
American cocker spaniel	Edema	Dominant?	527
Basenji	Edema	ND	350
Beagle	Lipid	ND	350, 527, 903
Bearded collie	Lipid	ND	903
Bichon frisé	Lipid	ND	903
Boston terrier	Edema	ND	350, 527, 827
Boxer	Bullae/erosions	ND	350, 827
Cavalier King Charles spaniel	Lipid	Polygenic suspected	527, 903
Chihuahua	Edema	ND	527, 903
Chow chow	Edema	ND	350
Collie	Lipid	ND	903
Collie	Proliferative episcleritis	ND	827
Dachshund	Edema	ND	350, 903
English pointer	Lipid	ND	903
English toy spaniel	Lipid	ND	903
German shepherd dog	Lipid	ND	527
Golden retriever	Lipid	ND	527
Italian greyhound	Edema	ND	903
Lhasa apso	Lipid	ND	903
Norwich terrier	Lipid	ND	903
Pembroke Welsh corgi	Vascularization	ND	903
Poodle, miniature and toy	Lipid	ND	344
Poodle, miniature	Granular	Recessive suspected	903
Rottweiler	Lipid	ND	527
Rough collie	Lipid	ND	527
Samoyed	Lipid	Autosomal recessive	527
Shetland sheepdog	Lipid/ crystals	ND	363, 527
Siberian husky	Lipid	Autosomal recessive with variable expression	344, 363, 527, 1094
Weimaraner	Lipid	ND	903
Whippet	Lipid	ND	903
Yorkshire terrier	Geographic	ND	903

* ND = Not determined

American cocker spaniel (567, 597), American Staffordshire terrier (903), beagle (903), Chesapeake Bay retriever (597), curly-coated retriever (903), English bulldog (567, 903), English cocker spaniel (1002), flat-coated retriever (903), French bulldog (903), golden retriever (597), Lhasa apso (597), Pekingese (567, 827), pug (903), St. Bernard (827), Shetland sheepdog (597), shih tzu (597, 903), Sussex spaniel (903), Tibetan terrier (1002), and toy and miniature poodles (567, 597). The condition is suspected to be a genetic disorder, but the mode of inheritance is unknown. Some experts classify congenital distichiasis as an autosomal dominant trait (365).

Distichiasis may not be problematic if the hairs are soft and fine and float on the tear film of the eye. If the hairs are coarse and stiff, or if the eyes become dry, problems can develop. Corneal ulcer-

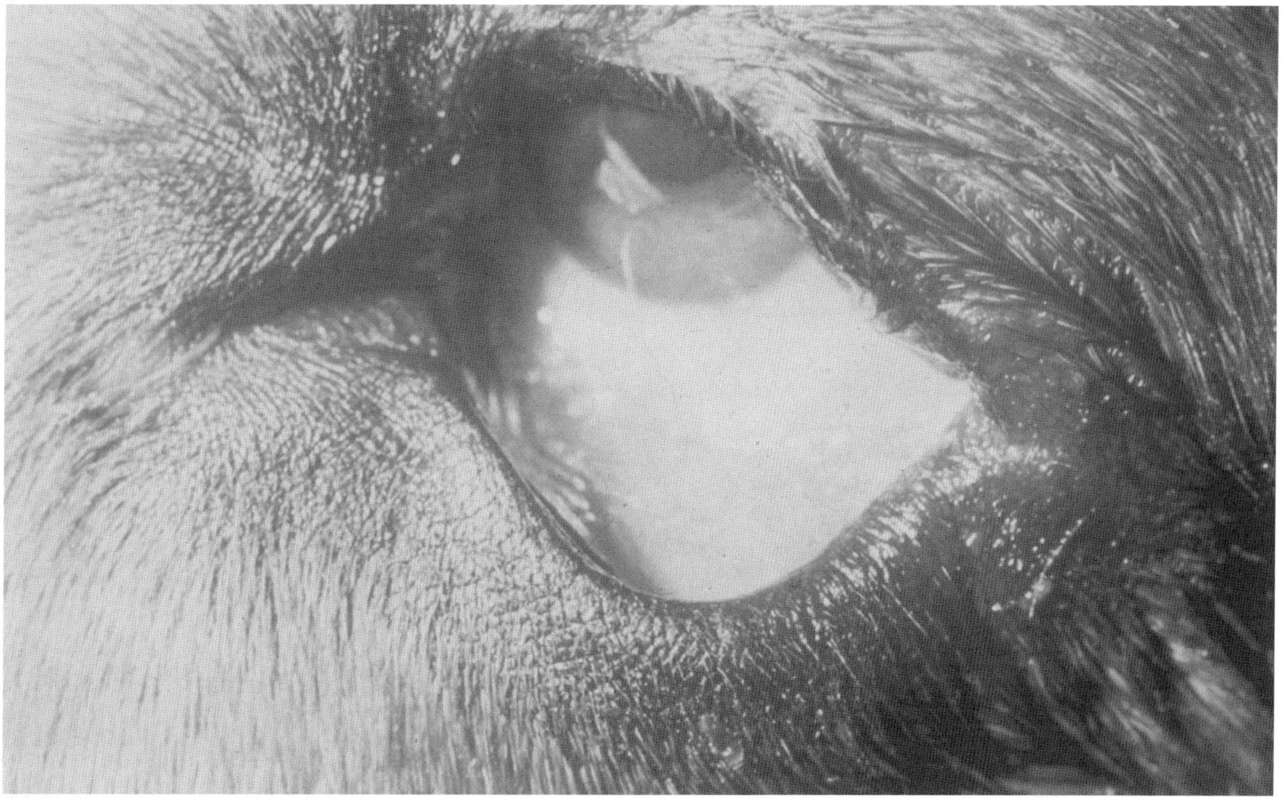

Figure 11-1 Ectropion
Courtesy of Dr. Dan Lavach, Eye Clinic for Animals, Garden Grove, California

ation, scarring, or pain can result from the hairs contacting the surface of the eye. Pain may be evident as dogs blink repeatedly (blepharospasm) or have weepy, runny eyes.

Distichiasis can be treated with a number of options. The abnormal hairs can be plucked periodically to provide temporary relief. Unfortunately, they often regrow. More sophisticated techniques such as radio wave surgery, electrocautery, or electroepilation can be used. Excision, laser techniques, or cryosurgery can be used in stubborn cases. Recurrence or scarring is possible with any of these procedures.

The hereditary basis for distichiasis has not been convincingly determined. In mildly affected animals, the decision on which animals are suitable for mating is considered a breeder option. In breeds in which distichiasis can be associated with significant clinical disease, such as the collie, English bulldog, and Weimaraner, breeding affected animals is discouraged.

ECTROPION

Ectropion refers to eyelids that are "turned out" and often have the appearance of drooping (Figure 11-1). This condition is seen most commonly in the lower lids. It is a breed characteristic in American and English cocker spaniels (597), basset hounds (597), bloodhounds (597, 903), boxers (903), Clumber spaniels (903), English bulldogs (597), mastiffs (597), Newfoundlands (597), St. Bernards (567, 597), and many other breeds. It is also commonly seen as an ophthalmic problem in the bull terrier, chow chow, English setter, English springer spaniel, flat-coated retriever, Irish setter, and Labrador retriever (903). Because the lids don't conform to the eyeball, these dogs may be prone to conjunctivitis—for which there are many other causes as well.

When problems arise, the surgical treatment for ectropion often involves removing a wedge of tissue from the lid margin (674). This is done only if the ectropion is resulting in conjunctival or corneal diseases. Additional "tightening" procedures may be used for best cosmetic results. These surgeries are performed to provide relief to affected dogs and are not meant to alter conformation in dogs used for show purposes. Minor problems can be treated with topical lubricating ointments. Guidelines do not exist regarding suitability of dogs with ectropion for breeding.

ENTROPION

Entropion occurs when the eyelids "turn in" toward the eye, often resulting in abrasive damage to the cornea. The lower lids are the ones most commonly involved. A heritable/conformational form is considered to be a polygenic trait with three subtypes (597):

1. Medial canthal entropion, involving the medial eyelids
2. Lateral canthal entropion, which involves the lateral upper and lower eyelids
3. Lower eyelid entropion

The heritable form of entropion is believed to be associated with poor canthal tension and excessive lid length, causing an inward rolling of the eyelids. The exact mode of inheritance has not been determined (567, 700). Dogs with mesaticephalic head types may have a lateral canthal tendon that renders the eye more prone to lid margin involution (880). Table 11-3 lists the forms of entropion by breed.

Entropion surgery involves complicated techniques to properly reposition the lids (723). A special procedure is recommended for dogs with lateral canthal entropion (881). In pups, temporary sutures are often necessary to evert the lids. This is often done at 3 to 4 weeks of age and is often referred to as "tacking." The final surgery is not performed until 5 to 12 months of age, when the dog reaches adult dimensions of the eyelid and head.

The most common procedure is to remove an ellipse of tissue parallel to the lid margin so the lid then returns to a more normal location. These surgeries are performed to provide relief to affected dogs. They are not meant to alter conformation in dogs used for show purposes. Because this form of entropion is believed to have a heritable component, affected dogs should not be used for breeding.

In breeds in which entropion is associated with pronounced clinical problems, such as the bullmastiff, Chinese shar pei, chow chow, and mastiff, breeding is not recommended (350). In some breeds, such as the vizsla, the national breed club has been instrumental in recognizing entropion as an unacceptable problem in the breed. In most breeds, however, this is considered a breeder option rather than a hard rule. The Institute for Genetic Disease Control in Animals (GDC) maintains an open registry of inherited eye diseases for all breeds.

GLAUCOMA

One of the leading causes of blindness in animals, glaucoma is caused by an increase in fluid pressure within the eye. Anything that interferes with drainage of fluid inside the eye can result in glaucoma, and not all cases have a genetic basis. Nevertheless, primary glaucoma does occur in several breeds, and inherited glaucoma is of three distinct types (558):

1. Narrow-angle (as seen in American cocker spaniels and miniature poodles)
2. Open-angle (as seen in beagles)
3. Goniodysgenesis (as seen in American cocker spaniels and chow chows).

In Siberian huskies, glaucoma seems to be associated with fibral dysplasia of the pectinate ligament (170). The type of abnormality and associated breed are given in Table 11-4.

With glaucoma, the eyes are often red and painful. The diagnosis is confirmed with a tonometer, an instrument that measures the pressure within the eye (998). The normal range of intraocular pressure varies with tonometrist, tonometer, conversion table, breed, and age (692). Gonioscopy is a technique used to visually inspect the drainage angle within the eye and determine the exact cause of the problem. Ultrasound biomicroscopy may yield more cross-sectional information on the iridocorneal filtration angle (355). Eventually, direct DNA tests will be available to diagnose most forms of hereditary glaucoma. A gene that causes primary open-angle glaucoma in humans has already been identified (1010) and can serve as a candidate gene for studies in canine glaucoma.

Treatment can involve medical or surgical options depending on the severity of the disorder (194, 364, 559). Screening all animals used in breeding programs can reduce the incidence of hereditary glaucoma. Affected animals, and those that have previously produced dogs with glaucoma, should not be bred. The Institute for Genetic Disease Control in Animals (GDC) maintains an open registry of inherited eye diseases for all breeds, which includes glaucoma in Chinooks and pigmentary glaucoma in Cairn terriers.

HEMERALOPIA

Hemeralopia is an inherited trait characterized by degeneration of the cones in the retina. It is reported most often in the Alaskan malamute, miniature poodle, and standard poodle and is believed to be autosomal recessive in the Alaskan malamute and miniature poodle (222, 350, 903, 904, 1108). It also has been reported in the Great Dane (1119).

The cones are responsible for vision in bright light, and in affected dogs they begin to deteriorate

Table 11-3 Entropion

Breed	Form of Entropion	Reference
Airedale	Lower eyelid	903
Akita	Lower eyelid	350, 903
American cocker spaniel	Lateral canthal	903
Bedlington terrier	Lower eyelid	903
Bichon frisé	Medial canthal	597
Black and tan coonhound	Lower eyelid	1119
Boston terrier	Medial canthal	1112
Bouvier des Flandres	Lateral canthal	903
Bullmastiff	Lateral canthal	597
Bull terrier	Lateral canthal	903
Chesapeake Bay retriever	Lateral canthal	1119
Chinese shar pei	Lateral canthal	597
Chow chow	Lateral canthal	567, 597, 881
Collie	Lower eyelid	903
Curly-coated retriever	Lower eyelid	903
Dachshund, miniature longhaired	Lower eyelid	903
Dalmatian	Lower eyelid	350
English bulldog	Lateral canthal	567, 597, 881
English cocker spaniel	Lower eyelid	1119
English pointer	Lower eyelid	597
English springer spaniel	Lower eyelid	350
Flat-coated retriever	Lower eyelid	903
French bulldog	Lower eyelid	903
German shorthaired pointer	Lower eyelid	1119
German wirehaired pointer	Lower eyelid	903
Golden retriever	Lower eyelid	597
Gordon setter	Lower eyelid	350
Great Dane	Lower eyelid	903
Great Pyrenees	Lateral canthal	903
Irish setter	Lower eyelid	350, 567
Irish wolfhound	Lower eyelid	903
Japanese chin	Medial canthal	350
Kerry blue terrier	Lateral canthal	903
Labrador retriever	Lower eyelid	597
Lhasa apso	Medial canthal	597
Mastiff	Lateral canthal	350, 881
Newfoundland	Lateral canthal, lower	350, 597
Norwegian elkhound	Lower eyelid	903
Old English sheepdog	Lower eyelid	903
Pekingese	Medial canthal	597
Pomeranian	Medial canthal	903
Poodle	Medial canthal	597
Pug	Medial canthal	567, 597
Rhodesian ridgeback	Lateral canthal	903
Rottweiler	Lateral canthal, lower	350, 597, 881
St. Bernard	Lateral canthal	567, 597
Shih tzu	Medial canthal	597
Siberian husky	Lower eyelid	903
Tibetan spaniel	Lower eyelid	903
Vizsla	Lateral canthal	903

Table 11-4 Glaucoma

Breed	Age of Onset (Years)	Genetics	Abnormality	References
Afghan hound	3+	ND	Goniodysgenesis	110, 1119
Akita	3+	ND	Goniodysgenesis	835
Alaskan malamute	3+	ND	Goniodysgenesis	350, 835
American cocker spaniel	3+	Familial	Narrow, Goniodysgenesis	111, 557, 826, 827, 835
Basset hound	3+	Familial	Goniodysgenesis	111, 557, 826, 827, 835
Beagle	1–3	AR	Open	347, 350, 557, 558, 826
Bedlington terrier	<9	ND	Narrow	110, 802
Bouvier des Flandres	3+	ND	Goniodysgenesis, Narrow	350, 826, 835, 905
Brittany	<9	ND	Narrow	110, 802
Cairn terrier	>5	ND	Open, melanosis	826, 903
Chihuahua	3+	ND	Goniodysgenesis	557, 558
Chinese shar pei	3+	Familial	Narrow, Goniodysgenesis	827, 835
Chow chow	3+	Familial	Narrow, Goniodysgenesis	200, 826, 827, 835
Dachshund	4+	ND	Narrow	110, 903
Dalmatian	4+	ND	Narrow	110, 903
Dandie Dinmont terrier	3+	Familial	Goniodysgenesis	903, 1119
English cocker spaniel	3+	ND	Narrow, Goniodysgenesis	557, 558, 826, 835
English springer spaniel	1–3	ND	Narrow	110, 111, 802
Entlebucher mountain dog	3+	ND	Goniodysgenesis	997

(continued on next page)

at 6 weeks of age and are essentially gone by 6 months of age. Actually, there is some breed variability, with Alaskan malamutes typically affected by 8 weeks of age, miniature poodles by 3 months of age, and standard poodles by 1 year of age (1108). This leaves dogs "blind" in bright light but still able to see in dim light because the rods are not affected.

The diagnosis is usually strongly suspected based on the breed and the description of being blind in bright light but not in dim light. Examination with an ophthalmoscope will not provide a diagnosis. Electroretinography (ERG) is necessary to pinpoint the problem. No treatment is available, but the condition does not progress to blindness because the rods remain unaffected.

Until more information on hemeralopia is collected, the condition should be considered autosomal recessive in most breeds. When individuals are affected, both parents are obligate carriers of the trait. Accordingly, affected animals should not be bred and parents should be considered as obligate carriers of the trait. Siblings should be considered potential carriers for the hemeralopia mutation.

KERATOCONJUNCTIVITIS SICCA (KCS)

Keratoconjunctivitis sicca (KCS), or "dry eye," is a common condition in dogs. It results from reduction in the amount of watery tears produced by the lacrimal glands. The orbital lacrimal glands provide 70% of the tear film, and the nictitans gland, 30% (909). The underlying reasons for this condition are numerous. Some are congenital, some

Table 11-4 Glaucoma (continued)

Breed	Age of Onset (Years)	Genetics	Abnormality	References
Great Dane	3+	ND	Goniodysgenesis	110
Keeshond	3+	ND	Narrow	557, 558
Maltese	6+	ND	Narrow	835, 903
Miniature pinscher	3+	ND	Narrow	557, 558
Miniature poodle	3+	ND	Open, Narrow	826, 835
Norwegian elkhound	3+	Familial	Narrow, Open, Goniodysgenesis	284, 350, 826, 835
Saluki	3+	ND	Goniodysgenesis	110
Samoyed	3+	Familial	Narrow, Goniodysgenesis	285, 557, 826, 835
Schnauzer, giant	3+	ND	Goniodysgenesis	557, 558
Schnauzer, miniature	<9	ND	Open, Narrow	692, 802
Sealyham terrier	3+	ND	Narrow	110, 903
Shih tzu	ND	ND	Narrow	835
Siberian husky	1+	Autosomal recessive suspected	Narrow, Goniodysgenesis	516, 766, 826, 835, 903
Standard poodle	3+	ND	Narrow	692
Toy poodle	6+	ND	Narrow	110, 558
Welsh springer spaniel	10 wk.–10 yrs.	Presumed autosomal dominant	Narrow, Goniodysgenesis	207, 350, 835
Welsh terrier	5+	ND	Narrow	903
West Highland white terrier	>5	ND	Open, melanosis	826
Wire fox terrier	<9	ND	Narrow	110, 692, 802

**ND = Not determined

result from toxins (including drugs), some from infection (e.g., chronic conjunctivitis), some from hypothyroidism, and some from abnormal immunologic reactions. The breeds most commonly affected with keratoconjunctivitis sicca (KCS) are:

American cocker spaniel (521, 909)
Bloodhound (909)
Boston terrier (1119)
Bull terrier (1119)
Chihuahua (1119)
Chinese pug (909)
Chinese shar pei (909)
Chow chow (520)
English bulldog (521)
English cocker spaniel (521, 909)
English setter (1119)
Gordon setter (1119)
Kerry blue terrier (1119)
Lhasa apso (521, 909)
Miniature dachshund (1119)
Miniature poodle (909)
Miniature schnauzer (909)
Pekingese (909)
Pug (520)
Sealyham terrier (520)
Shih tzu (521)
West Highland white terrier (909)
Yorkshire terrier (1119)

Most cases of KCS are immune-mediated, meaning that there is an abnormal immune response targeting the lacrimal glands. Regardless of cause, the condition should be recognized early and treated appropriately while it can still be corrected.

In keratoconjunctivitis sicca, the lack of corneal tear film results in patchy, dry areas on the corneal surface. The dried cornea, deprived of oxygen and nutrients from the tear film, rapidly undergoes destructive changes. This can result in brown pigmentation, scarring, ulceration, and growth of blood vessels on the surface of the eye. Mucus may accumulate in the eyes, and they then become painful and inflamed. The eyes are not necessarily observed to be "dry." With long-term loss of tears, vision is progressively lost because of "clouding" or opacification of the cornea, and the eyes may be permanently damaged.

Although the diagnosis of KCS is relatively straightforward, finding the underlying cause can be more difficult. The amount of tear film being produced can be measured with a Schirmer Tear Test. A thin strip of paper is placed inside the lower eyelid for 1 minute. It absorbs tears, which then can be measured to determine whether tear production is normal. Additional tests, such as antinuclear antibody (ANA) and rheumatoid factor (RF) tests, are typically run in a patient with KCS and no history of drug administration. The ANA and RF tests may be positive in 25%–30% of cases (504).

The goal of therapy is to restore or supplement tear production. This may be as basic as discontinuing a certain drug, or as sophisticated as using medications to restore normal tear production. Some surgical options reroute salivary ducts to provide saliva as a tear substitute. Antibiotics also may be necessary because the dry eye syndrome tends to promote the overgrowth of microbes on and around the eyes and in the mucus that accumulates.

Cyclosporine A has been extremely useful in arresting further loss of tear production in dogs with immune-mediated KCS (76, 186, 771, 865). The best responses are seen in dogs that have only mild or moderate tear loss, and breeds vary considerably in their responses to cyclosporine therapy. Cyclosporine should be used for at least 3 weeks before the long-term benefits are evaluated. Artificial tears may have to be applied to the eyes until tear production approaches normal levels. Pilocarpine, a drug used to treat glaucoma, is sometimes used in the management of KCS. It can be applied to the food and given orally, or it may be administered topically. Neither route seems to be consistently successful, and if too much drug is given, side effects might be observed.

A surgical option called parotid duct transposition is sometimes used with animals that do not respond to medical therapy. It involves surgically rerouting salivary ducts to the eye via a subcutaneous tunnel (51). In this way, saliva replaces tears in lubricating the eyes. Dogs that have had this procedure usually require little medication afterward. For dogs with immune KCS associated with salivary deficiency as well (known as Sjøgren's Syndrome in people), however, this option is not satisfactory.

Although keratoconjunctivitis sicca is believed to have a familial component, there is still no solid evidence that the trait is passed to future generations. Until more is known, though, affected animals should not be used for breeding. Information is insufficient to comment on the appropriateness of using the parents or siblings in a breeding program.

LENS LUXATION

Lens luxation refers to abnormal positioning of the lens and is often subdivided into partial (subluxation) or complete luxation depending on the extent of the process and whether the process is a primary or secondary event. Although the exact pathophysiology in not known, primary lens luxation is believed to be a heritable trait (293). In contrast, secondary lens luxation is not heritable and can result from a variety of other ocular diseases. Primary lens luxation is most commonly reported in the border collie, Brittany, Chinese shar pei, fox terrier (smooth and wire), Jack Russell terrier, miniature bull terrier, Sealyham terrier, Tibetan terrier, and Welsh terrier (293, 329, 350, 1002).

Although primary lens luxation is believed to be heritable, clinical problems are not typically detected until adulthood. The most common clinical signs include ocular pain, redness, corneal clouding, and blepharospasm of sudden onset. Complete ocular examination, with or without ultrasonography, allows confirmation of the diagnosis.

Treatment of lens luxation depends on the extent of damage. Control of intraocular pressure is critical, since glaucoma is a common sequel. Miotic therapy (e.g., pilocarpine) may be beneficial for mild cases, but lens extraction is the treatment of choice in most cases.

Affected animals should not be bred, but there is insufficient evidence on which to base more comprehensive breeding restrictions.

MICROPHTHALMIA

Microphthalmia denotes the condition of a congenitally small eye. In the Australian shepherd it is associated with merle coat color and a defect in retinal pigmented epithelium (RPE) development and seems to be inherited as an autosomal recessive trait with incomplete penetrance (350, 827, 1002). About 90% of cases also have heterochromia irides (344).

The condition has been reported to be familial in the Samoyed (827), Tibetan spaniel (903), and some collie lines (903). It is inherited as an autosomal recessive trait in the English toy spaniel (903) and in the West Highland white terrier (903). In the Doberman pinscher, it is associated with persistent hyperplastic tunica vasculosa lentis and persistent hyperplastic primary vitreous (193) and is believed to have an autosomal recessive form of inheritance (590). In the Akita, microphthalmia is associated with multiple defects such as cataracts, posterior lenticonus, and retinal dysplasia (350). In the Lakeland terrier and mastiff, the condition seems to be autosomal recessive and associated with persistent pupillary membranes (903). In the American cocker spaniel, beagle, borzoi, Cavalier King Charles spaniel, dachshund, Dalmatian, English springer spaniel, Irish terrier, Labrador retriever, Old English sheepdog, Portuguese water dog, St. Bernard, Siberian husky, and soft-coated wheaten terrier, microphthalmia is associated with multiple ocular anomalies (350, 1119). In the standard poodle, it can occur alone or with cataracts, persistent pupillary membranes, and keratopathy (350, 903, 1061, 1119). In the miniature schnauzer, microphthalmia and congenital cataracts are inherited together as an autosomal recessive trait (193, 350).

Cataract and microphthalmia has also been reported in a litter of Russian terriers (609). In the collie, dachshund, and Great Dane, there is an association between microphthalmia, partial albinism, and deafness (350). This condition has also been reported in the Bedlington terrier, Dalmatian, Great Dane, miniature and toy poodles, rottweiler, and West Highland white terrier (1119).

Clinically, the condition is not hard to identify because the eye appears small and the third eyelid is quite prominent. Entropion can occur and brush up against the cornea, causing irritation and ulceration. Often, an accumulation of discharge is apparent because of the space created between the small eye and the conjunctivae. Although the diagnosis can be made visually, it is important to look for associated abnormalities (34).

Microphthalmia obviously has no cure. Periodic flushing of the conjunctival sac is usually adequate for removing accumulated discharge. If the lids brushing up against it chronically traumatize the cornea, it may have to be removed surgically or the eyelids surgically altered. Genetic counseling should be individualized for each breed condition, as described above.

OPTIC NERVE COLOBOMAS

Optic nerve colobomas are pits on the optic disc, most often associated with collie eye anomaly or the multiple ocular anomalies as seen in the Australian shepherd (348) and basenji (365). The condition is also seen in the American cocker spaniel and Labrador retriever (903). Affected animals should not be bred.

OPTIC NERVE HYPOPLASIA AND MICROPAPILLA

Optic nerve hypoplasia is a congenital underdevelopment of the optic nerve, causing blindness, and micropapilla is a small optic disk not associated with blindness. Optic nerve hypoplasia seems to be inherited, but a mode of transmission has not been determined in most breeds. In the miniature poodle, the condition is transmitted as an autosomal recessive trait (187). Optic nerve aplasia, the complete absence of an optic nerve, has been reported in the poodle (1108). Table 11-5 presents these conditions, along with the breeds in which they appear.

Diagnosis is made by indirect or direct ophthalmoscopy, and evaluating pupillary light responses. No treatments are available for any of the conditions, but they are not progressive.

Because optic nerve hypoplasia and aplasia are believed to be inherited, affected animals should not be bred. In the miniature poodle, if not other breeds, both parents should be considered obligate carriers and apparently unaffected siblings should be considered as suspect carriers. Insufficient information is available on micropapilla in other breeds to make breeding recommendations.

PANNUS

Pannus, also known as chronic superficial keratitis, refers to a condition in which pigment and blood vessels grow across the cornea, appearing like a dark film (Figure 11-2). The cause of the condition is still a matter of much debate. It is believed that genetics may play some role, at least in the German shepherd dog (527), Belgian Tervuren (879), dachshund (1119), and greyhound (527), but studies have not shown how the condition passes from generation to generation. An autosomal recessive mode of inheritance has been postulated but not proven for the German shepherd dog (903). Other breeds affected include the Airedale, Australian

Table 11-5 Optic Nerve Hypoplasia and Micropapilla

Breed	Condition	Reference
Afghan	Optic nerve hypoplasia	903
American cocker spaniel	Optic nerve hypoplasia	1119
Beagle	Micropapilla	1119
Beagle	Optic nerve hypoplasia	187, 365, 1119
Belgian sheepdog	Micropapilla	1108
Belgian Tervuren	Micropapilla	903, 1108, 1119
Borzoi	Optic nerve hypoplasia	85, 903
Collie	Optic nerve hypoplasia	365, 1108, 1119
Dachshund	Micropapilla	1108
Dachshund	Optic nerve hypoplasia	365, 1108, 1119
English cocker spaniel	Optic nerve hypoplasia	1108
English springer spaniel	Optic nerve hypoplasia	1119
Flat-coated retriever	Micropapilla	903
German shepherd dog	Optic nerve hypoplasia	365, 1108, 1119
German shepherd dog	Micropapilla	903
Golden retriever	Micropapilla	903
Golden retriever	Optic nerve hypoplasia	1119
Gordon setter	Micropapilla	903
Great Pyrenees	Optic nerve hypoplasia	365, 461
Greyhound	Optic nerve hypoplasia	1119
Irish setter	Optic nerve hypoplasia	1119
Irish wolfhound	Micropapilla	1108
Keeshond	Optic nerve hypoplasia	1119
Labrador retriever	Optic nerve hypoplasia	903
Labrador retriever	Micropapilla	903
Miniature poodle	Micropapilla	1108
Miniature poodle	Optic nerve hypoplasia	365, 1108, 1119
Miniature poodle	Optic nerve aplasia	1108
Miniature schnauzer	Optic nerve hypoplasia	85, 1119
Norfolk terrier	Micropapilla	903
Old English sheepdog	Micropapilla	903
Old English sheepdog	Optic nerve hypoplasia	903
Pekingese	Optic nerve hypoplasia	85
Puli	Micropapilla	903
Russian wolfhound	Optic nerve hypoplasia	187, 365
St. Bernard	Optic nerve hypoplasia	187, 365
Shetland sheepdog	Optic nerve hypoplasia	1119
Soft-coated wheaten terrier	Optic nerve hypoplasia	1119
Standard poodle	Optic nerve hypoplasia	1119
Tibetan spaniel	Micropapilla	903
Toy poodle	Micropapilla	1108
Toy poodle	Optic nerve hypoplasia	377, 1108, 1119
Whippet	Micropapilla	903

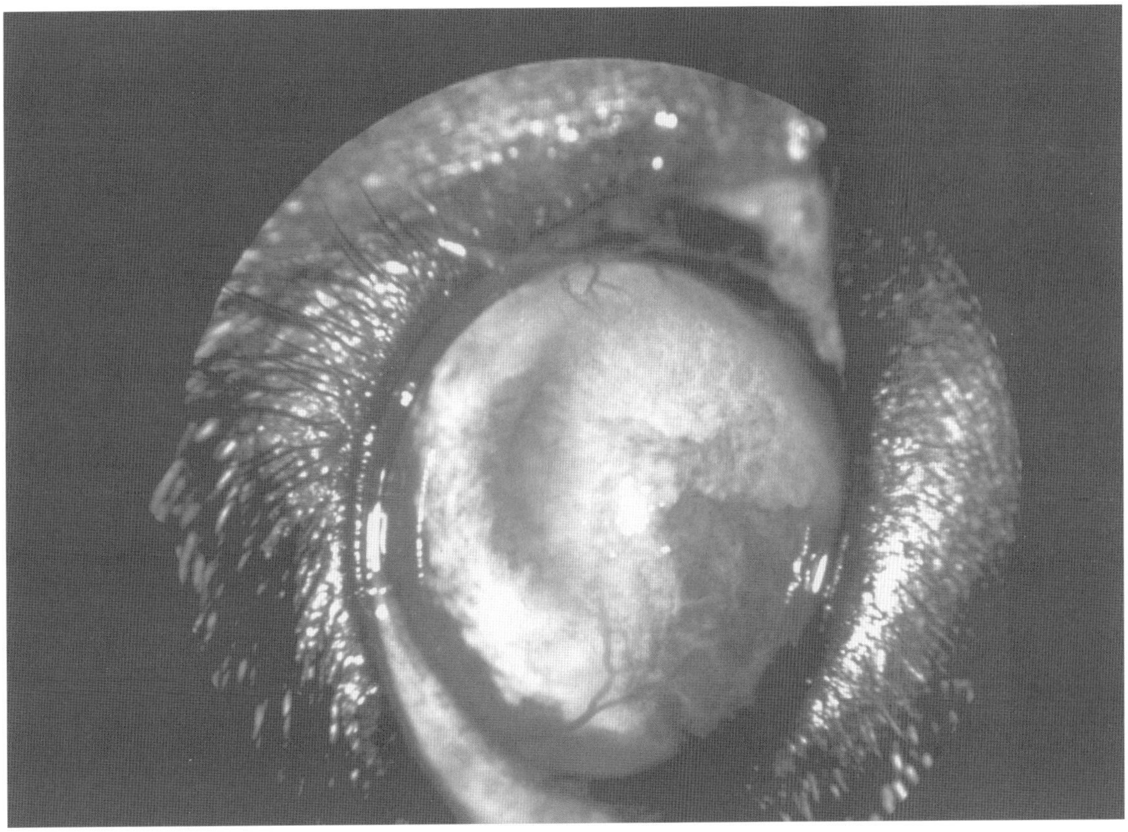

Figure 11-2 Pannus
Courtesy of Dr. Dan Lavach, Eye Clinic for Animals, Garden Grove, California

shepherd, Belgian sheepdog, border collie, Dalmatian, English pointer, miniature pinscher, and Siberian husky (344, 879, 903).

Dogs living at elevations higher than 5,000 feet are more likely to develop pannus, and this risk increases with increasing altitude (879). The roles of ultraviolet light and immune reactivity are being considered. A recent European study found virus-like particles in the eyes of affected dogs, but actual viruses could not be recovered (861). Most researchers now believe that pannus results from a genetic susceptibility to environmental factors that culminates in an immune-mediated inflammatory process (185).

In most cases, the condition involves dark pigment infiltrating the clear cornea, usually starting at the outer edge and moving inward. In time, blood vessels grow into the cornea where none existed previously. The end result is a dark, scarring eye disease, which, fortunately, is not usually too painful.

Although diagnosis is not difficult, consultation with a veterinary ophthalmologist may be warranted when considering treatment options. Some owners have even had opticians customize UV-protecting clear polycarbonate sunglasses for their pets. Commercial varieties are also available (e.g., Doggles™). Topical cyclosporine seems to be the best medical treatment option (865).

Affected dogs should ideally not be used for breeding even though genetic studies have not yet proven that the condition is heritable. The Institute for Genetic Disease Control in Animals (GDC) maintains an open registry of inherited eye diseases for all breeds, which includes pannus for the Belgian sheepdogs (Groenendael, Belgian Tervuren, Belgian Malinois, and Belgian Laeken).

PERSISTENT PRIMARY VITREOUS

Persistent primary vitreous (persistent hyperplastic tunica vasculosa lentis and persistent hyperplastic primary vitreous) refers to vascular remnants of the hyaloid artery or primary vitreous that persist (1001). It is an inherited trait in the Bouvier des Flandres (mode of inheritance unknown), Doberman pinscher (multiple locus inheritance pattern postulated), and Staffordshire bull terrier (mode of inheritance unknown), and usually is detected during the first year of life (293, 350, 365, 584). A breed predisposition has been suggested in the English toy spaniel (903), Siberian husky (798), Staffordshire bull terrier (903), and standard schnauzer (365). The condition often causes visual impairment and may be associated with other ophthalmic anomalies, such as lens colobomas, microphakia, and hemorrhage behind or within the lens.

The heritability is not known in most affected breeds (827). In the Bouvier des Flandres, the condition is associated with retinal dysplasia and detachment, optic nerve hypoplasia, lenticonus, cataract, and congenital blindness (350). In the bloodhound, persistent hyperplastic tunica vasculosa lentis and persistent hyperplastic primary vitreous can be associated with multiple ocular anomalies (1076). In the Irish setter, Labrador retriever, and soft-coated wheaten terrier, a persistent hyaloid artery can persist as a vascular strand or as a nonvascular remnant (350). Other affected breeds include the German shorthaired pointer (350), Labrador retriever (350), basset hound (1077), and Siberian husky (798).

The diagnosis is confirmed by slit lamp biomicroscopy, indirect ophthalmoscopy, and/or ultrasonography (69). Affected animals should not be used for breeding.

PERSISTENT PUPILLARY MEMBRANES

Persistent pupillary membranes (PPM) are remnants of fetal eye tissue that, before birth, cover the pupil and provide a blood supply for the developing lens. Typically this tissue disappears after birth, and certainly before 4 to 5 weeks of age. PPM is seen most commonly in the Australian cattle dog, Australian shepherd, basenji, bichon frisé, Cardigan Welsh corgi, collie, chow chow, Doberman pinscher, mastiff, miniature longhaired dachshund, Pembroke Welsh corgi, Scottish terrier, and standard poodle, but the mode of inheritance is still undefined (229, 350, 903, 1119). In the Australian shepherd, persistent pupillary membranes are believed to be inherited as an autosomal recessive trait (1119).

Clinically, PPM appears as strands of tissue visible within the eye and typically spanning the pupil. Most don't cause problems unless the strands are large or numerous, in which case they can interfere with vision. If the strands connect the iris to either the cornea or the lens, other vision problems may result, as well as pigment deposition on the cornea or lens. In many breeds, iris-to-iris PPM is classified as a "breeder option" because there is no evidence that this condition is hereditary. In other breeds, such as the basenji, chow chow, mastiff, Pembroke Welsh corgi, and Yorkshire terrier, in which PPM is known or strongly suspected to be inherited, affected animals will not receive certification and breeding them is discouraged (350). The condition in some breeds, such as the collie, English cocker spaniel, Labrador retriever, miniature bull terrier, Nova Scotia duck tolling retriever, Samoyed, and West Highland white terrier, is serious, with visual impairment commonplace, yet the American College of Veterinary Ophthalmologists still considers perpetuation as a breeder option.

The diagnosis is straightforward, and clinicians will want to trace the origins of the strands to the iris collarette. Even though few other congenital anomalies can be mistaken for PPM, it is important to carefully evaluate for other potential congenital eye disorders that might be associated with PPM.

In most cases, PPM requires no treatment unless it interferes with vision or is causing damage to the lens or cornea. In these extreme cases, surgery (synechiotomy, cataract extraction, and synechiotomy) may be performed to correct the situation. Severely affected animals should not be used for breeding. At this point, insufficient information is available on which to base breeding recommendations for parents and siblings.

PROGRESSIVE RETINAL ATROPHY, CENTRAL (CPRA)

Central progressive retinal atrophy is a disorder of retinal pigmented epithelium resulting in progressive retinal degeneration and photoreceptor degeneration. The condition is believed to be inherited as an autosomal dominant trait (with variable expressivity) in the border collie (1108), Labrador retriever (1108), and Shetland sheepdog (827), and as an autosomal recessive trait in the briard, English springer spaniel, golden retriever, and Irish setter (903, 1108). Other breeds affected include the black and tan coonhound, boxer, Cardigan Welsh corgi, Chesapeake Bay retriever, collie, English cocker spaniel, English setter, German shepherd dog, keeshond, pointer, red bone coonhound, and Shetland sheepdog (222, 724, 903, 1108, 1119).

The condition is reported most commonly in Great Britain, and few cases are documented in the United States. The condition bears some resemblance to retinal degeneration associated with vitamin E deficiency (230). Clinically, most dogs develop problems with day vision between 1.5 and 3.5 years of age, which can progress to total blindness. Retinal changes are seen early in the disease. Late in the course of the disease, it is impossible to distinguish between central and generalized PRA. The electroretinogram (ERG) remains normal until late in the course of the disease. Affected animals should not be used for breeding, and parents and siblings should be considered for breeding based upon the breed-specific modes of inheritance described above.

PROGRESSIVE RETINAL ATROPHY, GENERALIZED (PRA)

Progressive retinal atrophy (PRA) refers to several inherited disorders affecting the retina and resulting in blindness. PRA is thought to be inherited, with each breed demonstrating a specific age of onset and pattern of inheritance. For example, a blind collie with PRA (*rcd2*) bred to a blind Irish setter with PRA (*rcd1*) will produce pups with eyesight but as carriers for both forms of the disorder. The condition is potentially even more confusing because certain breeds may be prone to more than one form of PRA. For example, in the collie, both early-onset and late-onset forms of PRA have been recognized.

In the Irish setter, the gene mutation (W807X) causes the protein the gene produces to be shorter than normal, and nonfunctional, consequently resulting in retinal atrophy. The gene involved is the beta-subunit of cyclic guanosine monophosphate (GMP) phosphodiesterase, which encodes a protein of the visual transduction cascade (299, 833). Identification of the mutation has allowed the development of molecular tests that can detect normal, carrier, and affected individuals (863) with virtual certainty. In Cardigan Welsh corgis, the gene involved is the alpha-subunit of cyclic GMP phosphodiesterase, and DNA tests also allow precise diagnosis. It is hoped that this same technology will soon be used to determine the causes and allow diagnostic testing for PRA in other breeds. A marker linked to progressive rod-cone degeneration (*prcd*), which is similar to retinitis pigmentosa in humans, has been discovered and a DNA linkage-based test has been developed for applicable breeds (8, 397, 833).

Progressive retinal atrophy affects many breeds of dogs, each in a specific manner. Some breeds at increased risk include the Akita, Cairn terrier, collie, cocker spaniel, dachshund, golden retriever, Irish setter, Labrador retriever, miniature poodle, miniature schnauzer, Norwegian elkhound, and Samoyed. Because incidence data are not available in most cases, determining the exact prevalence of PRA in some breeds is difficult.

All of the conditions described as progressive retinal atrophy have one thing in common: progressive atrophy or degeneration of the retinal tissue. Visual impairment occurs slowly but progressively. Therefore, animals often adapt to their reduced vision until it is compromised to near blindness. Because of this, owners may not notice any visual impairment until the condition has progressed significantly.

Three of the early onset forms of PRA—*rcd1* in Irish setters, *rcd2* in collies, and *erd* in Norwegian elkhounds—are known to represent different, nonallelic, gene mutations (5, 7). Progressive rod-cone degeneration (*prcd*) is a late-onset form of PRA that has been identified in at least five breeds of dog (American and English cocker spaniels, miniature poodle, Labrador retriever, Portuguese water dog) and is known to be a mutation of the same, as yet unidentified, gene (5). X-linked PRA in Siberian huskies is the only form of PRA so far discovered to be transmitted as an X-linked trait. Miniature schnauzers have yet another form of PRA called photoreceptor dysplasia (PD). Affected dogs have defects in the differentiation of rods and cones after birth. The result is rapid degeneration of the rods and cones, although they maintain their vision longer than other breeds. Borzois develop a unique focal degeneration of the retina that seems to be transmitted as an autosomal recessive trait (171).

In most breeds, the exact type of PRA has not been determined. In at least one study (340), PRA in poodles seemed to be associated with coat color, to the extent that the incidence of PRA in poodles of darker color is higher than in poodles with a lighter coat color (339).

Because of the many different forms of PRA reported, PRA is subdivided further based on age of onset and pattern of progression. In its broadest terms, PRA variants can be described as early-onset or late-onset, although the distinction is somewhat arbitrary. In early-onset forms, night blindness is present from birth and total blindness occurs at 1 to 5 years of age. In late-onset forms, night blindness occurs after 1 year of age and total blindness occurs somewhat later. There is also considerable overlap with funduscopic examination. With electroretinography, in the early-onset forms, rod dysfunction is present at birth. Given all of these different overlapping criteria, it is good to know that DNA testing is capable of detecting not just affected animals but also carriers and normal individuals with near certainty.

The disease manifests in different ways in different breeds. For example, rough collies usually develop rod-cone dysplasia (type 2) before they are

1 year of age. The dogs are often night-blind by 6 weeks of age and functionally blind by 6 to 8 months of age. The miniature poodle develops a rod-cone degeneration, typically starting as night blindness, at 3–5 years of age. In between, the Norwegian elkhound may develop rod dysplasia and cone degeneration, with night-blindness evident by 6 weeks of age and day vision preserved until 2 to 3 years of age. Because progressive retinal atrophy differs with each breed, recommendations for ophthalmic evaluation differ for each breed.

Clinically, changes to the eyes rarely can be seen externally. That's what makes the condition so pernicious. In time, dogs will become blind, and then the condition is obvious. In early stages of PRA, night blindness occurs first (except in the greyhound). Affected dogs may have difficulty navigating at night or once the lights have been turned off. With progression, some pet owners may notice a characteristic shine from the eye, as a result of increased reflectivity of the back of the eye. Because dogs have many other well-developed senses, such as smell and hearing, their lack of sight is usually not evident immediately. The loss of vision is slow, but progressive, and blindness eventually results. Table 11-6 lists the breeds along with the forms, onset, and mode of inheritance.

PRA can be diagnosed in three ways:

1. Direct visualization of the retina
2. Electroretinography (ERG)
3. DNA testing.

An ophthalmoscope can be used to visualize the retinal tissue for characteristic changes. Use of indirect ophthalmoscopy requires a great deal of training and expertise. When viewing the retina with this instrument, one frequently can see changes in the pattern of retinal blood vessels, the optic nerve, and the reflective tapetum that provides "eye shine." In some breeds, however, the early changes may not be clearly visible and the eyes may appear normal until later stages of the disease. Cataracts may form as a consequence of progressive retinal atrophy in some dogs, especially late in the course of the disease. These cataracts may interfere with direct visualization of the retina and thereby confound an accurate diagnosis. Fortunately, other diagnostic options are available.

An additional highly sensitive test is electroretinography (ERG) , which measures electrical patterns in the retina in the same way that an electrocardiogram (ECG) measures electrical activity of the heart. The procedure is painless but usually is available only from specialty centers. Pattern ERGs are sensitive enough to detect even the early onset of disease (540). Although heterozygotes that appear "normal" usually cannot be distinguished, one study demonstrated impaired retinal function in young Labrador retrievers heterozygous for late-onset rod-cone degeneration (541).

Genetic testing is the future for diagnosing PRA. To date, only *rcd1* PRA in Irish setters and early-onset PRA in Cardigan Welsh corgis is detectable by direct DNA tests, but the search is on for other genes and other forms of PRA in different breeds. Progressive rod-cone degeneration (prcd) can be detected by marker testing in several different breeds. A random amplified polymorphic DNA (RAPD) marker linked to prcd has already been detected (398).

No treatment is available for progressive retinal atrophy. Fortunately, PRA is not a painful condition and dogs do have other keen senses upon which they can depend. In time, they will acclimate to their living environment and can do quite well with their owners' help. They can continue to go for walks, albeit always on a lead or halter. Indoors, they are usually fine, especially if owners are content not to constantly rearrange the furniture.

There has been much speculation about the role of nutrition in managing PRA in dogs. Undoubtedly this is because research has determined that taurine retinopathy in cats, a related condition, can be managed successfully with taurine supplementation. Other research in dogs has shown that vitamin E deficiency can result in conditions similar to PRA. At this time, however, no association has been made between any nutrient (or drug, for that matter) and the successful resolution of PRA. Once the genetics of PRA become known with certainty in breeds, gene therapy may be a possible mode of therapy. For example, in affected dogs, it may be possible to introduce a virus into the back of the eye that carries the normal gene so the retina does not atrophy.

Identification of affected breeding animals is essential to prevent the condition from spreading within the breed. Potential breeding dogs from breeds at increased risk should be examined annually by a veterinary ophthalmologist. Ideally, pups should be screened at 6 to 8 weeks of age, before being sold. Screening exams that don't involve DNA testing are not a sensitive method for early detection in many breeds. The Institute for Genetic Disease Control in Animals (GDC) maintains an open registry of inherited eye diseases for all breeds.

Table 11-6 Progressive Retinal Atrophy

Breed	Form	Onset (years)	Inheritance	Reference
Afghan	early-onset	2	ND	903, 1122
Airedale	early-onset	2	Recessive?	903, 1122
Akita	early-onset	1–3	ND	724, 903, 1122
Alaskan malamute	early–mid-onset	2–4	Recessive?	903, 1119
American cocker spaniel	prcd	2–3; 5	Autosomal recessive	5, 724, 1122
American Staffordshire terrier	early-onset	1.5	ND	1122
Australian cattle dog	late-onset (prcd?)	3–5; 6	Autosomal recessive?	5, 350, 903, 1122
Australian kelpi	early-onset	1.5+	ND	903
Australian shepherd	early/late-onset	2–7	ND	1119, 1122
Australian terrier	early-onset	1–5	Recessive suspected	903, 1122
Basenji	prcd?	2–6	ND	903, 1122
Basset hound	late-onset	3; 6–8	ND	903, 1122
Beagle	mid–late-onset	3–5; 10–13	Autosomal recessive	1119, 1122
Bearded collie	early-onset	1	ND	903, 1122
Bedlington terrier	early-onset	1.5	ND	903, 1122
Belgian Malinois	late-onset	ND	ND	5
Belgian sheepdog	ND	ND	Autosomal recessive?	350, 1122
Belgian Tervuren	mid-onset	3–5	ND	1122
Bernese mountain dog	early-onset	1	ND	903, 1122
Black and tan coonhound	early-onset	1.5	ND	903, 1122
Border collie	early-onset	2–5	ND	1119, 1122
Border terrier	ND	ND	ND	903, 1122
Borzoi	Focal retinal degeneration	0.5	Autosomal recessive?	171, 724, 827, 903, 1122
Boston terrier	late-onset	5+	ND	903, 1122
Boxer	mid/late-onset	3+	ND	903, 1122
Briard	prcd	4	ND	350
Briard	rped	0.2	ND	595, 903
Brittany spaniel	late-onset	4	ND	903, 1122
Brussels griffon	late-onset	4–9	ND	1122
Bull terrier	ND	ND	ND	1122
Cairn terrier	early-onset	1	Recessive	724, 1119, 1122
Cavalier King Charles spaniel	early-onset	1–5	ND	1122
Chesapeake Bay retriever	prcd	0.75–1; 4–7	ND	350, 1122
Chihuahua	late-onset	7–8	ND	903, 1122
Chow chow	early-onset	0.5	Familial	1119, 1122
Collie, rough & smooth	rcd2	0.5	Autosomal recessive	5, 724, 1122
Collie	late-onset	5–7	ND	350, 1122
Curly-coated retriever	late-onset	3–5	ND	903, 1122
Dachshund, miniature longhaired	early-onset	0.5–1	Autosomal recessive	5, 182, 224, 724, 1122

(continued on next page)

Table 11-6 Progressive Retinal Atrophy (continued)

Breed	Form	Onset	Inheritance	Reference
Dachshund	late-onset	4	Recessive suspected	1119, 1122
Dalmatian	late-onset	4–7	ND	903, 1122
Doberman pinscher	early-onset	1	ND	903, 1122
English cocker spaniel	prcd	4	Autosomal recessive	5, 724, 1122
English setter	early/late-onset	1.5; 7–8	ND	5, 724, 903, 1122
English springer spaniel	early/late-onset	2; 5	ND	724, 903, 1122
Entlebucher mountain dog	rod/cone abiotrophy	3	Autosomal recessive	997, 1002
Field spaniel	late-onset	4	ND	903, 1122
German shepherd dog	early-onset	1.5	ND	724, 1122
Giant schnauzer	late-onset	3–4	ND	903, 1122
Golden retriever	early-onset	2	ND	724, 1122
Gordon setter	early-onset	.3–1	Autosomal recessive	222, 724, 827, 1122
Great Dane	early-onset	0.5–2	ND	903, 1122
Greyhound	Retinal degeneration	1.5	ND	350, 724, 827, 1122
Irish setter	rcd1	.25; 4–5	Autosomal recessive	5, 724, 1122
Irish setter	late-onset	4–10	Sex-linked?	903
Irish terrier	ND	ND	ND	1122
Irish water spaniel	adult onset	5+	ND	903, 1122
Italian greyhound	early-onset (prcd?)	2–4	ND	350, 903
Japanese chin	ND	ND	ND	1122
Keeshond	late-onset	4–5	ND	724, 1122
Kerry blue terrier	late-onset	5–6	ND	903, 1122
Labrador retriever	prcd	4	Autosomal recessive	5, 1122
Lhasa apso	early/late-onset	2–5; 10	ND	903, 1122
Maltese	early/late onset	2–5; 10	ND	1122
Manchester terrier	late-onset	5+	ND	1122
Mastiff	prcd	2	Autosomal recessive?	802
Miniature pinscher	late-onset	5+	ND	903, 1122
Miniature schnauzer	pd	3–5	Autosomal recessive	5, 724, 1122
Miniature schnauzer	late-onset	10–13	ND	1122
Norwegian elkhound	rd	0.5	Autosomal recessive	5, 724, 1122
Norwegian elkhound	erd	0.25	Autosomal recessive	5, 724, 1122
Nova Scotia duck tolling retriever	late-onset (prcd?)	3–5	ND	5, 1122
Old English sheepdog	late-onset	4–6	ND	903, 1122
Papillon	late-onset (prcd?)	5–6	Autosomal recessive	350, 408, 757
Pekingese	late-onset	5–6	ND	903, 1122
Pit bull terrier	ND	ND	ND	1122

(continued on next page)

Table 11-6 Progressive Retinal Atrophy (continued)

Breed	Form	Onset	Inheritance	Reference
Pointer	late-onset	5–6	ND	724, 903, 1122
Pomeranian	late-onset	5–6	ND	903, 1122
Poodle, miniature	prcd	3–5	Autosomal recessive	5, 724, 1122
Poodle, miniature	hemeralopia		ND	724
Poodle, standard	late-onset	5–6	Recessive suspected	1119
Portuguese water dog	prcd	3–6	Autosomal recessive	5, 350
Puli	late-onset	9–10	ND	1122
Queensland blue heeler	ND	ND	ND	1122
Rottweiler	early/late-onset	3	ND	5, 1122
Saluki	early-onset	2	ND	724, 1122
Samoyed	early/late-onset	3–5	Recessive suspected	724, 1119, 1122
Schipperke	late-onset	5–6	Recessive suspected; X-linked?	903, 1122
Scottish terrier	ND	ND	ND	903, 1122
Sealyham terrier	late-onset	5–6	ND	1122
Shetland sheepdog	early- and late-onset	2–3; 5–6	ND	903, 1122
Shih tzu	late-onset	5–6	ND	1122
Siberian husky	XLPRA	2–3; 5–6	X-linked	5, 6, 724, 1122
Silky terrier	late-onset	5+	ND	903, 1122
Smooth fox terrier	early-onset	2	ND	903
Soft-coated wheaten terrier	early-onset	1–2	ND	903, 1122
Swiss hound	ND	ND	ND	724, 1122
Tibetan spaniel	late-onset	3–7	Autosomal recessive	5, 60
Tibetan terrier	PRA	0.9–4	Autosomal recessive	5, 702, 724, 1122
Tibetan terrier	Night blindness	1–4	ND	350, 1119
Toy Havanese	ND	ND	ND	1122
Vizsla	early/late-onset	3–6	ND	903, 1122
Welsh corgi, Cardigan	early-onset	1	Autosomal recessive	350, 724, 1119, 1122
Welsh corgi, Pembroke	late-onset	5–6	ND	1122
Welsh springer spaniel	late-onset	5–7	ND	903, 1119
Whippet	late-onset	5+	ND	903, 1122
Wire fox terrier	rped	2	Autosomal recessive suspected	169, 903, 1122
Yorkshire terrier	late-onset	5–11	ND	724, 1119, 1122

erd = early retinal degeneration; pd = photoreceptor degeneration; PRA = progressive retinal atrophy; prcd = progressive rod-cone degeneration; rcd1 = rod cone dysplasia 1; rcd2 = rod cone dysplasia 2; XLPRA = X-linked progressive retinal atrophy; rped = retinal pigmented epithelium dystrophy; ND = not determined.

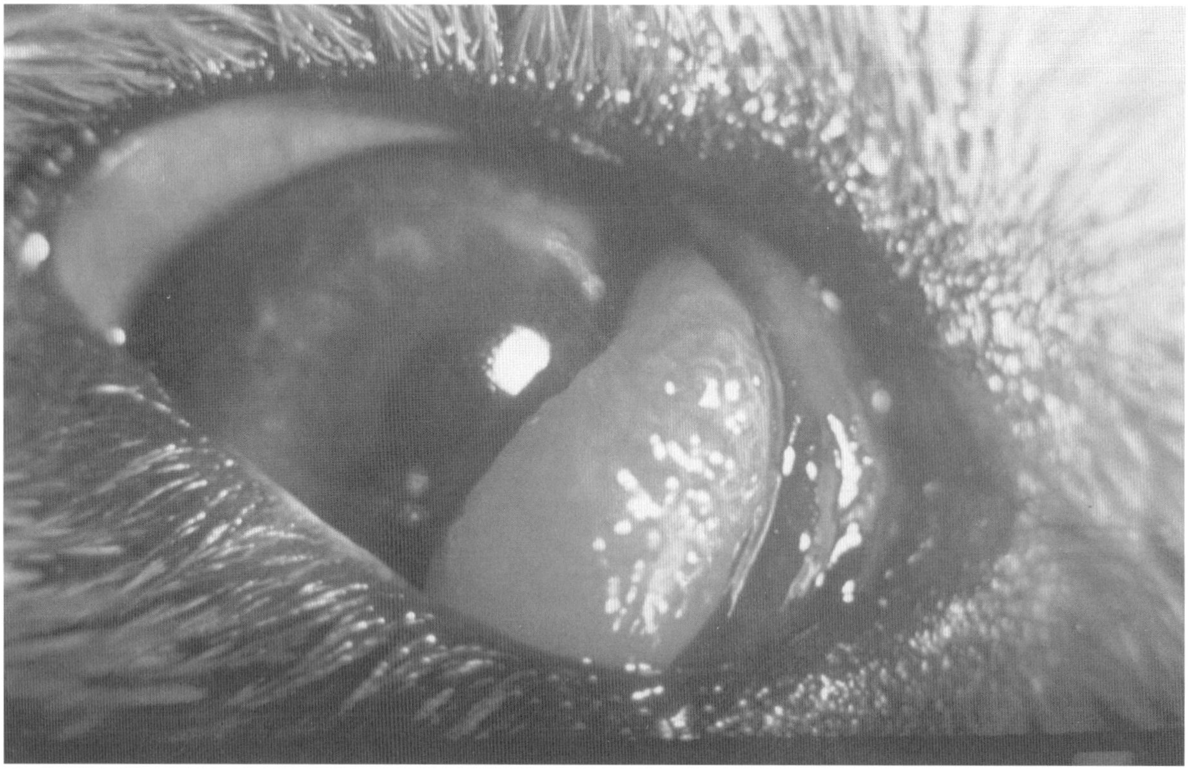

Figure 11-3 Prolapsed gland of the nictitans
Courtesy of Dr. Dan Lavach, Eye Clinic for Animals, Garden Grove, California

PROLAPSED GLAND OF THE NICTITANS (CHERRY EYE)

Prolapsed gland of the nictitans (which breeders frequently call "cherry eye" or "haw") refers to an enlarged gland at the base of the nictitating membrane that is displaced from its normal position (Figure 11-3). It is seen as a red mass above the margin of the nictitating membrane. It is seen commonly in the American cocker spaniel (722, 734), basset hound (722), beagle (722, 903, 1119), bloodhound (350), Boston terrier (722, 903), boxer (1119), bull terrier (903), Chinese shar pei (722), English bulldog (722, 734), Lhasa apso (722, 734), miniature poodle (722), Neapolitan mastiff (1119), St. Bernard (903), and shih tzu, as well as other breeds. Although there seems to be a clear-cut breed predisposition, a heritable nature has not been proven. Most dogs are quite young when this condition develops, and both eyes can be affected simultaneously.

The old treatment for prolapsed gland of the nictitans was to surgically remove it. Now it is known that this gland produces a significant amount of tear film, so it should be preserved whenever possible. Most surgeries today conserve the gland and "tack it down" into its normal location. The problem can recur with any of the surgical techniques, at which time the surgery will have to be repeated. There is insufficient information on which to base breeding recommendations.

RETINAL DYSPLASIA

Retinal dysplasia is an abnormal development of the retina, which is evident at birth. Invagination of the outer retinal layers affects retinal function and vision, depending on the amount of retina affected (1108). Abnormal arrangements of neural cells can occur in the retina, resulting in folding, palisading, or clustering of focal areas of neuroretina, which can cause visual impairment and blindness (724). Retinal folds are considered the mildest form of the condition.

In some breeds, such as the Labrador retriever, German shepherd dog, and Samoyed, the condition is associated with skeletal achondrodysplasia (855, 1108). Studies in the Labrador retriever and Samoyed suggest that the syndrome is caused by one abnormal gene, which has recessive effects on the skeleton and incompletely dominant effects on the eye (155, 350, 855). In most breeds, the inheritance of retinal dysplasia alone is believed to be autosomal recessive (1108). Retinal dysplasia also

Table 11-7 Retinal Dysplasia

Breed	Extent	Inheritance	Reference
Afghan	Detachment	ND	1108
Airedale terrier	Detachment	ND	1108
Akita	Multifocal folds, geographic, detachment	ND	903, 1119
American cocker spaniel	Multifocal folds	Autosomal recessive	724, 1108
American water spaniel	Multifocal folds	ND	903, 1119
Australian shepherd	Multifocal folds	Associated with color dilution	724, 1108
Australian terrier	Multifocal folds	Recessive suspected	903, 1119
Basenji	Detachment, optic disk colobomas	ND	724, 903
Beagle	Multifocal folds	ND	724, 1108
Bearded collie	Multifocal folds, detachment	ND	1108
Bedlington terrier	Vitreoretinal dysplasia, multifocal folds, geographic, detachment	Autosomal recessive	350, 724, 827, 1108
Belgian Malinois	Multifocal folds	ND	350
Belgian sheepdog	Multifocal folds	ND	1119
Bichon frisé	Multifocal folds	ND	350
Border collie	Multifocal folds, geographic, detachment	Autosomal recessive suspected	903, 1108
Border terrier	multifocal folds	ND	903, 1119
Borzoi	Retinal degeneration	Familial?	350, 724, 1119
Brittany	Multifocal folds	Recessive suspected	903
Bull mastiff	Multifocal folds	Recessive suspected	903, 1108
Cairn terrier	Multifocal folds, geographic	Autosomal recessive	903
Cavalier King Charles spaniel	Multifocal folds, geographic	ND	1108
Chesapeake Bay retriever	Multifocal folds, geographic	ND	903, 1119
Clumber spaniel	Multifocal folds	ND	350
Collie	Multifocal folds	ND	903, 1108
Dachshund	Detachment	ND	724, 903
Doberman pinscher	Multifocal folds	ND	903, 1108
English bulldog	Multifocal folds	ND	903, 1108
English cocker spaniel	Multifocal folds	ND	1108
English springer spaniel	Multifocal folds, geographic, detachment	Autosomal recessive	724, 827, 1108
English toy spaniel	Multifocal folds	ND	1119
Field spaniel	Multifocal folds	ND	350, 903, 1119
German shepherd dog	Multifocal folds	ND	1108
German wirehaired pointer	Multifocal folds	ND	1119
Giant schnauzer	Multifocal folds	ND	903
Golden retriever	Multifocal folds, geographic, detachment	ND	1108
Gordon setter	Multifocal folds	ND	350

(continued on next page)

Table 11-7 Retinal Dysplasia (continued)

Breed	Extent	Inheritance	Reference
Great Dane	Dysplasia	Associated with Harlequin	1119
Havanese, toy	Detachment	ND	1119
Irish wolfhound	Geographic	ND	1108
Labrador retriever	Multifocal folds, geographic, detachment	Autosomal recessive	724, 827, 855, 1108
Maltese	Multifocal folds	ND	1119
Mastiff	Multifocal folds	ND	1108
Newfoundland	Multifocal folds	ND	1108
Norwegian elkhound	Multifocal folds	ND	350, 1108
Old English sheepdog	Multifocal folds	ND	350, 1108
Petite basset griffon vendeen	Multifocal folds	ND	350, 1108
Poodle (miniature and toy)	Detachment	ND	1119
Poodle, standard	Multifocal folds	ND	903
Puli	Multifocal folds	ND	1108
Rottweiler	Multifocal folds, detachment	ND	724, 1108
St. Bernard	Multifocal folds	ND	724
Samoyed	Multifocal folds, geographic	ND	724, 1108
Schnauzer, giant	Multifocal folds	ND	1108
Schnauzer, miniature	Multifocal folds	ND	724
Schnauzer, standard	Multifocal folds	ND	1108
Shetland sheepdog	Multifocal folds	ND	1119
Sealyham terrier	Multifocal folds, geographic, detachment	Autosomal recessive	724, 827, 1108
Shih tzu	Detachment	ND	1119
Siberian husky	Multifocal folds	ND	1119
Soft-coated wheaten terrier	Multifocal folds	ND	350, 1108
Sussex spaniel	Multifocal folds	ND	903
Tibetan terrier	Multifocal folds	Familial	903, 1108
Welsh corgi, Cardigan	Multifocal folds	ND	724, 1108
Welsh corgi, Pembroke	Multifocal folds, geographic	ND	1108
West Highland white terrier	Multifocal folds, detached	ND	350, 1119
Whippet	Vitreous degeneration	ND	350
Yorkshire terrier	Geographic, detachment	Recessive suspected	724, 1108, 1119

can occur as a secondary event to viral infections, irradiation, certain drugs, and intrauterine trauma (701). Table 11-7 lists the breeds involved along with the variation and hereditary factors.

The condition is congenital and is best documented at 12 to 16 weeks of age, when the retina is mature. It can be inapparent or can result in blindness, depending on the extent of the damage. The condition can be localized (multifocal retinal folds) or generalized (geographic, detachment) as judged by ophthalmoscopy, and inherited retinal dysplasia cannot be distinguished funduscopically from acquired retinal dysplasia (1108).

Animals with retinal detachments, geographic retinal dysplasia, skeletal abnormalities, or concurrent vitreous degeneration should not be bred (1108). The presence of retinal folds is more controversial when it comes to certification. In breeds that are subject to devastating retinal dysplasia, such as the Labrador retriever, Samoyed, and

English springer spaniel, retinal folds are enough to disqualify an animal from certification. More severe forms of retinal dysplasia will prohibit certification in all breeds. The Institute for Genetic Disease Control in Animals (GDC) maintains an open registry of inherited eye diseases for all breeds, which includes retinal detachment in the Chinook.

Tapetal degeneration is a recessively inherited condition in the beagle (350). Degeneration of the tapetum does not affect vision in any way and, therefore, is not associated with ophthalmic problems.

STATIONARY NIGHT BLINDNESS

Congenital stationary night blindness, also known as hereditary retinal dystrophy, is a poorly understood condition in which nonprogressive night blindness is apparent by 5 to 6 weeks of age. There is marked early rod degeneration while the cones remain unaffected (173). The condition is autosomal recessive in the briard (10, 350, 759, 766), and presumed to be autosomal recessive in the Shetland sheepdog (903) and standard poodle (903). In the briard, a four nucleotide deletion in the RPE65 gene is responsible (10, 1079). There seems to be some variability between the clinical presentation in American and European briards (1145). It is uncertain whether congenital night blindness in the Tibetan terrier is distinct from progressive retinal atrophy or merely represents a different stage of the same disorder (365). Day vision is variably affected.

The disorder is diagnosed by electroretinography. In the affected briard, plasma levels of arachidonic acid are often elevated (903). DNA-based testing is available for the briard. This allows identification of unaffected, carrier, and affected animals. Treatment is unsuccessful.

Presuming that stationary night blindness in most other breeds is also autosomal recessive, affected animals should not be bred and parents should be considered obligate carriers of the trait. Siblings are suspect carriers and should be used cautiously in breeding programs.

UVEAL HYPOPIGMENTATION

Blue irides, heterochromia irides, and iris hypoplasia are related to coat-color genetics and may be seen in Alaskan malamutes, Australian shepherds, beagles, blue merle collies, Dalmatians, harlequin Great Danes, Shetland sheepdogs, and Siberian huskies, and may be associated with deafness (827). White or merle coats are inherited as autosomal dominant traits, and heterochromia iridis and deafness are autosomal dominant with incomplete penetrance (827). Selection of dogs with uveal hypopigmentation for breeding programs is a breeder option.

CHAPTER 12

Reproductive Problems

Although reproductive problems are common in purebred dogs, most have not been intensively studied. There are no registries for reproductive disorders, and no tests for carriers.

CRYPTORCHIDISM

Cryptorchidism refers to testicles that have not descended into the scrotum. During fetal development, the testicles migrate from within the abdomen through an opening into the scrotum. In some cases, however, the transition is incomplete and one or both testicles remain within the abdomen. Results of studies suggest that testicular descent is accelerated by dihydrotestosterone and testosterone secretory function of Leydig cells, increasing after 54 days of gestation (507).

Cryptorchidism is believed to be at least partially hereditary, and it is commonly seen in the border collie (181), boxer (461, 890), Cairn terrier (461, 890), Chihuahua (334, 461, 890), English bulldog (461, 890), greyhound (976), Lakeland terrier (181), Maltese (461, 890), miniature dachshund (461, 890), miniature schnauzer (334, 461, 890), Old English sheepdog (890), Pekingese (461, 890), Pomeranian (334, 461, 890), Shetland sheepdog (334, 461, 890), Siberian husky (334, 890), silky terrier (181), toy and miniature poodles (334, 461, 890), whippet (181), and Yorkshire terrier (334, 461, 890). Although the actual cause is still a matter of some debate, it is thought that insufficient stimulation of sex organs during fetal development may be partially to blame.

Originally it was thought that cryptorchidism was a simple recessive trait (211). Now, though, it is believed that the condition is more likely polygenic (334, 890). It has also been suggested that, although the condition is seen only in males, the genes involved can be inherited from either parent (46).

Cryptorchidism is either unilateral or bilateral, depending on whether one or both testicles, respectively, have failed to descend into the scrotum. The right testicle is involved nearly twice as often as the left, and most cryptorchid cases (75%) are unilateral (890). As a general rule, if the testicles have not descended fully into the scrotum by 4 months of age, they are unlikely to do so.

Dogs that are cryptorchid have a much higher incidence (approximately 10 times) of testicular cancer (890), presumably because the testicle is exposed to higher temperatures in the abdomen than it would be in the scrotum. Also, dogs with cryptorchidism are not suitable for show purposes.

Cryptorchidism can be determined, in most cases, by 4 months of age (334). Before then the testicles may be present in the scrotum but can also be retracted into the abdomen. In these cases, it is important to determine if the testicle can be manipulated through the inguinal ring into the scrotum. If this can be accomplished, the pup is not likely cryptorchid. On the other hand, attempts to relocate the testes manually into the scrotum are unsuccessful in cryptorchid puppies.

Evidence on which to base breeding recommendations for animals closely related to affected individuals is insufficient.

Cryptorchidism

Dogs that are cryptorchid should be neutered. This is important for two reasons:

1. If this dog is bred, it likely will pass on the trait to future generations.
2. If the testicles aren't removed, the dog is at increased risk for testicular cancer.

ABNORMALITIES IN SEXUAL DIFFERENTIATION

Normal sexual differentiation depends on a series of three steps under genetic control: the establishment of chromosomal, gonadal, and then phenotypic sex. Thus, abnormalities of sexual differentiation can also be determined based on the step at which the trait differs from normal (i.e., a chromosomal, gonadal, or phenotypic error).

Chromosomal sex is determined at the time of fertilization. For males, the Tdy gene encodes a testis-determining factor that is a genetic switch for development of male gonads. Male phenotypic sex is determined by Mullerian-inhibiting substance and testosterone. In the absence of a Y chromosome and Tdy gene, the default pathway is female gonadal sex.

Chromosomal intersex, resulting from abnormalities in chromosomal sexual differentiation, is rare in dogs and is thought not to have a genetic basis. Examples include Klinefelter syndrome (XXY), Turner syndrome (X0), X trisomy (XXX), chimeras, and mosaics. The XXY genotype causes testicular hypoplasia and azoospermia, so affected dogs may have abnormally small testes. The XO genotype has been reported in dogs, and these affected animals are often smaller than their siblings and do not possess Barr bodies or drumsticks (174). Most XO individuals die before birth. The diagnosis, in living animals, is suspected when females haven't cycled by 24 months of age, and is confirmed by karyotyping (685). This condition has been reported in the Doberman pinscher (461, 977). Presence of the XXX genotype, also referred to as superfemales, is likely to remain undetected unless someone happens to notice two drumsticks per mature neutrophil on a hemogram. Affected dogs may have training difficulties but otherwise appear phenotypically normal (174). The condition has been reported in the Airedale (461).

True hermaphrodism can reveal chimeras with XX/XY or XX/XXY chromosome combinations, the external appearance of a female, and both testicular and ovarian tissue internally. In other cases, the testicle-determining gene may be translocated to cause development of both ovarian and testicular tissue from the indifferent gonads (174). These animals usually have ambiguous genitalia, such as an enlarged clitoris or a small penis, with phenotype varying from near-normal female to near-normal male (944). Gonadal sex in chimeras and mosaics depends upon the distribution of the cell populations within the gonadal primordium (685).

Gonadal intersex, resulting from sexual differentiation abnormalities in the gonads, includes XX sex reversal, which is autosomal recessive in cocker spaniels, but is limited to dogs with an XX chromosome constitution. XY sex reversal has not been reported in the dog. Sexual reversal refers to animals in which chromosomal sex and gonadal sex differ. This can be associated with true hermaphrodism, in which the testicular and ovarian tissues are combined into ovotestes (both ovary and testis in the same animal), or pseudohermaphrodism (the dog has the gonads of one sex and the external genitalia of another), or actual sex reversal (a female (XX) karyotype but testes retained in the abdominal cavity). It has been shown that a sex-determining region on the Y chromosome (Sry) is needed to initiate normal male sexual development.

True hermaphrodites with an XX chromosome complement (hereditary XX sex reversal) can have the external appearance of a female and ovotestes internally. Hereditary XX sex reversal has been documented in the American cocker spaniel (461, 684), German shorthaired pointer (461, 682), beagle (438, 461), basset hound (174), pug (174, 461), Kerry blue terrier (438, 461), and Weimaraner (46, 461). In the American cocker spaniel, the condition is transmitted as an autosomal recessive trait (46). The condition is inherited in the beagle, but the mode of transmission has not been determined (438). Sry-negative sex reversal has been documented in the American cocker spaniel (684), German shorthaired pointer (682), and Norwegian elkhound (667).

In the XX male syndrome, the phenotype is predominantly male and individuals are positive for the H-Y antigen, but there is an XX chromosome complement. In most cases, one of the X chromosomes has a small insertion from the Y chromosome, which includes the Sry gene. This condition has been reported in the cocker spaniel, pug, German shorthaired pointer, and Kerry blue terrier (438, 859). Males having an XX genotype have small poorly functioning testes that are often undescended (174). XY females may result when the Y chromosome has a Sry gene deletion, a mutant Sry allele, or lack of an androgen receptor (772).

Phenotypic intersex, resulting from sexual differentiation abnormalities in the phenotype, include persistent Mullerian duct syndrome and testicular feminization syndrome, which has not been conclusively demonstrated in the dog but is seen in the cat. Male pseudohermaphrodism is caused by inadequate synthesis of fetal testosterone and is seen in miniature schnauzers in association with persistent Mullerian duct syndrome, and it has also been reported in the poodle, Pekingese, and pug (281, 461). Female pseudohermaphrodism is caused primarily by environmental influences (exogenous androgens, metabolic errors), and no evidence suggests a genetic etiology. It is seen in many different breeds and has been reported in female Greyhound littermates (796).

Persistent Mullerian duct syndrome is a hereditary disorder in male miniature schnauzers, transmitted as an autosomal recessive trait (46). It is also seen in the basset hound (498, 776), in which the genetics are suspected to be the same. In this syndrome, normal-appearing XY males have oviducts, a uterus, and a cranial vagina in addition to their male sex organs (681). Affected dogs produce normal amounts of MIS, but the MIS receptor is absent or defective (46, 683). Both of the parents should be considered to be carriers of the trait, and normal-appearing siblings could be carriers as well.

> **Mullerian Ducts**
>
> The Mullerian ducts are prenatal structures that develop into oviducts, uterus, and cranial vagina in the normal female. In males, the testes produce Mullerian-inhibiting substance (MIS) to prevent development of this duct system.

The sexual differentiation anomalies are typically suspected with clinical abnormalities of external genitalia such as clitoral enlargement or abnormal penis or a history of infertility. Diagnosis requires karyotyping and evaluating both internal and external sex organs. Affected animals should be neutered. Until more evidence is gathered for XX sex reversal, both parents should be assumed to be potential carriers of the trait and should not be used for future breeding. Siblings should be considered to be potential carriers.

CHAPTER 13

Respiratory Disorders

Although many genetic disorders include a respiratory component, few entirely respiratory conditions have been studied extensively from a genetic standpoint.

BRACHYCEPHALIC SYNDROME

Brachycephalic syndrome consists of anatomic abnormalities that may include stenotic nares, tortuous turbinates, caudally displaced maxillae and elongated soft palate, everted laryngeal saccules, and hypoplastic trachea. All brachycephalic breeds likely have at least some degree of increased upper airway resistance, just based on their anatomy. Breeds commonly cited with brachycephalic syndrome include the Boston terrier, Chinese shar pei, English bulldog, pug, French bulldog, Lhasa apso, Pekingese, and shih tzu (424, 440, 658). Because the maxillae are shortened, the caudal aspect of the soft palate extends beyond the tip of the epiglottis and interferes with laryngeal function, resulting in inspiratory noise and dyspnea (647). Bulldogs often have repeated episodes of sleep-disordered breathing (440).

Increased negative inspiratory pressure to move air through narrow air passages can result in eversion of the mucosa that lines the lateral laryngeal ventricles, and eventually in collapse of the corniculate and cuneiform processes of the arytenoid cartilage (457). This typically results in exercise intolerance, noisy breathing, and coughing. Laryngoscopy is required for definitive assessment.

Short-term relief may be gained by judicious use of corticosteroids to reduce inflammation of the airway. Surgery may be needed to correct some anatomic faults that are impeding breathing. Animals with marked respiratory abnormalities should not be used for breeding.

HYPOPLASTIC TRACHEA

Tracheal hypoplasia is a congenital malformation that results in narrowing of the trachea, and a congenital or inherited pathogenesis is suspected (489). In some cases, it is associated with brachycephalic syndrome (658). There seems to be a higher incidence in the bulldog, Boston terrier, and boxer (489), and the condition has also been reported in black Labrador retrievers (424). Clinical signs include exercise intolerance, noisy breathing, and, sometimes, syncope.

The diagnosis is confirmed by radiographic assessment of tracheal diameter. Tracheal hypoplasia has no specific treatments other than managing secondary or associated problems. Affected animals should not be used for breeding.

LARYNGEAL PARALYSIS

Hereditary laryngeal paralysis is characterized by failure of vocal folds and arytenoid cartilage to abduct properly during inspiration. It has been described as a hereditary disorder in Bouvier des Flandres (385, 1075), Dalmatians (93), English bulldogs (62), bull terriers (62, 385), Rottweilers (83), and Siberian huskies and their crosses (385, 785). In the Bouvier des Flandre, and presumably the Siberian husky, the mode of inheritance is autosomal dominant (87, 385, 467, 784).

Clinical signs include exercise intolerance, stridor, dyspnea, coughing, retching, and even syncope (385). The age of onset is typically 4 to 6 months (87). Whereas Bouviers with laryngeal paralysis develop degeneration of recurrent laryngeal nerves as well as neurons in the nucleus ambiguus, Siberian huskies appear to experience degeneration of the recurrent laryngeal nerve only (467). In Dalmatians, laryngeal paralysis seems to be one sign of a more diffuse primary polyneuropathy that is believed to be autosomal recessive

Tracheal hypoplasia

Tracheal hypoplasia is diagnosed when the ratio of the tracheal lumen diameter at the thoracic inlet (TD) to the diameter of the thoracic inlet is less than 0.127 in the bulldog, 0.160 for other brachycephalic breeds, or 0.204 for other breeds (489).

in nature (90). In the Dalmatian, distal axonal degeneration is seen in medium- and large-diameter fibers in all peripheral nerves, including the recurrent laryngeal nerves (51). Megaesophagus is seen in more than 50% of affected Dalmatians (467). The prognosis for Dalmatians with laryngeal paralysis polyneuropathy complex is guarded to poor. Laryngeal paralysis and generalized polyneuropathy have also been reported in young rottweilers (281, 626).

The diagnosis of laryngeal paralysis is often made by performing laryngoscopy on a lightly anesthetized animal. Characteristic changes include medially and ventrally displaced arytenoid cartilages and vocal folds remaining in a paramedian position in both inspiratory and expiratory phases (385). Not all cases of laryngeal paralysis are hereditary in nature. Also, laryngeal paralysis can be a feature of other inherited disorders, such as giant axonal neuropathy in German shepherd dogs.

Clinical signs include voice change, stridor, respiratory distress, coughing, and exercise intolerance (457). Most affected dogs have respiratory distress. The diagnosis can be rendered with electromyographic evaluation. Although no treatments are considered universally successful, sedation and avoiding exertion may give temporary relief.

Affected animals should not be bred. In the Bouvier des Flandres and other breeds in which an autosomal dominant mode of inheritance is suspected, closely related relatives should be evaluated carefully for evidence of the problem. In Dalmatians and other breeds in which the mode of inheritance is autosomal recessive, parents should be considered obligate carriers and siblings as suspect carriers.

TRACHEAL COLLAPSE

Tracheal collapse results from reduction in the luminal diameter of the cervical or intrathoracic trachea, or both, and the pathogenesis is still a matter of debate. Some consider the entity to be a congenital or inherited problem, and it is reported most commonly in the Chihuahua, Pomeranian, poodle, and Yorkshire terrier (424, 489). Affected dogs often make a "honking" sound and may suffer from chronic, intermittent airway obstruction.

The diagnosis is suspected by evaluating both inspiratory and expiratory radiographs to detect the level of the tracheal collapse, and is confirmed with bronchoscopy. Palliative treatment of associated and complicating conditions is usually beneficial but won't correct the problem. Surgical placement of ring prostheses for cervical tracheal collapse can be corrective but is technically difficult (125). Affected animals ideally should not be used for breeding, but the decision remains a breeder option.

CHAPTER 14

Urinary System Disorders

In veterinary practice, disorders of the urinary system are common. Yet, relatively few cases are well-documented as having a genetic basis. The gene for cystinuria in Newfoundlands has been detected, and a genetic test is now available for that breed.

CONGENITAL RENAL DISEASE

Congenital kidney diseases are quite heterogeneous. The most common clinical signs are polyuria, polydipsia, lethargy, reduced appetite, and weight loss. Because the disease has several different subgroupings, they will be covered separately.

Renal agenesis is rarely recognized in dogs but seems to be familial in the beagle, Doberman pinscher, and Shetland sheepdog (551, 878). The mode of inheritance is not known. Bilateral agenesis is fatal, but unilateral agenesis may remain inapparent as long as the animal maintains adequate renal function.

The diagnosis may be made fortuitously when radiography or ultrasonography of the abdomen fail to reveal one of the kidneys, or if abnormal urogenital components are found during neutering. No treatment is necessary, but affected animals should not be bred.

Renal telangiectasia, a vascular anomaly characterized by multiple dilated renal blood vessels, has been reported in Pembroke Welsh corgis. Affected dogs present with episodes of hematuria during adulthood (725). The diagnosis is confirmed by pathologic examination of the kidneys. Affected animals should not be bred.

Renal dysplasia refers to abnormal differentiation of kidney tissue such that inappropriate or anomalous structures appear within the renal parenchyma. Renal dysplasia is presumed to be familial in the Lhasa apso, shih tzu (787), soft-coated wheaten terrier (570, 571, 760) (presumed autosomal recessive-[551]), and is suspected to be familial in the Alaskan malamute (570, 1082), American cocker spaniel (306), Bedlington terrier (551), chow chow (118, 570, 571), golden retriever (25, 251, 519, 570), keeshond (551), miniature schnauzer (551, 738), standard poodle (257, 570, 571), and Weimaraner (888).

The actual cause, pathogenesis, and mode of inheritance remain unknown in most cases, and familial trends have apparently not been reported in association with sporadic cases in the Airedale terrier, beagle, border terrier, Cavalier King Charles spaniel, English bulldog, Great Dane, Great Pyrenees, Irish wolfhound, New Foundland, Old English sheepdog, Pekingese, Rhodesian ridgeback, Swedish foxhound, and Yorkshire terrier (239, 255, 551, 607, 693).

Renal failure may appear as early as 3 to 6 months of age (570). The diagnosis is confirmed by light or electron microscopic evaluation of kidney biopsies. In Lhasa apsos and shih tzus, glucosuria also may be noted, although it is rare (570, 787). In the soft-coated wheaten terrier, the nephropathy may be associated with a protein-losing enteropathy as well. Eosinophilia, increased fecal alpha-1-protease inhibitor, and hypoglobulinemia may herald evidence of glomerulonephritis in this breed. A marker-based test is available for use in the Shih tzu, Lhasa apso, and soft-coated wheaten terrier. It appears to be about 80% predictive, despite the fact, that the genetics of the disorder in these breeds has not yet been confirmed.

Treatment is palliative and includes dietary modification, oral adsorbents, and dried aluminum hydroxide gel (707). Presuming that most cases are autosomal recessive in nature, affected animals should not be bred and their parents should be considered as likely carriers. Siblings are considered as potential carriers of the trait.

Primary hereditary nephritis results from the defective synthesis of type IV collagen, which is a major component of the glomerular basement membrane. This is a heterogeneous group of disorders with a final, common, end result. In the Samoyed, the defect has been fully characterized as an α5(IV) gene defect, with an X-linked inheritance similar to that of Alport syndrome in humans (570, 571). A nonsense mutation in exon 35 of the gene for the alpha-5 chain of basement membrane collagen is responsible (1022). Affected males develop proteinuria at 3 to 5 months of age, and it rapidly progresses to renal failure before 1 year of age (477). Carrier females develop proteinuria at about the same age but don't develop renal failure until middle age (570). Ultrastructural glomerular basement membrane changes can be detected in both affected and carrier animals (569).

Hereditary protein-losing glomerulopathies have no cure, although a high-quality, low-protein diet may be beneficial (615). Also, angiotensin-converting enzyme inhibitors (e.g., enalapril) may lower the blood pressure, delay the onset of azotemia, improve the effective renal plasma flow, slow the rate of increases in proteinuria, and delay the decline of glomerular filtration rate (392).

Affected animals should not be bred, and the dam should be considered as an obligate carrier. Female siblings should be screened for evidence of proteinuria at 1 year of age, before being considered for breeding.

An autosomal dominant form of hereditary nephritis has been described in bull terriers (366, 408, 458, 571). The clinical presentation differs in this breed in that age of onset is typically older than 2 years; in some cases, the clinical manifestations of kidney failure do not develop until the animal reaches 8 years of age. Proteinuria is a characteristic finding.

Affected animals should not be bred, and neither should the affected parent. Any related animal being considered for breeding should be screened for evidence of proteinuria even if the dog does not have obvious signs of hereditary nephritis.

Renal Disease Ratio

$$\frac{\text{Urine protein (mg/dl)}}{\text{Urine creatinine (mg/dl)}}$$

UP/Ucr > 1 indicates renal disease, urinary tract infection, and/or hematuria (M060)

In the English cocker spaniel, familial nephropathy is inherited as an autosomal recessive trait (571, 572, 573, 886). It is thought to be yet another form of Alport syndrome, caused by a mutation in one of the collagen IV genes (574). Once again, proteinuria is an important clinical finding and heralds a predictable sequence of changes including decreased growth, diminishing urine concentrating ability, and increased blood concentrations of urea and creatinine (572). Suspect cases can be screened for proteinuria when they are 4 to 5 months of age. Ultrastructural changes of the glomerular basement membrane zone are evident in affected animals, but not in carriers (569).

If persistent proteinuria is documented, a renal biopsy should be considered to more fully characterize the problem. Histopathologic evaluation typically reveals mesangial thickening, glomerular fibrosis, periglomerular fibrosis, and glomerular obsolescence (574). However, transmission electron microscopy (TEN) is needed to reveal the ultrastructural glomerular basement membrane changes characteristic of each condition (569). Affected animals should not be bred, and both parents should be considered as obligate carriers of the trait. Siblings should be considered as suspect carriers.

Other conditions, such as a familial nephropathy (membranoproliferative glomerulonephritis) in Doberman pinschers and miniature schnauzers, protein-losing nephropathy in soft-coated wheaten terriers, glomerulosclerosis/glomerulofibrosis syndrome in Newfoundland dogs, and an atrophic membranous glomerulopathy in rottweiler dogs have not been fully characterized (196, 472, 570, 836).

In *Doberman pinscher familial glomerulonephritis*, clinical signs of renal failure may be seen in weaned pups or not until old age. It is characterized by marked proteinuria and, variably, glucosuria. Concurrent unilateral renal aplasia is seen in some cases. The diagnosis is confirmed on histopathologic evaluation that reveals glomerular sclerosis and atrophy. Although the condition is presumed to be familial, a mode of inheritance has not been determined (551).

A similar condition reported in Newfoundland dogs is termed *glomerulosclerosis/glomerulofibrosis syndrome* (538). Atrophic membranous glomerulopathy in rottweiler dogs seems to be distinct from other glomerulopathies, and renal failure occurs between 6 and 12 months of age (196). Routine laboratory studies reveal isosthenuria and proteinuria. The diagnosis is confirmed by histopathologic assessment in which atrophic membranous glomerulopathy with secondary degenerative changes is prominent (551).

Tubulointerstitial nephropathy is a noninflammatory progressive renal disease reported as familial in Norwegian elkhounds (314). The mode of inheritance is not known, but there is a strong familial tendency (551, 571). The kidneys of affected dogs are normal at birth but undergo advancing irreversible interstitial fibrosis. The course is highly variable. Some dogs develop renal failure by 1 year of age, and others do not develop problems until several years of age (570).

Polycystic renal disease is reported in many breeds, and a strong familial tendency has been reported in Cairn terriers and beagles (551). In Cairn terriers, it is often associated with concurrent biliary cysts. The condition can progress to renal failure if the cysts enlarge and compress the renal parenchyma. Polycystic kidney and liver disease has also been reported in the West Highland white terrier and is suspected to be an autosomal recessive trait similar to autosomal recessive polycystic kidney disease (ARPKD) in humans (651). Since a polymorphism has been detected in the canine polycystic kidney disease 1 gene (606), a diagnostic test to detect carriers may be possible in the near future.

Pups affected with both liver and kidney disease may develop liver failure by the time they are weaned. The diagnosis is confirmed by finding renal cysts in collecting ducts and hepatic cysts within biliary ducts. Although affected animals typically don't live long enough to breed, their parents should be excluded from breeding programs and siblings should be considered suspect carriers.

FANCONI SYNDROME

Fanconi syndrome (or Fanconi's syndrome), also referred to as paradoxic glucosuria, is a collection of abnormalities associated with defective renal tubular function. The primary abnormalities are derangements of proximal renal tubular function causing reduced reabsorption of filtered solutes, such as glucose and amino acids (570). The result is a loss of glucose, sodium, potassium, phosphorus, bicarbonate, and amino acids into the urine.

About 75% of all cases of Fanconi syndrome have been observed in the basenji, in which the prevalence rate is estimated at 10% to 30%. That makes this disorder extremely significant in this breed. The disorder has also been reported in the border terrier (in association with renal dysplasia), Doberman pinscher, Labrador retriever, miniature schnauzer, Norwegian elkhound, Shetland sheepdog, and Yorkshire terrier (255, 285, 551, 654, 976).

Fanconi syndrome runs in families, but the specifics of inheritance have been elusive. It is hoped that the gene will be isolated in the near future so DNA testing can reveal carriers. Because affected dogs often appear phenotypically normal until they are 2 to 6 years of age, they may have contributed to future generations already, by the time of diagnosis (570).

The clinical signs are quite variable, depending in part on the extent of kidney dysfunction. Initially, the dog has polydipsia, polyuria, and weight loss. In most cases, the loss of glucose and amino acids into the urine doesn't cause clinical problems. Kidney failure is responsible for most clinical signs, but muscle weakness can occur as a result of profound potassium loss in the urine. Rickets in immature animals (osteomalacia in adults) can be seen as a consequence of marked loss of calcium and phosphorus. The ultimate cause of death is kidney failure, often associated with metabolic acidosis. Some dogs remain stable for years with therapy, and others go downhill rapidly. The course is extremely variable.

The diagnosis is suspected when a breed at risk (such as the basenji) develops detectable loss of glucose in the urine (glucosuria) without hyperglycemia (such as would be expected with diabetes mellitus). This still could be consistent with another disorder, primary renal glucosuria, but dogs with Fanconi syndrome also show evidence of amino acids and protein in the urine. The ability to produce acidic urine, despite a proximal tubular bicarbonate reabsorptive defect, is an important feature of Fanconi syndrome (119). Urinary clearance studies can be done, if necessary, to confirm a diagnosis.

Fanconi syndrome has no cure, although the clinical signs can be treated successfully as they arise. For example, potassium supplementation can be instituted in the dog with hypokalemia. Metabolic acidosis may be treated with sodium bicarbonate or potassium citrate. Compensated kidney failure can be treated with a high-quality, low-protein diet and special supplements. Because the specific mode of inheritance is still unknown, owners should be cautious in breeding dogs from families that have experienced Fanconi syndrome. Some breeders do not breed their basenjis until the dogs are at least 6 years of age, to be certain that those dogs are "clear."

IMMUNE-MEDIATED GLOMERULONEPHRITIS

Glomerulonephritis results in loss of protein into the urine and may be classified as membranous, mesangioproliferative, membranoproliferative, glomerulosclerosis, minimal change disease, and amyloidosis depending on the microscopic features (120, 162). Immune-mediated damage to the glomeruli has been documented in Bernese mountain dogs and soft-coated wheaten terriers (162, 571).

The Bernese mountain dog shows subendothelial deposits of immune complexes. Glomerulonephritis in this breed is postulated to be inherited as an autosomal recessive trait, with its expression influenced by a second gene locus with a sex-linked dominant exchange (869).

A membranoproliferative glomerulonephritis, sometimes associated with intestinal lesions, has been recognized in related soft-coated wheaten terriers (605). This condition must be differentiated from renal dysplasia, which is also reported in the breed. For both conditions, females seem to be affected slightly more than males (570).

The diagnosis is suspected with persistent proteinuria and must be differentiated from amyloidosis and renal dysplasia. Progression of glomerular disease is unpredictable, with no apparent correlation between survival time and biochemical parameters (172). Most cases of protein-losing glomerulonephritis carry a poor prognosis.

Until more is known about the genetics of immune-mediated glomerulonephritis, affected animals should not be bred and the mating that produced affected individuals should not be repeated. In the Bernese mountain dog, in which the trait is thought to have an autosomal recessive mode of inheritance, both parents should be considered to be carriers of the trait, and siblings to be suspect carriers.

PRIMARY RENAL GLUCOSURIA

Primary renal glucosuria refers to a defect in proximal renal tubular reabsorption of glucose that results in glucosuria without hyperglycemia. It has been reported in the Norwegian elkhound, Scottish terrier, and mixed-breed dogs, and it seems to be familial in the Norwegian elkhound (551). The condition is asymptomatic but may pose concerns for veterinarians who are trying to determine the cause of the glucosuria. Testing is required to differentiate this condition from diabetes mellitus, Fanconi syndrome, and renal dysplasia.

UROLITHIASIS

Urolithiasis is the condition caused when crystals combine to form "stones" in the urinary tract. These stones also are called calculi or uroliths. Uroliths can form in any part of the urinary tract. and can be found in the kidneys, ureters, bladder, or urethra. They collect most commonly in the bladder.

Several types of uroliths have been identified. These may contain magnesium ammonium phosphate hexahydrate (commonly called MAP stones, triple phosphate stones, or struvite stones), ammonium acid urate (also called urate stones), cystine, calcium oxalate, and others. The magnesium ammonium phosphate uroliths are by far the most common, accounting for about 50–60% of all uroliths.

Although calculi occur in all breeds of dogs, the breeds affected most commonly include basset hounds, bulldogs, cocker spaniels, corgis, dachshunds, Dalmatians, Pekingese, poodles, pugs, schnauzers, shih tzus, terriers, and Yorkshire terriers (613, 1100). The breeds definitely vary when it comes to individual types of uroliths. Prevalence of canine uroliths also differs significantly based on age and gender (599). The different types of uroliths are discussed individually following a general review of urolithiasis.

Approximately 90% of canine uroliths are detected in the urinary bladder or urethra and not in the kidneys. Breeds prone to nephroliths include the Lhasa apso, miniature schnauzer, miniature poodle, pug, shih tzu, and Yorkshire terrier (609, 800). In the female urinary tract, most small stones pass through the urethra because it is shorter, straighter, and wider than that of the male. In the male urinary tract, the stones commonly occlude or "plug" the urethra, causing a situation in which the dog cannot urinate until the stones are removed.

Although the exact cause of urolith formation cannot always be determined, some contributing factors to stone formation have been identified. These include:

1. Urinary tract infection with urea-splitting bacteria
2. Genetic or acquired metabolic abnormalities producing crystals
3. Infrequent urination so that urine accumulates in the bladder, allowing time for stones to form

Some clinical signs that may be evident in dogs with urolithiasis are hematuria, difficulty urinating (dysuria), inappropriate urination, and reduced size and force of the urine stream. Abdominal discomfort may result from straining, and signs of kidney failure (vomiting, loss of appetite, lethargy) may occur if calculi completely obstruct the outflow of urine.

Urolithiasis usually can be suspected by thoroughly examining the urine. Urine analysis (urinalysis) can be easily conducted with samples and often helps to detect the crystals that form uroliths. It also can aid in detecting conditions such as bacterial infections, tumors, and diabetes. Because bacterial infections are commonly associated with urolithiasis, culture and sensitivity testing of microbes may be helpful. Together with other tests, blood counts and organ profiles are often done to produce a more complete picture of the patient's overall health.

Many uroliths can be detected by appropriate radiography and ultrasonography. Radiographs of the abdomen are often taken in suspect cases because most stones are denser than the surrounding tissues and will show up on a radiograph. Some stones (most notably, urate uroliths) have the same density as the surrounding tissues and may not show up on survey radiographs; other methods, such as contrast studies, must be used to diagnose these radiolucent stones. Ultrasound examinations are helpful in detecting urinary tract "stones," regardless of their radiodensity. Sometimes, even careful palpation can reveal large stones.

If a urolith is found in the urine or is "passed," it can be analyzed to determine the chemical composition. Special laboratories can determine the actual makeup of "stones" by sophisticated tests such as optical crystallography, x-ray diffraction, or infrared spectroscopy. Knowing the chemical composition of the urolith helps determine how and why it occurred, the best methods of treatment, and how to prevent relapses. Approximately 50%–60% of uroliths in the general US dog population are MAP (struvite), 15%–30% are calcium oxalate, 6%–8% purines (e.g., uric acid), 1%–2% cystine, and most of the others are mixtures.

Treatment for canine urolithiasis can involve surgically removing the stones, or attempting to dissolve them so they can pass out in the urine, or ablating the stones with laser-induced shock-wave lithotripsy (1141). Surgery usually is preferred when a quick remedy is needed, such as when animals are in pain or when a stone is blocking the kidney or ureter. In these cases, uroliths should be sent to a laboratory to determine the type and the most appropriate way to prevent further occurrences. Retrograde urohydropropulsion should be used prior to surgery to flush uroliths, which may be in the urethra, back into the bladder.

Medical approaches to the problem center on causing the stones to dissolve in the urine so they can be passed more easily. Often the solubility can be increased by changing the pH of the urine; some uroliths are more prevalent in alkaline urine, and some in acidic urine. MAP (struvite) crystals tend to form in alkaline urine and are most readily dissolved if the urine can be made more acidic. Other stones may be more prevalent in acidic urine and, therefore, can be dissolved if the urine can be made more alkaline. Changing the pH of the urine can be accomplished with medications, certain nutritional supplements, or special diets. The special diets tend to limit the specific mineral found in the urolith and reduce the urine concentration of urea in addition to changing the pH of the urine. These diets often produce more urine so the crystals become diluted and dogs urinate more frequently. This frequent urination is important so crystals can be excreted before they become large enough to cause problems.

Reducing the number of stone-forming crystals in the urine usually means that fewer stones are likely to form. Increasing the volume of urine produced is more likely to dilute the crystal concentration. Accordingly, feeding canned diets with a high water content is preferred, or mixing dry food with water prior to feeding.

Treating bladder infections with antibiotics is often necessary because bacterial infections are commonly associated with these conditions. Antibiotics are often continued during the entire time the uroliths are being dissolved because, as the stones form, bacteria are trapped within the stone and will become released and start new infections as the various layers of the stone dissolve. A urease inhibitor, acetohydroxamic acid, is sometimes used to dissolve struvite uroliths that are resistant to antibiotic and dietary treatment.

When medical management rather than surgery is used, periodic radiographs and urinalyses should be done to check progress. If successful, medical management is usually continued for at least 1 month after the stones are no longer visible on the radiograph, to make sure they have been completely dissolved. To dissolve uroliths completely sometimes takes several months.

Urolithiasis—Magnesium Ammonium Phosphate (MAP)

Frequently referred to as struvite, or triple phosphate, "stones," MAP uroliths are the most common type of stones seen in dogs. They are most often reported in beagles, dachshunds, English cocker spaniels, miniature schnauzers, poodles, Scottish terriers, and Welsh corgis (616).

Struvite uroliths occur when the urine is supersaturated with magnesium, ammonium, and phosphate ions (613). Metabolic, dietary, and familial factors are involved in the formation of struvite, and the uroliths can be dissolved medically or removed surgically. Prevention includes control and early eradication of urinary tract infections, along with dietary intervention. Dissolution of MAP uroliths is dependent on their surface porosity. Stones that have low porosity or contain more apatite than struvite are less amenable to dissolution by dietary intervention (270). Calcium phosphate uroliths are commonly found as a component of struvite or calcium oxalate and are not amenable to medical treatments.

Although struvite urolithiasis is common, not much is known about the genetics of the condition and prevention through genetic counseling. Although it seems reasonable to recommend that severely affected individuals not be bred, little information is available on which to base sound breeding strategies.

Urolithiasis—Calcium Oxalate

Calcium oxalate crystals (the most common type in people) are seen most often in the bichon frisé, Cairn terrier, Dalmatian, Lhasa apso, miniature poodle, miniature schnauzer, shih tzu, and Yorkshire terrier (78, 600, 613, 614, 616, 617). Calcium oxalate uroliths are usually associated with metabolic factors promoting hypercalciuria (614). For example, in dogs with urolithiasis, those that had hyperadrenocorticism were 10 times as likely to have calcium-containing uroliths (446). Hypercalciuria, however, does not imply hypercalcemia, and normocalcemic hypercalciuria is to be expected in most cases (614).

The diagnosis is confirmed by identifying calcium oxalate urolithiasis, usually associated with urinary tract infection. Urolithiasis can be problematic even with an absence of calcium oxalate crystals in the urine. Although normocalcemia is to be expected, serum calcium concentrations should be measured in patients suspected of having calcium oxalate urolithiasis and hypercalciuria. Dogs should not be fasted prior to measuring urinary calcium levels, as this may artificially lower the results (614). Uroliths are radiodense and usually obvious on radiography.

> **Urate Uroliths**
>
> If urine samples cannot be assessed promptly for uric acid levels, the sample should be diluted 1:10 or 1:20 with deionized water and stored at –20°C (59).

Medical dissolution of calcium oxalate uroliths has not been successful. In human medicine, high dietary calcium intake has been shown to actually decrease the risk of symptomatic kidney stones (186). The principal recommended treatment is to remove uroliths by voiding urohydropropulsion, lithotripsy, and cystotomy (581). To some extent, occurrence or reoccurrence of calcium oxalate urolithiasis is prevented by feeding canned food, encouraging drinking (but not with supplementation of sodium chloride), and supplementing with potassium citrate. Severely affected individuals should not be bred, although little information is available on which to base sound breeding strategies.

Urolithiasis—Urate

Approximately 60% of urate uroliths are seen in Dalmatians, and the odds that uroliths retrieved from Dalmatians are composed of urate are more than 160 times greater than for other breeds (38). Dalmatians have a defective hepatic urate transport system and a membrane transport defect in the kidneys that causes reduced reabsorption of filtered urate in the renal tubules, which in turn results in a urinary urate excretion 4 to 8 times more than other breeds (601, 993). Nevertheless, urate stones are not inevitable, because uric acid secretion in renal tubules is higher than in other dog breeds (370). Predisposing factors for urate urolith formation include hyperuricemia, hyperuricosuria, hyperammonemia, hyperammonuria, aciduria, and genetic predisposition (37).

Hyperuricuria in Dalmatians is transmitted as an autosomal recessive trait (551, 915, 1010). The gene pair responsible for urate excretion is separate from, but genetically linked to, the gene pair responsible for the absence of white hairs in spots (993). Possibly, when breeders selected dogs with well-delineated black spots, they inadvertently also selected dogs with high urate excretion (993). Other than Dalmatians, the bulldog is the breed most commonly afflicted with urate urolithiasis (41, 600).

The diagnosis is not always straightforward, as urate uroliths may not be strongly radiopaque and can be radiolucent. Urate crystalluria cannot be used as a predictor of urolithiasis because it is present in the urine of many dogs that never develop urate urolithiasis (992). Contrast radiography and ultrasonography appear to be the most useful techniques for detecting urate uroliths within the body (188). Analysis of uroliths is the most precise method of confirming the diagnosis.

Many Dalmatians with urate urolithiasis remain inapparent unless they are fed meals high in purines. The worst offenders are organ meats (e.g., liver, kidney, brain, sweetbreads), fish (mackerel, herring, sardines, anchovies), and wild game (e.g., venison, rabbit). Treatment is most effective when the diet is altered to contain mainly low-purine items (not just low protein) such as eggs, cheese, cottage cheese, vegetables, and breads and cereals (but not whole grain).

If dietary change is insufficient to correct the problem, drugs such as allopurinol can be used. If the diet is not changed concurrently, allopurinol can result in the formation of xanthine crystals instead of urate (194). Because the rate of absorption and excretion of allopurinol varies significantly among Dalmatians, as does the extent of hyperuricosuria, an oral dose must be titrated to the needs of each dog (598). Measuring urine urate-to-creatinine ratios is a practical way to monitor treatment (723). Dalmatians with a tendency to form uroliths should be removed from breeding programs.

Prevention of urate urolithiasis is an elusive goal. The best strategy involves promoting urine of low specific gravity. The use of long-term low-purine diets and urinary alkalinizers is controversial (992).

Urolithiasis—Cystine

Cystinuria results from a kidney disorder that allows cystine crystals and "stones" (uroliths) to form in the urine and potentially to block the urinary tract. Studies performed in the Newfoundland breed strongly suggest that the disorder is transmitted as an autosomal recessive trait (158), and researchers at the University of Pennsylvania School of Veterinary Medicine have identified the causative gene. A recessive mode of inheritance is also suspected in the Irish terrier and Scottish terrier (551). About 29 other breeds seem to be overrepresented, including the Australian cattle dog, Australian shepherd dog, basenji, bichon frisé, bullmastiff, Chihuahua, dachshund, English bulldog, mastiff, miniature pinscher, Pembroke Welsh corgi, pitbull terrier, Scottish deerhound, silky terrier, and Staffordshire terrier (38, 41, 158, 565, 600).

The disorder is one of an inherited defect in the renal proximal tubular transport system, which allows excessive urinary excretion of cystine (and, to a lesser extent, ornithine, lysine, and arginine) in the urine. Although cystinuria occurs in both male and female dogs, cystine calculi develop almost exclusively in males.

Clinically, the condition is seen most commonly in males, where the crystals can form stones in acidic urine and block the urinary tract. Affected dogs have difficulty urinating, because of the presence of cystine uroliths, and may have blood in the urine. Females are also affected, but they have a shorter and wider urethra, so blockage is less likely. They can still experience painful urination and blood in the urine, though. In other dog breeds, cystinuria is not clinically evident until 4 to 6 years of age, but in the Newfoundland, clinical signs may be apparent at less than 1 year of age.

All affected dogs (male and female) have cystine crystals in the urine, although the crystals are apparent only in acidic urine. Dogs that are on heavily vegetarian diets and are producing alkaline urine should have the urine acidified to detect the crystals. Otherwise, a cyanide nitroprusside spot test can be conducted at special metabolic laboratories. Animals with cystinuria can be detected in the first 2 months of life by examining acidic urine for typical crystals; confirmation requires metabolic testing (156).

A DNA test for cystinuria in Newfoundlands is now available. For the first time, this has allowed identification of clear, affected, and carrier animals. Running combinations of the urine and DNA tests is advisable for dogs experiencing hematuria or urolithiasis, as well as for Newfoundlands intended for breeding.

Cystinuria has no cure, but it usually can be effectively managed. Because cystine uroliths tend to form in acidic urine, the urine should be alkalinized by feeding diets with more vegetable protein and supplemental sodium bicarbonate, if necessary, to raise the urine pH above 7.4. In addition, D-penicillamine will reduce the concentration of cystine in the urine. Although daily doses of 2-mercaptoproprionylglycine (2-MPG) will dissolve cystine uroliths, a safe and effective regimen has not been completely standardized (158).

Dogs with cystinuria should not be bred because all offspring will be carriers or affected, depending on the status of the other parent. Carriers can now be detected, even though cystine is not detectable in their urine. This will eventually allow us to rid Newfoundlands and other breeds of the trait. In populations that have many carriers, breeding carriers to clear animals may be necessary at first. To breed two carriers or any affected animals is ill-advised.

Urolithiasis—Silica

Most silicate uroliths are seen in German shepherd dogs, Labrador retrievers, golden retrievers, and Old English sheepdogs; males seem to be more commonly affected than females (8, 565). Silica uroliths are most often associated with diets containing substantial quantities of corn gluten feed or soybean hulls. A mode of inheritance has not been determined and it is quite likely that the condition is not heritable. Severely affected individuals should not be bred, but little information is available on which to base sound breeding strategies.

Urolithiasis—Xanthine

Primary xanthinuria is seen in the Cavalier King Charles spaniel (1073) and perhaps the dachshund (535) and can occur secondarily in dogs treated with allopurinol. In the Cavalier King Charles spaniel, a deficiency of the enzyme xanthine oxidase causes increased excretion of hypoxanthine and xanthine (30–60× normal) (1072). The family history of affected individuals is consistent with an autosomal recessive mode of inheritance (1073). Therefore, affected animals should not be bred and parents are considered to be obligate carriers. Siblings are suspect carriers.

APPENDIX

The Major Players

The Animal Health Trust

The Animal Health Trust is a charitable organization that provides specialty veterinary clinical, diagnostic, and surgical services in Great Britain. They sponsor and conduct research in many different fields and disciplines as well as perform genetic screening tests. For more information on their activities, visit their Web site at www.aht.co.uk or contact them at Lanwades Park, Kentford, Newmarket, Suffolk CB8 7UU.

Canine Eye Registration Foundation (CERF)

The Canine Eye Registration Foundation (CERF) is an international organization devoted to eliminating hereditary eye diseases from purebred dogs. CERF is a nonprofit organization that cooperates with the American College of Veterinary Ophthalmologists (ACVO) to maintain a registry of purebred dogs that have been examined by board-certified veterinary ophthalmologists and found to be unaffected by major heritable eye disease. A database of all the information generated by CERF examinations serves as a resource to help breeders and ophthalmologists identify trends in eye disease and breed susceptibility. The goal is to identify purebreds without heritable eye problems so they can be used for breeding. Dogs being considered for breeding programs should be screened and certified by CERF annually because not all problems are evident in puppies. CERF registration has no minimum age requirement and is good for 12 months from the examination date.

The advantage of CERF is that it is a recognized entity in the purebred dog world and the evaluation by Diplomates of the ACVO lends great credibility to the registration process and the breeding advice given. A disadvantage—no fault of CERF—is that a dog can be registered with CERF, be used for breeding, and then develop a genetic problem that can be passed on to the offspring. When giving breeding advice to clients, it is, therefore, imperative to check that the CERF evaluation was done within the previous 12 months and that family history is known for conditions such as glaucoma, progressive retinal atrophy and even cataracts that might not be evident until later in life. General practice veterinarians, or those board-certified in other related specialties, might have expertise in eye diseases but are not permitted to certify dogs under the current evaluation process.

CERF is located at the Purdue University's School of Veterinary Medicine and is a subsidiary of the Veterinary Medical Data Base (VMDB), which compiles animal data from nearly all North American veterinary medicine colleges.

For more information on CERF, write to CERF, 1248 Lynn Hall, Purdue University, West Lafayette, IN 47907; (765) 494-8179; fax (765) 494-9981; http://www.prodogs.com//chn/cerf/.

Canine Reference Family DNA Distribution Center (Genetics Reference Center)

The Canine Reference Family DNA Distribution Center supports the development of a marker map by maintaining DNA from selected dog families and distributing it to scientists around the world. The Center will be located at the Purina facilities in the St. Louis, Missouri, area and will be supported by Ralston Purina. The Center will be a major resource for scientists investigating canine genetics, making DNA from reference families available to researchers worldwide. Purina also plans to maintain a related Web site devoted to canine genome research.

Canine Health Foundation

The American Kennel Club created the Canine Health Foundation to devote significant resources to canine research with an emphasis on canine genetics and breed-related health programs. In addition to AKC involvement, a scientific advisory committee was assembled to make recommendations for grant allocation to new research projects. The Foundation has made grants to various institutions for genetic disease research, as well as funds for developing a map of the canine genome.

For more information, contact the Canine Health Foundation, 251 W. Garfield Road, Suite 160, Aurora, OH 44202-8856; 330-995-0807; www.akcchf.org.

Dog Genome Project

The Dog Genome Project is a collaborative study involving scientists at the University of California, the University of Oregon, and the Fred Hutchinson Cancer Research Center, aimed at producing a map of all of the chromosomes in dogs, which can be used to map the genes causing disease and genes controlling morphology and behavior. A goal of the project is to develop a map that will be useful to the entire scientific community for the purpose of mapping genes that cause inherited disease in dogs. The genetic map being created will allow more effective breeding practices to eliminate many genetic diseases from breeds currently afflicted.

For more information, visit the Dog Genome Project web site at http://mendel.berkeley.edu/dog.html or the Fred Hutchinson Cancer Research Center Dog Genome Project at http://www.fhcrc.org/science/dog_genome/dog.html

DogMap

DogMap is an international collaboration of labs from many different countries that are working toward a low-resolution canine marker map. This work is being done under the auspices of the International Society for Animal Genetics (ISAG).

Participants are using microsatellites as markers to provide the backbone for the genome map. Part of the effort focuses on standardization of the canine karyotype, and special attention is paid to determining information of use in the diagnosis and management of hereditary diseases.

For more information on DogMap, visit its web site at http://ubeclu.unibe.ch/itz/dogmap.html

GeneSearch

GeneSearch LLC was founded in 1997 to provide cost-effective DNA-based genetic tests for hereditary problems afflicting purebred dogs. They also do original research to identify gene mutations and assess candidate genes based on genetic disorders already determined in other species. Tests currently available include those for progressive retinal atrophy in the Irish Setter, congenital stationary night blindness in the briard, phosphofructokinase deficiency in the American Cocker spaniel and English springer spaniel, and pyruvate kinase deficiency in the basenji. GeneSearch also asserts that their test results are accepted by the Orthopedic Foundation for Animals DNA-based Genetic Registry.

For more information on GeneSearch, visit their web site at www.genesearch.net, or contact them at: GeneSearch, 11014 Schuylkill Rd., Rockville, MD 20852, 301-770-6970, info@genesearch.net

Institute for Genetic Disease Control in Animals (GDC)

The Institute for Genetic Disease Control in Animals (GDC), a nonprofit organization founded in 1990, maintains an open registry of genetic problems. In an open registry like GDC, owners, breeders, veterinarians, and scientists can trace the genetic history of any dog once that dog and close relatives have been registered. The information about each dog automatically becomes linked in the open registry with relatives of that animal. An open registry delivers information on specific animals to breeders (for a fee) so the breeder can make knowledgeable selection of mates whose bloodlines indicate a reduced risk of producing genetic disease. Closed registries tell only if an individual animal is free of clinical signs of the disease and do not provide information about parents, siblings, or half siblings.

GDC operates both registries and databases, depending on the amount of information known about a specific disorder. To be included in a registry, the mode of inheritance and age of onset must be known and there must be an accepted method of diagnosis. A research database includes information on both affected and unaffected individuals and converts to an open registry once sufficient data exist to establish inheritance.

At present, the GDC operates several orthopedic registries. The diagnosis of all conditions is by radiographic evaluation. All films are read by at least two persons, a board-certified veterinary radiologist (Diplomate of the American College of Veterinary Radiology) and a board-certified surgeon (Diplomate of the American College of Veterinary Surgeons). In cases where there is question, a radiologist makes an additional blind evaluation for a final consensus.

GDC Registries and Databases

System	Breed(s)	Categories	Status	Opened
Eye	All	Unaffected, retinal dysplasia, PRA, corneal dystrophy, entropion, cataract	Registry	09-1994
Eye	Belgian sheepdogs	Above plus micropapilla, pannus, retinopathy	Registry	12-1996
Eye	Chinooks	Above plus glaucoma, retinal detachment, optic nerve coloboma, lens luxation/subluxation, PHPV/PTUL	Registry	07-1997
Eye	Cairn terriers	Pigmentary glaucoma, optic nerve coloboma	Database	06-1997
Orthopedic	All	Hips, elbows, shoulders and hocks	Registry	07-1990
Orthopedic	Miniature and toy poodles	Medial patellar luxation, Legg-Perthes	Registry	10-1994
Orthopedic	Cairn terrier	Hip dysplasia, Legg-Perthes, medial patellar luxation, craniomandibular osteopathy	Registry	11-1993
Orthopedic	All terriers	Hip dysplasia, Legg-Perthes, medial patellar luxation, craniomandibular osteopathy	Registry	03-1997
Orthopedic	Great Pyrenees	Chondrodysplasia	Database	07-1993
Circulatory	Labrador retriever	Tricuspid valve dysplasia	Registry	01-1997
Circulatory	Cairn terrier	Portosystemic shunt	Database	04-1994
Circulatory	All terriers	Portosystemic shunt	Database	03-1997
Cancer	Bernese mountain dog	Histiocytosis; mastocytoma	Registry	07-1994
Cancer	Bernese mountain dog	Other tumors	Database	07-1994
Skin	Standard poodles	Sebaceous adenitis	Registry	07-1992
Neurologic	All	Deafness	Registry	11-1997
Neurologic	Labrador retriever	Idiopathic epilepsy	Database	07-1993
Neurologic	Irish setter	Idiopathic epilepsy	Database	04-1996
Neurologic	Bernese mountain dog	Idiopathic epilepsy	Database	04-1998
Neurologic	Cairn terrier	Globoid cell leukodystrophy	Registry	11-1995
Neurologic	West Highland white terrier	Globoid cell leukodystrophy	Registry	03-1997

Diplomates of the American College of Veterinary Ophthalmologists do all eye examinations for GDC. These can be requested on a CERF form. The owner's copy of the examination form is sent to GDC with an application. A "certificate of unaffected" is valid for 1 year. Animals with ophthalmic disorders are registered in the database.

For more information, contact the Institute for Genetic Disease Control in Animals, PO Box 222, Davis, CA 95617; phone and fax (530) 756-6773; www.vetmed.ucdavis.edu/gdc/gdc.html

International Elbow Working Group (IEWG)

The International Elbow Working Group (IEWG) is a group of veterinary surgeons, radiologists, geneticists, and dog breeders who work with all aspects of elbow dysplasia. They have developed a standard protocol for the radiographic screening of elbows, which has proven effective for genetic disease control and for coordination of data for international study.

For more information, contact the Secretary of the IEWG at 12640 La Cresta Drive, Los Altos

Hills, CA 94022, 650-941-7848, www.vetmed.ucdavis.edu/iewg/iewg.html

OptiGen

OptiGen LLC is a service and research company established to provide DNA-based diagnoses and information about inherited diseases of purebred dogs. Currently, OptiGen offers a DNA test for progressive retinal atrophy (PRA) in the Irish setter, a marker test for PRA in the Portuguese water dog, and testing for congenital stationary night blindness in the briard. It is anticipated that PRA testing will soon become available for toy and miniature poodles, English cocker spaniels, American cocker spaniels, Labrador retrievers, and Australian cattle dogs.

For more information, contact OptiGen LLC, Cornell Business and Technology Park, 33 Thornwood Drive, Suite 102, Ithaca, NY 14850, 607-257-0301, www.optigen.com

Orthopedic Foundation for Animals (OFA)

Many dogs are prone to developing inherited problems of the bones and joints. The most common of these are hip dysplasia and elbow dysplasia. Because these traits are often hereditary, an impartial registry was needed to record dogs that had no such problems so they could be used for breeding. The OFA is a nonprofit organization established in 1966 to collect and disseminate information concerning orthopedic diseases of animals and to establish control programs intended to lower the incidence of orthopedic diseases in animals. In the recent past, the OFA has extended its mandate to include other genetic diseases. Currently, the OFA functions as a voluntary diagnostic service and registry for:

- Hip dysplasia
- Elbow dysplasia
- Patellar luxation
- Craniomandibular osteopathy
- Copper toxicosis in Bedlington terriers
- Heart disease
- Hypothyroidism
- von Willebrand's disease in Shetland sheepdogs, Doberman pinschers, Scottish terriers, Pembroke Welsh corgis, poodles, and Manchester terriers
- Phosphofructokinase deficiency in cocker spaniels and English springer spaniels
- Progressive retinal atrophy (PRA) in Irish setters
- Pyruvate kinase deficiency in basenjis
- Cystinuria in Newfoundlands
- Congenital stationary night blindness in briards
- Renal dysplasia in Shih tzu, Lhasa apso, and soft-coated wheaten terriers

Hip dysplasia is a common developmental disease in which the hip joints do not form correctly. The diagnosis is made by radiography. To standardize radiographic examination of dogs for dysplasia, the Orthopedic Foundation for Animals (OFA) formed a Hip Dysplasia Registry. Any veterinarian can take the radiographs, but, if they are to be certified, they have to be sent to the OFA. Although puppy radiographs can be evaluated, a registry number can be assigned only to dogs older than 2 years of age. Each hip radiograph submitted to the OFA is evaluated by veterinary radiologists and the hip joint conformation is classified. Classifications of excellent, good, and fair are considered to be within normal limits, and if the dog is 2 years of age or older, a breed registry number is assigned.

Elbow dysplasia is also a common orthopedic problem of dogs and may result from ununited anconeal process, fragmented medial coronoid process, osteochondritis of the medial humeral condyle, or a combination of these. Like hip dysplasia, although problems may be evident earlier, certification cannot be made until 24 months of age. Dogs with normal elbows upon evaluation are given a breed registry number and are reported periodically to the parent breed club. Abnormal findings are reported only to the owner and submitting veterinarian.

The ultimate purpose of OFA certification is to provide information to dog owners that will assist in the selection of good breeding animals. Therefore, attempts to get an unsuitable dog certified will only hurt the breed by perpetuating the disease.

For more information, contact the Orthopedic Foundation for Animals, 2300 E. Nifong Blvd., Columbia, MO 65201-3856; (573)-442-0418; www.offa.org

PE AgGen

Perkin-Elmer is the world leader in the development, manufacture, and marketing of analytical instruments and life science systems used in markets such as pharmaceuticals, biotechnology, environmental testing, food, agriculture, and chemical manufacturing. Its agricultural division, PE AgGen, was formed in July 1997, combining the efforts of the Applied Biosystems Division of the Perkin-Elmer Corporation with PE Zoogen and Linkage Genetics Inc. to deliver DNA diagnostic, automated genotyping, gene discovery, trait-specific analyses, and diagnostic screening.

Both the American Kennel Club and the United Kennel Club selected PE AgGen to provide DNA-based identity and parentage verification. The PE AgGen's DNA CheekSwab™ is used to collect samples. The PE AgGen's DNA PawPrint™ can provide genetic identification and parentage for dogs that can be certified with a confidence of over 99.9%. PE AgGen also offers a comprehensive canine DNA archiving program to preserve a complete copy of the unique hereditary information carried within each animal.

The American Kennel Club is offering a voluntary DNA certification program to preserve the integrity of the registry. In the compliance audit program, AKC inspectors will collect DNA samples at random during their kennel inspections, which will permit verification of parentage for litters observed. Participating clubs are also encouraged to have their members voluntarily provide DNA samples for identification, and to obtain reliable estimates of genetic marker variability within each breed. The United Kennel Club offers a DNA-VIP (Verified Identified Parentage) Program, which is also provided by PE AgGen.

For more information, contact PE AgGen at 1756 Picasso Avenue, Davis, CA 95616-0549; (800) 995-2473 or 530-297-3000; www2.perkin-elmer.com/ab/aggen/

PennHip

The University of Pennsylvania Hip Improvement Program (PennHip®) was formed to evaluate a dog for its susceptibility to develop hip dysplasia. To do the evaluation, the dog is heavily sedated or anesthetized and measurements on hip laxity are taken from a series of three radiographs. The degree of looseness, or laxity, in the hip joints when the muscles are completely relaxed is an important factor in determining susceptibility to develop hip dysplasia and degenerative joint disease (arthritis) later in life. In addition, unlike other screening tests, PennHip® can predict susceptibility to hip dysplasia in dogs as young as 16 weeks of age. Only PennHip® trained and certified veterinarians can participate in the program. That program is administered by Synbiotics Corporation of San Diego, California.

PennHip® Evaluation provides some interesting information for pet owners, veterinarians, and breeders. A Distraction Index (DI) is determined, expressed as a number between 0 and 1. The closer the number to 0, the tighter the hips and the lower the risk of hip dysplasia. The closer the number to 1, the looser the hips and the higher the risk of hip dysplasia. The database also supplies breed-specific information to help in selecting dogs for breeding. A dog receiving a ranking in the 70th percentile means that 30% of the breed members have hips that are tighter and 70% have hips that are looser. This allows breeders to easily identify animals with tighter hips within the breed, which in turn are less likely to develop hip dysplasia and pass on that genetic tendency to future generations.

For more information on PennHip®, contact Synbiotics Corporation, 11011 Via Frontera, San Diego CA 92127; www.synbiotics.com/pennhip.html

VetGen

In 1998, a team of molecular geneticists from Michigan State University School of Veterinary Medicine and University of Michigan's Department of Human Genetics began researching canine genetic disease as a team. With the assistance of the American Kennel Club (AKC), the Morris Animal Foundation (MAF), and the Orthopedic Foundation for Animals (OFA), the team began researching genetic diseases with the goal of developing disease-detection tests. In the process, they detected some 625 markers that formed the Canine Molecular Genetics Resource™ (CMGR™), the world's most comprehensive collection of canine genetic markers. Based on one of the markers in the CMGR™, the team first developed the linkage-based test for copper toxicosis in Bedlington terriers.

In 1995, the research team merged into a commercial enterprise dedicated to researching and developing genetic tests for purebred dogs, which became VetGen. The team also established a diagnostic laboratory to evaluate samples, created DNA profiling to provide positive identification of tested dogs, and provided DNA storage for long-term handling of samples.

VetGen currently provides DNA testing for the following conditions:

- Copper toxicosis in Bedlington terriers
- Pyruvate kinase deficiency in basenjis
- Progressive retinal atrophy (PRA) in Irish setters
- von Willebrand's disease in Doberman pinschers, Shetland sheepdogs, Pembroke Welsh corgis, poodles, Scottish terriers, and Manchester terriers
- Phosphofructokinase deficiency in springer and cocker spaniels

- Renal dysplasia in Shih tzu, Lahsa apso, and soft-coated wheaten terriers.

Current research projects include tests for: PRA of the progressive rod-cone degeneration (prcd) type, such as seen in cocker spaniels, Labrador retrievers, Portuguese water dogs and poodles; hip dysplasia; inherited epilepsy, skeletal muscle myopathy in Labrador retrievers; elbow dysplasia in Labrador retrievers; inherited thyroid disease I; and many others.

For more information, contact VetGen at: 3728 Plaza Drive, Suite One, Ann Arbor MI 48108; www.vetgen.com

Veterinary Genetics Laboratory

Veterinary Genetics Laboratory, a division of the School of Medicine, University of California, Davis, uses microsatellite markers to determine identification and parentage. Karyotyping is also available for the rare instances of chromosomal abnormality.

For more information on Veterinary Genetics Laboratory, contact the School of Veterinary Medicine, University of California, Davis, CA 95616-8744; http://www.vgl.ucdavis.edu/Service/Canine/

Breed Table

The following table lists breeds, the conditions that affect them, and where to find appropriate information in this book. The table is not meant to be all-inclusive and it does not reflect true prevalence of traits. It should be considered a starting point when evaluating heritable conditions of specific purebreds. Conditions reported in italics are anecdotally reported to be important in the breed, but have not been documented in peer-reviewed scientific literature.

Breed	AKC Rank* (1998)	Disorder†	Inheritance‡	Page
Abyssinian sand terrier				
		Hairlessness	AD	48
Affenpinscher	121			
		Anasarca	AR	47
		Cataracts	ND	147
		Cleft lip/palate	ND	73
		Cryptorchidism	ND	173
		Dermoid	ND	52
		Elongated soft palate	ND	177
		Hip dysplasia	Polygenic	116
		Hypothyroidism	ND	69
		Inhalant allergies	ND	93
		Keratoconjunctivitis sicca	ND	156
		Legg-Calvé-Perthes disease	ND	120
		Oligodontia	ND	41
		Patellar luxation	ND	127
		Patent ductus arteriosus	ND	34
		Progressive retinal atrophy	ND	163
		Retained primary teeth	ND	42
		Seasonal flank alopecia	ND	71
		Tracheal collapse	ND	178
		X-linked myopathy	XR	121
Afghan hound	85			
		Amyloidosis	ND	101
		Brachygnathism	ND	39
		Cataracts	AR	147
		Corneal dystrophy	ND	150
		Deafness	ND	132
		Demodicosis	ND	50
		Distichiasis	ND	151
		Elbow dysplasia	ND	113
		Exocrine pancreatic insufficiency	ND	75
		Fanconi syndrome	ND	181
		Gastric dilatation-volvulus	ND	76
		Glaucoma	ND	154
		Hereditary myelopathy	AR	133
		Hip dysplasia	Polygenic	116

Breed	AKC Rank* (1998)	Disorder†	Inheritance‡	Page
		Hypothyroidism	ND	69
		Intervertebral disk disease	ND	136
		Laryngeal paralysis	AD	177
		Megaesophagus	ND	75
		Mitral valve disease	ND	33
		Narcolepsy	ND	144
		OCD–shoulder	ND	124
		Oligodontia	ND	41
		Optic nerve hypoplasia	ND	159
		Patellar luxation	ND	127
		Perineal hernia	ND	111
		Persistent pupillary membranes	ND	162
		Prognathism	ND	42
		Progressive retinal atrophy	ND	163
		Pulmonic stenosis	ND	34
		Retinal dysplasia	ND	168
		Seborrhea	ND	61
		Umbilical hernia	ND	111
		von Willebrand disease	AID?	89
		Wobbler syndrome	ND	130
Ainu				
		Uveodermatological syndrome	ND	99
Airedale terrier	50			
		Atrial septal defect	ND	30
		Cardiomyopathy	ND	30
		Cataracts	ND	147
		Cerebellar abiotrophy	Familial	129
		Chromasomal intersex	ND	174
		Corneal dystrophy	XR	150
		Cryptorchidism	ND	173
		Demodicosis	ND	50
		Distichiasis	ND	151
		Elbow dysplasia	ND	113
		Entropion	Polygenic	154
		Epilepsy	ND	143
		Exocrine pancreatic insufficiency	ND	75
		Factor IX deficiency	XR	83
		Gastric dilatation-volvulus	ND	76
		Hemophilia B	XR	83
		Hip dysplasia	Polygenic	116
		Hyperlipoproteinemia	ND	106
		Hypoadrenocorticism	ND	69
		Hypothyroidism	ND	69
		Intervertebral disk disease	ND	136
		Laryngeal paralysis	ND	177
		Myasthenia gravis	ND	139
		Narcolepsy	ND	144
		Pancreatitis	ND	78
		Panosteitis	ND	126
		Pannus	ND	159
		Polycystic kidney disease	ND	181
		Portosystemic shunt	ND	78
		Progressive retinal atrophy	AR?	163
		Pulmonic stenosis	ND	34
		Retinal dysplasia	ND	168
		Saddle alopecia	ND	54
		Seasonal flank alopecia	ND	71
		Sebaceous adenitis	ND	60
		Seborrhea	ND	61
		Subaortic stenosis	ND	29
		Tricuspid valve dysplasia	ND	36
		Umbilical hernia	ND	111
		Ventricular septal defect	ND	37
		von Willebrand disease	AID?	89

Breed	AKC Rank* (1998)	Disorder†	Inheritance‡	Page
Akbash dog				
		Cardiomyopathy	ND	30
		Entropion	ND	154
		Epilepsy	ND	143
		Gastric dilatation-volvulus	ND	76
		Hip dysplasia	Polygenic	116
		Hypertrophic osteodystrophy	ND	120
		Hypothyroidism	ND	69
		Panosteitis	ND	126
		Prognathism	ND	42
		Umbilical hernia	ND	111
Akita	36			
		Brachygnathism	ND	39
		Cataracts	ND	147
		Central PRA	ND	162
		Deafness	ND	132
		Entropion	Polygenic	154
		Epilepsy	ND	143
		Epidermolysis bullosa	ND	52
		Fragmented coronoid process	ND	114
		Gastric dilatation-volvulus	ND	76
		Glaucoma	ND	154
		Glycogen storage disease III	AR	105
		Hip dysplasia	Polygenic	116
		Hypothyroidism	ND	69
		IgA deficiency	ND	99
		Microcytosis	ND	85
		Microphthalmia	ND	158
		OCD–shoulder	ND	124
		OCD–stifle	ND	124
		Osteochondrodysplasia	ND	126
		Patellar luxation	ND	127
		Pemphigus foliaceus	ND	97
		Peripheral vestibular disease	ND	132
		Portosystemic shunt	ND	78
		Prognathism	ND	42
		Progressive retinal atrophy	ND	163
		Pseudohyperkalemia	ND	86
		Renal dysplasia	ND	179
		Retinal dysplasia	ND	168
		Sebaceous adenitis	ND	60
		Uveodermatological syndrome	ND	99
		Vestibular disease	ND	132
		von Willebrand disease	AID?	89
Alaskan malamute	46			
		Cataracts	AR?	147
		Corneal dystrophy	ND	150
		Cryptorchidism	ND	173
		Cutaneous lupus erythematosus	ND	96
		Diabetes mellitus	ND	65
		Distichiasis	ND	151
		Epilepsy	ND	143
		Factor VII deficiency	AR	82
		Factor VII deficiency	AR	82
		Factor VIII deficiency	XR	82
		Factor IX deficiency	XR	83
		Factor IX deficiency	XR	83
		Fragmented coronoid process	ND	114
		Gastric dilatation-volvulus	ND	76
		Glaucoma	ND	154
		Hemeralopia	AR	154
		Hemivertebra	ND	135
		Hemolytic anemia	AR	85

Breed	AKC Rank* (1998)	Disorder†	Inheritance‡	Page
		Hip dysplasia	Polygenic	116
		Hypothyroidism	ND	69
		Keratoconjunctivitis sicca	ND	156
		Macrocytosis/Stomatocytosis	ND	85
		Megaesophagus	ND	75
		Muscular dystrophy	XR	121
		Myelodysplasia	ND	140
		Narcolepsy	ND	144
		OCD–shoulder	ND	124
		Optic nerve hypoplasia	ND	159
		Osteochondrodysplasia	AR	126
		Panosteitis	ND	126
		Patellar luxation	ND	127
		Persistent pupillary membranes	ND	162
		Polyneuropathy	AR	141
		Portosystemic shunting	ND	78
		Progressive retinal atrophy	AR?	163
		Pulmonic stenosis	ND	34
		Renal dysplasia	ND	179
		Retained primary teeth	ND	42
		Ulcerative keratitis	ND	151
		Uveal hypopigmentation	ND	171
		Uveodermatological syndrome	ND	99
		Ventricular septal defect	ND	37
		von Willebrand disease	AID?	89
		Wooly syndrome	ND	54
		Zinc-responsive dermatosis	ND	63
American bulldog				
		Cystinuria	XR	185
		Hip dysplasia	Polygenic	116
		Hypothyroidism	ND	69
American Eskimo dog	96			
		Anasarca	AR	47
		Cataracts	ND	147
		Cryptorchidism	ND	173
		Epilepsy	ND	143
		Hemivertebra	ND	135
		Hip dysplasia	Polygenic	116
		Hypothyroidism	ND	69
		Laryngeal paralysis	ND	177
		Megaesophagus	ND	75
		Methemoglobin reductase deficiency	ND	85
		Narcolepsy	AR?	144
		Patellar luxation	ND	127
		Patent ductus arteriosus	ND	34
		Prognathism	ND	42
		Progressive retinal atrophy	ND	163
		Pyruvate kinase deficiency	AR	86
		Sebaceous adenitis	ND	60
		Zinc-responsive dermatosis	ND	63
American hairless terrier (rat terrier)				
		Hairlessness	AR	48
		Lens luxation	ND	158
		Patellar luxation	ND	127
American pit bull terrier				
		Cleft lip/palate	ND	73
		Hip dysplasia	Polygenic	116
		Hypothyroidism	ND	69
		Ichthyosis	ND	56
		Inhalant allergies	ND	93
		Patellar luxation	ND	127
		Zinc-responsive dermatosis	ND	63
American Staffordshire terrier	68			
		Cataracts	ND	147

Breed	AKC Rank* (1998)	Disorder†	Inheritance‡	Page
		Cleft lip/palate	ND	73
		Compulsive tail chasing	ND	131
		Cruciate ligament rupture	ND	112
		Cryptorchidism	ND	173
		Cystinuria	ND	185
		Deafness	ND	132
		Demodicosis	ND	50
		Distichiasis	ND	151
		Fragmented coronoid process	ND	114
		Hip dysplasia	Polygenic	116
		Hypothyroidism	ND	69
		Ichthyosis	ND	56
		Patent ductus arteriosus	ND	34
		Progressive retinal atrophy	ND	163
		Subaortic stenosis	ND	29
		Wobbler syndrome	ND	130
American water spaniel	117			
		Allergic inhalant dermatitis	ND	93
		Cataracts	ND	147
		Cleft lip/palate	ND	73
		Cryptorchidism	ND	173
		Diabetes mellitus	ND	65
		Epilepsy	ND	143
		Follicular dysplasia	ND	53
		Hermaphrodism	ND	174
		Growth hormone-responsive dermatosis	ND	67
		Hip dysplasia	Polygenic	116
		Hypothyroidism	ND	69
		Inguinal hernia	ND	111
		Osteochondrodysplasia	ND	126
		Patent ductus arteriosus	ND	34
		Progressive retinal atrophy	ND	163
		Retinal dysplasia	ND	168
Anatolian shepherd dog	126			
		Distichiasis	ND	151
		Elbow luxation	ND	113
		Hip dysplasia	Polygenic	116
		Hypothyroidism	ND	69
		Renal dysplasia	ND	179
Argentino Dogo				
		Deafness	ND	132
		Glaucoma	ND	154
		Hip dysplasia	ND	116
		Hypothyroidism	ND	69
Australian blue heeler				
		Ceroid lipofuscinosis	AR?	102
		Deafness	ND	132
		Pelger-Huet anomaly	AID?	85
		Progressive retinal atrophy	ND	163
Australian cattle dog (Queensland Heeler)	67			
		Cataracts	ND	147
		Ceroid lipofuscinosis	AR?	102
		Cystinuria	ND	185
		Deafness	ND	132
		Dermatomyositis	AID?	51
		Fragmented coronoid process	ND	114
		Hip dysplasia	Polygenic	116
		Hypothyroidism	ND	69
		Lens luxation	ND	158
		OCD–hock	ND	124
		Patellar luxation	ND	127
		Pelger-Huet anomaly	ND	85
		Persistent pupillary membranes	ND	162

Breed	AKC Rank* (1998)	Disorder†	Inheritance‡	Page
		Polioencephalomyelopathy	ND	137
		Portosystemic shunting	ND	78
		Progressive retinal atrophy	AR?	163
		von Willebrand disease	AID?	89
Australian kelpie				
		Cerebellar abiotrophy	AR	129
		Cutaneous asthenia	ND	49
		Hip dysplasia	ND	116
		Hypothyroidism	ND	69
		Pannus	ND	159
		Progressive retinal atrophy	ND	163
Australian shepherd	40			
		Anterior crossbite	ND	41
		Brachygnathism	ND	39
		Cataracts	ND	147
		Cerebellar vermian hypoplasia	AR	130
		Choroidal hypoplasia	ND	147
		Collie eye anomaly	AR?	147
		Cryptorchidism	ND	173
		Cutaneous lupus erythematosus	ND	96
		Cystinuria		185
		Deafness	ND	132
		Diabetes mellitus	ND	65
		Epilepsy	ND	143
		Factor VIII deficiency	ND	82
		Fragmented coronoid process	ND	114
		Hip dysplasia	Polygenic	116
		Hypothyroidism	ND	69
		Microphthalmia	ND	158
		Optic nerve coloboma	ND	159
		Osteochondrodysplasia	XR	126
		Pannus	ND	159
		Panosteitis	ND	126
		Patent ductus arteriosus	ND	34
		Pelger-Huet anomaly	AID?	85
		Persistent pupillary membranes	ND	162
		Persistent right aortic arch	ND	36
		Portosystemic shunting	ND	78
		Prognathism	ND	42
		Progressive retinal atrophy	ND	163
		Pulmonic stenosis	ND	34
		Retinal dysplasia	ND	168
		Uveal hypopigmentation	ND	171
		von Willebrand disease	ND	89
Australian terrier	101			
		Allergic inhalant dermatitis	ND	93
		Cataracts	ND	147
		Cleft lip/palate	ND	73
		Cryptorchidism	ND	173
		Diabetes mellitus	ND	65
		Epilepsy	ND	143
		Glucocerebrosidosis	ND	104
		Hypothyroidism	ND	69
		Inhalant allergies	ND	93
		Juvenile cellulitis	ND	56
		Legg-Calvé-Perthes disease	ND	120
		Megaesophagus	ND	75
		Patellar luxation	ND	127
		Patent ductus arteriosus	ND	34
		Portosystemic shunting	ND	78
		Progressive retinal atrophy	AR?	163
		Retinal dysplasia	AR?	168

Breed	AKC Rank* (1998)	Disorder†	Inheritance‡	Page
Azawakh				
		Hypothyroidism	ND	69
		von Willebrand disease	AID?	89
Basenji	70			
		Cataracts	ND	147
		Corneal dystrophy	ND	150
		Cystinuria	ND	185
		Epilepsy	ND	143
		Fanconi syndrome	Familial	181
		Hip dysplasia	ND	116
		Hypothyroidism	ND	69
		Immunoproliferative enteropathy	Familial	77
		Intestinal lymphangiectasia	ND	79
		Optic nerve coloboma	ND	159
		Pelger-Huet anomaly	AID?	85
		Persistent pupillary membranes	ND	162
		Progressive retinal atrophy	ND	163
		Pyruvate kinase deficiency	AR	86
		Retinal dysplasia	ND	168
		Umbilical hernia	ND	111
Basset hound	21			
		Allergic inhalant dermatitis	ND	93
		Black hair follicular dysplasia	ND	53
		Brachygnathism	ND	39
		Cataracts	ND	147
		Cervical vertebral instability	Familial	130
		Combined immunodeficiency	XR	100
		Corneal dystrophy	ND	150
		Cystinuria	XR	185
		Dermatomyositis	AID?	51
		Dilated cardiomyopathy	ND	30
		Elongated soft palate	ND	177
		Gastric dilatation-volvulus	ND	76
		Glaucoma	Familial	154
		Globoid cell leukodystrophy	AR?	103
		Hemivertebra	ND	135
		Hypoadrenocorticism	ND	69
		Hypothyroidism	ND	69
		Hypotrichosis	ND	48
		Intervertebral disk disease	ND	136
		Lafora body disease	AR?	106
		Malassezia dermatitis	ND	58
		Mycobacterial susceptibility	ND	96
		Panosteitis	ND	126
		Patellar luxation	ND	127
		Persistent Mullerian duct syndrome	AR?	175
		Progressive retinal atrophy	ND	163
		Prolapsed gland of nictitans	ND	168
		Pulmonic stenosis	ND	34
		Sebaceous adenitis	ND	60
		Seborrhea	ND	61
		Subaortic stenosis	ND	29
		Thrombopathia	AD, VE	87
		Ununited anconeal process	ND	115
		von Willebrand disease	AID?	89
		Wobbler syndrome	ND	130
		XX sex reversal	ND	174
Beagle	6			
		Black hair follicular dysplasia	ND	53
		Brachygnathism	ND	39
		Cataracts	AID?	147
		Cerebellar abiotrophy	ND	129
		Cervical vertebral instability	ND	130
		Cleft lip/palate	ND	73

Breed	AKC Rank* (1998)	Disorder†	Inheritance‡	Page
		Copper hepatopathy	ND	74
		Corneal dystrophy	ND	150
		Cryptorchidism	ND	173
		Cutaneous asthenia	ND	49
		Deafness	ND	132
		Demodicosis	ND	50
		Diabetes mellitus	ND	65
		Dilated cardiomyopathy	ND	30
		Distichiasis	ND	151
		Dysfibrinogenemia	ND	81
		Ectodermal defect	ND	52
		Elongated soft palate	ND	177
		Epilepsy	Familial	143
		Factor VII deficiency	AR	82
		Factor VIII deficiency	XR	82
		Glaucoma	AR	154
		Globoid cell leukodystrophy	AR?	103
		GM-1 gangliosidosis	AR	105
		Hip dysplasia	Polygenic	116
		Hound ataxia	ND	138
		Hyperlipidemia	ND	106
		Hypothyroidism	ND	69
		Hypotrichosis	ND	48
		IgA deficiency	ND	99
		Intervertebral disk disease	ND	136
		Lafora body disease	AR	106
		Lissencephaly	ND	138
		MAP urolithiasis	ND	183
		Micropapilla	ND	159
		Microphthalmia	ND	158
		Mitral valve disease	ND	33
		Narcolepsy	AR	144
		Nonspherocytic hemolytic anemia	AR?	85
		Optic nerve hypoplasia	ND	159
		Pain syndrome	ND	139
		Panosteitis	ND	126
		Peripheral vestibular disease	ND	132
		Prognathism	ND	42
		Progressive retinal atrophy	AR	163
		Prolapsed gland of nictitans	ND	168
		Pulmonic stenosis	Polygenic	34
		Pyruvate kinase deficiency	AR	86
		Renal agenesis	Familial	179
		Renal amyloidosis	ND	101
		Retinal dysplasia	ND	168
		Shaker syndrome	ND	144
		Small intestinal bacterial overgrowth	ND	80
		Spina bifida	ND	145
		Uveal hypopigmentation	ND	171
		Vasculitis	ND	88
		Vertebral stenosis	ND	146
		Vestibular syndrome	AR	132
		XX sex reversal	ND	174
Bearded collie	90			
		Black hair follicular dysplasia	ND	53
		Brachygnathism	ND	39
		Cataracts	ND	147
		Cleft lip/palate	ND	73
		Corneal dystrophy	ND	150
		Cryptorchidism	ND	173
		Epilepsy	ND	143
		Fragmented coronoid process	ND	114
		Hip dysplasia	Polygenic	116
		Hypoadrenocorticism	ND	69

Breed	AKC Rank* (1998)	Disorder†	Inheritance‡	Page
		Hypothyroidism	ND	69
		Oligodontia	ND	41
		Patellar luxation	ND	127
		Patent ductus arteriosus	ND	34
		Pemphigus foliaceus	ND	97
		Prognathism	ND	42
		Progressive retinal atrophy	ND	163
		Retinal dysplasia	ND	168
		Seasonal flank alopecia	ND	71
		Subaortic stenosis	ND	29
		Systemic lupus erythematosus	ND	95
		von Willebrand disease	AID?	89
Beauceron shepherd				
		Dermatomyositis	AID?	51
		Epidermolysis bullosa	ND	52
		Hip dysplasia	ND	116
		Hypothyroidism	ND	69
		Inhalant allergies	ND	93
Bedlington terrier	124			
		Cataracts	AR	147
		Chronic inflammatory hepatic disease	ND	73
		Copper hepatopathy	AR	74
		Distichiasis	ND	151
		Entropion	Polygenic	154
		Epilepsy	ND	143
		Glaucoma	ND	154
		Imperforate nasolacrimal puncta	ND	156
		Inhalant allergies	ND	93
		Keratoconjunctivitis sicca	ND	156
		Microphthalmia	ND	158
		Oligodontia	ND	41
		Osteogenesis imperfecta	ND	126
		Progressive retinal atrophy	ND	163
		Renal dysplasia	ND	179
		Retinal dysplasia	AR	168
Belgian Laekenois				
		Fragmented coronoid process	ND	114
		Hip dysplasia	ND	116
		Hypothyroidism	ND	69
Belgian Malinois	92			
		Cataracts	ND	147
		Epilepsy	ND	143
		Exertional myositis	ND	115
		Fragmented coronoid process	ND	114
		Gastric dilatation-volvulus	ND	76
		Hip dysplasia	Polygenic	116
		Hypothyroidism	ND	69
		Prognathism	ND	42
		Progressive retinal atrophy	ND	163
		Retinal dysplasia	ND	168
Belgian sheepdog (Belgian Groenendael)	106			
		Cataracts	ND	147
		Ectodermal defect	ND	52
		Epilepsy	ND	143
		Fragmented coronoid process	ND	114
		Gracilis or semitendinosus myopathy	ND	115
		Hypothyroidism	ND	69
		Hypotrichosis	ND	48
		Micropapilla	ND	159
		Muscular dystrophy	XR	121
		Pannus	ND	159
		Prognathism	ND	42
		Progressive retinal atrophy	AR?	163

Breed	AKC Rank* (1998)	Disorder†	Inheritance‡	Page
		Retinal dysplasia	ND	168
		Subaortic stenosis	ND	29
		Vitiligo	ND	62
Belgian Tervuren	100			
		Anasarca	AR	47
		Anterior crossbite	ND	41
		Atrial septal defect	ND	30
		Cataracts	ND	147
		Epilepsy	Familial	143
		Fragmented coronoid process	ND	114
		Hypothyroidism	ND	69
		Level bite	ND	40
		Lymphedema	ND	85
		Micropapilla	ND	159
		Oligodontia	ND	41
		Optic nerve hypoplasia	ND	159
		Pannus	ND	159
		Prognathism	ND	42
		Progressive retinal atrophy	ND	163
		Vitiligo	ND	62
		Wry mouth		41
Bern running dog				
		Cerebellar abiotrophy	ND	129
Bernese mountain dog	63			
		Aseptic meningitis	ND	138
		Cataracts	ND	147
		Cerebellar abiotrophy	Familial	129
		Color dilution alopecia	AR?	48
		Dysmyelinogenesis	AR	134
		Epilepsy	ND	143
		Fibrinoid leukodystrophy	ND	137
		Fragmented coronoid process	ND	114
		Gastric dilatation-volvulus	ND	76
		Glomerulonephritis	Familial	181
		Hip dysplasia	Polygenic	116
		Histiocytosis	Familial	58
		Hypertrophic osteodystrophy	ND	120
		Hypoadrenocorticism	ND	69
		Hypothyroidism	ND	69
		Sebaceous adenitis	ND	60
		Vasculitis	ND	88
		von Willebrand disease	AID?	89
Bichon frisé	25			
		Allergic inhalant dermatitis	ND	93
		Brachygnathism	ND	39
		Calcium oxalate urolithiasis	ND	184
		Cataracts	ND	147
		Ciliary dyskinesia	ND	98
		Corneal dystrophy	ND	150
		Cryptorchidism	ND	173
		Cystinuria	ND	185
		Deafness	ND	132
		Entropion	Polygenic	154
		Epilepsy	ND	143
		Factor IX deficiency	XR	83
		Fragmented coronoid process	ND	114
		Hip dysplasia	Polygenic	116
		Hypotrichosis	ND	48
		Legg-Calvé-Perthes disease	ND	120
		Patent ductus arteriosus	Polygenic	34
		Persistent pupillary membranes	ND	162
		Portosystemic shunting	ND	78
		Prognathism	ND	42
		Progressive retinal atrophy	ND	163

Breed	AKC Rank* (1998)	Disorder†	Inheritance‡	Page
		Retinal dysplasia	ND	168
		Shaker syndrome	ND	144
		Ventricular septal defect	ND	37
		von Willebrand disease	AID?	89
Black and tan coonhound	116			
		Cataracts	ND	147
		Central PRA	ND	162
		Cryptorchidism	ND	173
		Entropion	Polygenic	154
		Factor IX deficiency	XR	83
		Gastric dilatation-volvulus	ND	76
		Hip dysplasia	Polygenic	116
		Hypothyroidism	ND	69
		Patellar luxation	ND	127
		Pelger-Huet anomaly	AID?	85
		Progressive retinal atrophy	ND	163
Bloodhound	51			
		Brachygnathism	ND	39
		Cryptorchidism	ND	173
		Ectropion	ND	153
		Elbow dysplasia	ND	113
		Entropion	ND	154
		Gastric dilatation-volvulus	ND	76
		Hip dysplasia	Polygenic	116
		Hypothyroidism	ND	69
		Keratoconjunctivitis sicca	ND	156
		Prolapsed gland of nictitans	ND	168
		Spinal muscular atrophy	ND	145
		Ununited anconeal process	ND	115
Bluetick coonhound				
		Cataracts	ND	147
		Gastric dilatation-volvulus	ND	76
		Globoid cell leukodystrophy	AR?	103
		Hip dysplasia	ND	116
		Hock luxation	ND	125
		Hypothyroidism	ND	69
		Pelger-Huet anomaly	ND	85
Border collie	71			
		Cataracts	Familial	147
		Central PRA	AD, VE	162
		Cerebellar abiotrophy	AR?	129
		Ceroid lipofuscinosis	AR	102
		Ciliary dyskinesia	ND	98
		Cobalamin malabsorption	AR?	109
		Collie eye anomaly	AR?	147
		Corneal dystrophy	ND	150
		Cyclic hematopoiesis	ND	94
		Deafness	AID?	132
		Epilepsy	ND	143
		Fragmented coronoid process	ND	114
		Hip dysplasia	Polygenic	116
		Lens luxation	ND	158
		Malignant hyperthermia	ND	107
		Neuroaxonal dystrophy	ND	140
		OCD–stifle	ND	124
		Pannus	ND	159
		Patent ductus arteriosus	ND	34
		Pelger-Huet anomaly	AID?	85
		Progressive retinal atrophy	ND	163
		Retinal dysplasia	AR?	168
		Sensory neuropathy	ND	142

Breed	AKC Rank* (1998)	Disorder†	Inheritance‡	Page
Border terrier	87			
		Brachury	AR	177
		Cataracts	ND	147
		Craniomandibular osteopathy	AR	112
		Cryptorchidism	ND	173
		Fanconi syndrome	ND	181
		Legg-Calvé-Perthes disease	ND	120
		Oligodontia	ND	41
		Patellar luxation	ND	127
		Persistent atrial standstill	ND	35
		Prognathism	ND	42
		Progressive axonopathy	ND	141
		Progressive retinal atrophy	ND	163
		Retained primary teeth	ND	42
		Retinal dysplasia	ND	168
		Thrombopathia	ND	87
Borzoi (Russian wolfhound)	81			
		Cataracts	ND	147
		Cervical vertebral instability	AR	130
		Dysfibrinogenemia	ND	81
		Focal retinal degeneration	AR?	162
		Gastric dilatation-volvulus	ND	76
		Hypertrophic osteodystrophy	ND	120
		Hypothyroidism	ND	69
		Lymphedema	ND	85
		Methemoglobin reductase deficiency	ND	85
		Microphthalmia	ND	158
		OCD–stifle	ND	124
		Oligodontia	ND	41
		Optic nerve hypoplasia	ND	159
		Persistent pupillary membranes	ND	162
		Posterior crossbite	ND	41
		Retinal degeneration	Familial?	162
		Retinal dysplasia	ND	168
		Tricuspid valve dysplasia	ND	36
		Wobbler syndrome	ND	130
Boston terrier	19			
		Allergic inhalant dermatitis	ND	93
		Anasarca	AR	47
		Brachycephalic syndrome	ND	177
		Calcinosis circumscripta	ND	47
		Cataracts	AR	147
		Cerebellar vermian hypoplasia	ND	130
		Cleft lip/palate	ND	73
		Corneal dystrophy	ND	150
		Craniomandibular osteopathy	ND	112
		Cryptorchidism	ND	173
		Deafness	ND	132
		Demodicosis	ND	50
		Elongated soft palate	ND	177
		Entropion	Polygenic	154
		Fold dermatitis	ND	53
		Hemivertebra	ND	135
		Hydrocephalus	ND	135
		Hyperadrenocorticism	ND	67
		Hypoplastic trachea	ND	177
		Hypothyroidism	ND	69
		Keratoconjunctivitis sicca	ND	156
		Legg-Calvé-Perthes disease	ND	120
		Medial patellar luxation	ND	127
		Mitral valve disease	ND	33
		Pelger-Huet anomaly	AID?	85

Breed	AKC Rank* (1998)	Disorder†	Inheritance‡	Page
		Progressive retinal atrophy	ND	163
		Prolapsed gland of nictitans	ND	168
		Pyloric stenosis	ND	80
		Sacrocaudal dysgenesis	ND	142
		Spina bifida	ND	145
		Ulcerative keratitis	ND	151
		Wry mouth	ND	41
Bouvier des Flandres	72			
		Brachygnathism	ND	39
		Cataracts	ND	147
		Cleft lip/palate	ND	73
		Degenerative myopathy	ND	111
		Entropion	Polygenic	154
		Gastric dilatation-volvulus	ND	76
		Glaucoma	ND	154
		Hip dysplasia	Polygenic	116
		Hypothyroidism	ND	69
		Laryngeal paralysis	AID?	177
		Megaesophagus	ND	75
		Persistent primary vitreous	ND	161
		Portosystemic shunting	ND	78
		Prognathism	ND	42
		Seasonal flank alopecia	ND	71
		Subaortic stenosis	ND	29
Boxer	12			
		Allergic inhalant dermatitis	ND	93
		Atrial septal defect	ND	30
		Calcinosis circumscripta	ND	47
		Cardiomyopathy	ND	30
		Cataracts	ND	147
		Central PRA	ND	162
		Cervical vertebral instability	ND	130
		Corneal dystrophy	ND	150
		Cryptorchidism	ND	173
		Cutaneous asthenia	ND	49
		Cystinuria	XR	185
		Deafness	ND	132
		Degenerative myelopathy	ND	133
		Demodicosis	ND	50
		Dermoid sinus	ND	52
		Dysrhythmia	AD	29
		Elongated soft palate	ND	177
		Epilepsy	ND	142
		Factor II deficiency	AR	81
		Factor VII deficiency	AR	82
		Gastric dilatation-volvulus	ND	76
		Hip dysplasia	Polygenic	116
		Histiocytic ulcerative colitis	Familial	74
		Hyperadrenocorticism	ND	67
		Hypoplastic trachea	ND	177
		Hypothyroidism	ND	69
		Lupoid onychopathy	ND	57
		Nodular dermatofibrosis	ND	59
		OCD–stifle	ND	124
		Patellar luxation	ND	127
		Polydontia	ND	42
		Progressive axonopathy	AR	141
		Progressive retinal atrophy	ND	163
		Prolapsed gland of nictitans	ND	168
		Pyloric stenosis	ND	80
		Renal dysplasia	ND	179
		Seasonal flank alopecia	ND	71
		Sphingomyelinosis	AR?	109
		Spina bifida	ND	145

Breed	AKC Rank* (1998)	Disorder†	Inheritance‡	Page
		Subaortic stenosis	ND	29
		Supernumerary teeth	ND	42
		Tricuspid valve dysplasia	ND	36
		Vasculitis	ND	88
		von Willebrand disease	AID?	89
Boykin spaniel				
		Fragmented coronoid process	ND	114
		Hip dysplasia	Polygenic	116
		Hypothyroidism	ND	69
		Patellar luxation	ND	127
		Pulmonic stenosis	ND	34
Briard	110			
		Cataracts	ND	147
		Central PRA	AR	162
		Fragmented coronoid process	ND	114
		Gastric dilatation-volvulus	ND	76
		Hip dysplasia	Polygenic	116
		Hyperlipidemia	ND	106
		Hypothyroidism	ND	69
		Open bite	Familial	41
		Progressive retinal atrophy	ND	163
		Retinal pigmented epithelium dystrophy	ND	162
		Seasonal flank alopecia	ND	71
		Stationary night blindness	AR?	171
Brittany	32			
		Brachygnathism	ND	39
		C3 deficiency	AR	94
		Cataracts	ND	147
		Cerebellar abiotrophy	AR?	129
		Cleft palate	AR	73
		Cryptorchidism	ND	173
		Cutaneous lupus erythematosus	ND	96
		Epilepsy	ND	143
		Factor VIII deficiency	XR	82
		Fragmented coronoid process	ND	114
		Glaucoma	ND	154
		Hip dysplasia	Polygenic	116
		Hyperlipidemia	ND	106
		Incomplete ossification of humeral condyle	ND	114
		Lens luxation	ND	158
		OCD–shoulder	ND	124
		Oligodontia	ND	41
		Patellar luxation	ND	127
		Prognathism	ND	42
		Progressive retinal atrophy	ND	163
		Retinal dysplasia	AR?	168
		Spinal muscular atrophy	AD,VE	145
		Ventricular septal defect	ND	37
		Wry mouth	ND	41
Brussels Griffon (Belgian Griffon)	88			
		Cataracts	ND	147
		Cleft lip/palate	ND	73
		Corneal dystrophy	ND	150
		Hip dysplasia	ND	116
		Hypothyroidism	ND	69
		Patellar luxation	ND	127
		Progressive retinal atrophy	ND	163
		Retained primary teeth	ND	42
		Ulcerative keratitis	ND	151
Bull terrier	84			
		Cerebellar abiotrophy	ND	129
		Cerebellar vermian hypoplasia	ND	130
		Cleft lip/palate	ND	73
		Compulsive tail chasing	ND	131

Breed	AKC Rank* (1998)	Disorder†	Inheritance‡	Page
		Deafness	AR	132
		Deep pyoderma	ND	45
		Demodicosis	ND	50
		Ectropion	ND	153
		Entropion	Polygenic	154
		Fragmented caronoid process	ND	114
		Hip dysplasia	ND	116
		Hypothyroidism	ND	69
		Inguinal hernia	ND	111
		Keratoconjunctivitis sicca	ND	156
		Laryngeal paralysis	ND	177
		Lens luxation	ND	158
		Lethal acrodermatitis	AR	56
		Mitral valve disease	ND	33
		OCD–hock	ND	124
		OCD–stifle	ND	124
		Polycystic kidney disease	DN	181
		Prognathism	ND	42
		Progressive retinal atrophy	ND	163
		Prolapsed gland of nictitans	ND	168
		Retained primary teeth	ND	42
		Subaortic stenosis	Polygenic	29
		Wry mouth	ND	41
Bull terrier, miniature	133			
		Compulsive tail chasing	ND	131
		Lens luxation	ND	158
		Persistent pupillary membranes	ND	162
Bull terrier, Staffordshire	95			
		Brachycephalic syndrome	ND	177
		Cataracts	AR	147
		Compulsive tail chasing	ND	131
		Epilepsy	ND	143
		Hip dysplasia	Polygenic	116
		OCD–stifle	ND	124
		Persistent primary vitreous	ND	161
		Prognathism	ND	42
Bulldog, French	76			
		Anasarca	ND	47
		Brachycephalic syndrome	ND	177
		Cataracts	ND	147
		Cleft lip/palate	ND	173
		Cryptorchidism	ND	132
		Deafness	ND	73
		Distichiasis	ND	151
		Elongated soft palate	ND	177
		Entropion	Polygenic	154
		Factor VIII deficiency	XR	82
		Factor IX deficiency	XR	83
		Fold dermatitis	ND	53
		Hemivertebra	ND	135
		Histiocytic ulcerative colitis	Familial	74
		Hypothyroidism	ND	69
		Intervertebral disk disease	ND	136
		Patellar luxation	ND	127
		Spina bifida	ND	145
		Ununited anconeal process	ND	115
		von Willebrand disease	ND	89
Bullmastiff	52			
		Anasarca	ND	47
		Cardiomyopathy	ND	30
		Cerebellar abiotrophy	AR	129
		Cervical vertebral instability	Familial	130
		Cruciate ligament rupture	ND	112
		Cystinuria	ND	185

Breed	AKC Rank* (1998)	Disorder†	Inheritance‡	Page
		Elbow dysplasia	ND	113
		Entropion	Polygenic	154
		Epilepsy	ND	143
		Gastric dilation-volvulus	ND	76
		Hip dysplasia	Polygenic	116
		Hydrocephalus	ND	135
		Hypothyroidism	ND	69
		Neuroaxonal dystrophy	AR	140
		OCD–hock	ND	124
		Panosteitis	ND	126
		Retinal dysplasia	AR?	168
		Seasonal flank alopecia	ND	71
		Supernumerary teeth	ND	42
		Ununited anconeal process	ND	115
Cairn terrier	44			
		Allergic inhalant dermatitis	ND	93
		Base-narrow canines	ND	41
		Cataracts	ND	147
		Cleft lip/palate	ND	73
		Craniomandibular osteopathy	AR	112
		Cryptorchidism	ND	173
		Factor VIII deficiency	ND	82
		Factor IX deficiency	XR	83
		Glaucoma	ND	154
		Globoid cell leukodystrophy	AR	103
		Hydrocephalus	ND	135
		Legg-Calvé-Perthes disease	ND	120
		Pancreatitis	ND	78
		Patellar luxation		127
		Polycystic kidney disease	ND	181
		Portosystemic shunting	ND	78
		Progressive retinal atrophy	AR	163
		Pyruvate kinase deficiency	AR	86
		Retinal dysplasia	AR	168
		Vitamin A-responsive dermatosis	ND	62
		von Willebrand disease	AID?	89
		Wry mouth	ND	41
Canaan dog	135			
		Cryptorchidism	ND	173
		Epilepsy	ND	143
		Fragmented coronoid process	ND	114
		Hip dysplasia	ND	116
		Hypothyroidism	ND	69
		Progressive retinal atrophy	ND	163
Catahoula leopard dog				
		Cataracts	ND	147
		Deafness	ND	132
		Diabetes mellitus	ND	65
		Hip dysplasia	ND	116
		Hypothyroidism	ND	69
		OCD–shoulder	ND	124
		Panosteitis	ND	126
Caucasian mountain dog (Caucasian Ovcharka)		*Elbow dysplasia*	ND	113
		Hip dysplasia	ND	116
Cavalier King Charles spaniel	56			
		Brachygnathism	ND	39
		Cataracts	ND	147
		Corneal dystrophy	Polygenic?	150
		Diabetes mellitus	ND	65
		Elongated soft palate	ND	177
		Epilepsy	ND	143

Breed	AKC Rank* (1998)	Disorder†	Inheritance‡	Page
		Femoral artery occlusion	ND	33
		Hip dysplasia	Polygenic	116
		Hydrocephalus	ND	135
		Ichthyosis	ND	56
		Macrothrombocytopenia	ND	87
		Microphthalmia	ND	158
		Mitochondrial myopathy	ND	121
		Mitral valve disease	ND	33
		Patellar luxation	ND	127
		Prognathism	ND	42
		Progressive retinal atrophy	ND	163
		Renal dysplasia	ND	179
		Retinal dysplasia	ND	168
		Wry mouth	ND	41
		Xanthine urolithiasis	AR	186
Chesapeake Bay retriever	43			
		Anterior crossbite	ND	41
		Brachygnathism	ND	39
		Cataracts	AID?	147
		Central PRA	ND	162
		Degenerative myelopathy	ND	133
		Distichiasis	ND	151
		Elbow dysplasia	ND	113
		Entropion	Polygenic	154
		Gastric dilation-volvulus	ND	76
		Hip dysplasia	Polygenic	116
		Hypothyroidism	ND	69
		OCD–shoulder	ND	124
		Prognathism	ND	42
		Progressive retinal atrophy	AR?	163
		Retinal dysplasia	ND	168
		Ununited anconeal process	ND	115
		von Willebrand disease	AR	89
		Wry mouth	ND	41
Chihuahua	8			
		Brachygnathism	ND	39
		Ceroid lipofuscinosis	AR?	102
		Color dilution alopecia	AR?	48
		Corneal dystrophy	ND	150
		Cryptorchidism	ND	173
		Cystinuria	ND	185
		Demodicosis	ND	50
		Factor VIII deficiency	XR	82
		Glaucoma	ND	154
		Hydrocephalus	ND	135
		Keratoconjunctivitis sicca	ND	156
		Medial patellar luxation	ND	127
		Methemoglobin reductase deficiency	ND	85
		Mitral valve disease	ND	33
		Myelodysplasia	ND	140
		Neuroaxonal dystrophy	ND	140
		OCD–shoulder	ND	124
		Patent ductus arteriosus	Polygenic	34
		Prognathism	ND	42
		Progressive retinal atrophy	ND	163
		Pulmonic stenosis	ND	34
		Retained primary teeth	ND	42
		Spina bifida	ND	145
		Tracheal collapse	ND	178
		Wry mouth	ND	41
Chinese crested	69			
		Brachygnathism	ND	39

Breed	AKC Rank* (1998)	Disorder†	Inheritance‡	Page
		Hairlessness	AD	48
		Oligodontia	ND	41
		Prognathism	ND	42
Chinese shar-pei	35			
		Allergic inhalant dermatitis	ND	93
		Amyloidosis	ND	101
		Brachycephalic syndrome	ND	177
		Brachygnathism	ND	39
		Ciliary dyskinesia	ND	98
		Cleft lip/palate	ND	73
		Demodicosis	ND	50
		Entropion	Polygenic	154
		Factor XII deficiency	ND	84
		Familial benign pemphigus	AID?	53
		Fold dermatitis	ND	53
		Fragmented coronoid process	ND	114
		Gastric dilatation-volvulus	ND	76
		Glaucoma	Familial	154
		Hip dysplasia	Polygenic	116
		Hypothyroidism	ND	69
		IgA deficiency	ND	99
		Immune deficiency	ND	94
		Keratoconjunctivitis sicca	ND	156
		Lens luxation	ND	158
		Megaesophagus	ND	75
		Mucinosis	ND	58
		OCD–shoulder	ND	124
		Patellar luxation	ND	127
		Prognathism	ND	42
		Progressive retinal atrophy	ND	163
		Prolapsed gland of nictitans	ND	168
		Seborrhea	ND	61
		Subaortic stenosis	ND	29
Chinook				
		Hip dysplasia	ND	116
		Hypothyroidism	ND	69
Chow chow	39			
		Adrenal sex hormone imbalance	ND	65
		Cataracts	ND	147
		Cervical vertebral instability	ND	130
		Ciliary dyskinesia	ND	98
		Color dilution alopecia	AR?	48
		Corneal dystrophy	ND	150
		Dermatomyositis	AID?	51
		Diabetes mellitus	ND	65
		Dysmyelinogenesis	Familial	134
		Ectropion	ND	153
		Entropion	Polygenic	154
		Epilepsy	ND	143
		Fragmented coronoid process	ND	114
		Gastric dilatation-volvulus	ND	76
		Glaucoma	Familial	154
		Growth hormone-responsive dermatosis	ND	67
		Hip dysplasia	Polygenic	116
		Hypoadrenocorticism	ND	69
		Hypothyroidism	ND	69
		IgA deficiency	ND	99
		Keratoconjunctivitis sicca	ND	156
		Myotonia	AR?	122
		OCD–stifle	ND	124
		Pemphigus foliaceus	ND	97
		Persistent pupillary membranes	ND	162
		Progressive retinal atrophy	ND	163
		Renal dysplasia	ND	179

Breed	AKC Rank* (1998)	Disorder†	Inheritance‡	Page
		Sebaceous adenitis	ND	60
		Tyrosinase deficiency	ND	109
		Uveodermatological syndrome	ND	99
		Ventricular septal defect	ND	37
Clumber spaniel	115			
		Distichiasis	ND	151
		Epilepsy	ND	143
		Hip dysplasia	Polygenic	116
		Hypothyroidism	ND	69
		Mitochondrial myopathy	Mitochondrial?	121
		Oligodontia	ND	41
		Portosystemic shunting	ND	78
		Prognathism	ND	42
		Retinal dysplasia	ND	168
		Wry mouth	ND	41
Cocker spaniel, American	13			
		Allergic inhalant dermatitis	ND	93
		Black hair follicular dysplasia	ND	53
		Brachygnathism	ND	39
		Cardiomyopathy	ND	30
		Cataracts	AR?	147
		Ceroid lipofuscinosis	AR?	102
		Chronic inflammatory hepatic disease	ND	73
		Cleft lip/palate	ND	73
		Cryptorchidism	ND	173
		Cyclic hematopoiesis	ND	94
		Deafness	ND	132
		Distichiasis	ND	151
		Ectodermal defect	ND	52
		Entropion	Polygenic	154
		Epilepsy	ND	143
		Factor IX deficiency	XR	83
		Factor X deficiency	AD, VE	84
		Fold dermatitis	ND	53
		Glaucoma	Familial	154
		Hip dysplasia	Polygenic	116
		Hypothyroidism	ND	69
		Hypotrichosis	ND	48
		IgA deficiency	ND	99
		Incomplete ossification of humeral condyle	ND	114
		Intervertebral disk disease	ND	136
		Keratoconjunctivitis sicca	ND	156
		Malassezia dermatitis	ND	58
		Malignant hyperthermia	ND	107
		Microphthalmia	ND	158
		Narcolepsy	ND	144
		Neuronal degeneration	AR	133
		Optic nerve colobomas	ND	159
		Optic nerve hypoplasia	ND	159
		Patellar luxation	ND	127
		Pelger-Huet anomaly	AID?	85
		Phosphofructokinase deficiency	AR	108
		Platelet δ granule deficiency	AR?	87
		Portosystemic shunting	ND	78
		Prognathism	ND	42
		Progressive retinal atrophy	AR	163
		Prolapsed gland of nictitans	ND	168
		Proliferative episcleritis	ND	151
		Pulmonic stenosis	ND	34
		Renal dysplasia	ND	179
		Retinal dysplasia	AR	168
		Sebaceous adenitis		60
		Seborrhea	ND	61

Breed	AKC Rank* (1998)	Disorder†	Inheritance‡	Page
		Vascular ring anomaly	ND	36
		Vitamin A-responsive dermatosis	ND	62
		von Willebrand disease	AID?	89
		XX sex reversal	AR	174
Cocker spaniel, English	77			
		Brachygnathism	ND	39
		Cardiomyopathy	ND	30
		Cataracts	Familial	147
		Ceroid lipofuscinosis	ND	102
		Distichiasis	ND	151
		Entropion	ND	154
		Factor II deficiency	ND	81
		Factor VIII deficiency	XR	82
		Factor IX deficiency	XR	83
		Glaucoma	ND	154
		Hip dysplasia	Polygenic	116
		Hypothyroidism	ND	69
		Keratoconjunctivitis sicca	ND	156
		MAP urolithiasis	ND	183
		Optic nerve hypoplasia	ND	159
		Patellar luxation	ND	127
		Peripheral vestibular disease	ND	132
		Persistent pupillary membranes	ND	162
		Prognathism	ND	42
		Progressive retinal atrophy	AR	163
		Retained primary teeth	ND	42
		Retinal dysplasia	ND	168
		von Willebrand disease	AID?	89
Collie	31			
		Brachygnathism	ND	39
		Bullous pemphigoid	ND	97
		Cataracts	ND	147
		Central PRA	ND	162
		Cerebellar abiotrophy	ND	129
		Collie eye anomaly	AR	147
		Corneal dystrophy	ND	150
		Cyclic hematopoiesis	AR	94
		Deafness	ND	132
		Degenerative myelopathy	ND	133
		Demodicosis	ND	50
		Dermatomyositis	AID?	51
		Dysfibrinogenemia	ND	81
		Entropion	Polygenic	154
		Epilepsy	ND	143
		Exocrine pancreatic insufficiency	ND	75
		Factor VIII deficiency	XR	82
		Gastric dilatation-volvulus	ND	76
		Lupus erythematosus	ND	95
		Microphthalmia	Familial	158
		Neuroaxonal dystrophy	AR?	140
		Nodular panniculitis	ND	59
		OCD–stifle	ND	124
		Optic nerve colobomas	ND	159
		Optic nerve hypoplasia	ND	159
		Patent ductus arteriosus	Polygenic	34
		Pemphigus erythematosus	ND	97
		Persistent pupillary membranes	ND	162
		Posterior crossbite	ND	41
		Prognathism	ND	42
		Progressive retinal atrophy	AR/ND	163
		Proliferative episcleritis	ND	151
		Retinal dysplasia	ND	168
		Sebaceous adenitis		60

Breed	AKC Rank* (1998)	Disorder†	Inheritance‡	Page
		Supernumerary teeth	ND	42
		Ulcerative dermatosis	ND	62
		Uveal hypopigmentation	ND	171
		von Willebrand disease	AID?	89
Curly-coated retriever	128			
		Cataracts	ND	147
		Coat dilution alopecia	ND	48
		Corneal dystrophy	ND	150
		Distichiasis	ND	151
		Ectropion	ND	153
		Elbow dysplasia	ND	113
		Entropion	ND	154
		Follicular dysplasia	ND	53
		Hip dysplasia	Polygenic	116
		Hypothyroidism	ND	69
		Persistent pupillary membranes	ND	162
		Progressive retinal atrophy	ND	163
		Retinal dysplasia	ND	168
		von Willebrand disease	ND	89
Dachshund	5			
		Acanthosis nigricans	AR?	45
		Black hair follicular dysplasia	ND	53
		Brachygnathism	ND	39
		Bullous pemphigoid	ND	97
		Calcinosis circumscripta	ND	47
		Ceroid lipofuscinosis	AR?	102
		Cleft lip/palate	ND	73
		Color dilution alopecia	AR?	48
		Corneal dystrophy	ND	150
		Cryptorchidism	ND	173
		Cutaneous asthenia	ND	49
		Cystinuria	ND	185
		Deafness	ND	132
		Demodicosis	ND	50
		Dermoid	AR	151
		Entropion	Polygenic	154
		Epilepsy	Familial	143
		Glaucoma	ND	154
		Heterochromia iridis	AID?	171
		Hip dysplasia	Polygenic	116
		Hyperadrenocorticism	ND	67
		Hypothyroidism	ND	69
		IgA deficiency	ND	99
		Intervertebral disk disease	ND	136
		Juvenile cellulitis	ND	56
		Keratoconjunctivitis sicca	ND	156
		MAP urolithiasis	ND	183
		Micropapilla	ND	159
		Microphthalmia	ND	158
		Mitral valve disease	ND	33
		Narcolepsy	AR	144
		Nodular panniculitis	ND	59
		Optic nerve hypoplasia	ND	159
		Pannus	ND	159
		Persistent pupillary membranes	ND	162
		Portosystemic shunting	ND	78
		Pneumoncystosis	ND	97
		Progressive retinal atrophy	AR	163
		Retinal dysplasia	ND	168
		Seasonal flank alopecia	ND	71
		Sebaceous adenitis	ND	60
		Sensory neuropathy	AR	142
		Ununited anconeal process	ND	115
		Vasculitis	ND	88

Breed	AKC Rank* (1998)	Disorder†	Inheritance‡	Page
		von Willebrand disease	AID?	89
		Xanthine urolithiasis	ND	186
Dalmatian	30			
		Allergic inhalant dermatitis	ND	93
		Brachygnathism	ND	39
		Bronzing syndrome	ND	49
		Calcium oxalate urolithiasis	ND	184
		Cardiomyopathy	ND	30
		Ceroid lipofuscinosis	AR?	102
		Ciliary dyskinesia	ND	98
		Deafness	AR	132
		Deep pyoderma	ND	45
		Demodicosis	ND	50
		Dermoid	ND	151
		Diabetes mellitus	ND	65
		Dysmyelinogenesis	ND	134
		Entropion	Polygenic	154
		Glaucoma	ND	154
		Globoid cell leukodystrophy	AR?	103
		Hip dysplasia	ND	116
		IgA deficiency	ND	99
		Laryngeal paralysis	AR	177
		Leukodystrophy	AR	137
		Microphthalmia	ND	158
		Muscular dystrophy	ND	121
		Myelodysplasia	ND	140
		Pannus	ND	159
		Polyneuropathy	ND	141
		Prognathism	ND	42
		Progressive retinal atrophy	ND	163
		Sebaceous adenitis	ND	60
		Spina bifida	ND	145
		Urate urolithiasis	ND	184
		Uveal hypopigmentation	ND	171
		Wry mouth	ND	41
Dandie Dinmont terrier	138			
		Brachygnathism	ND	39
		Cataracts	ND	147
		Glaucoma	Familial	154
		Hyperadrenocorticism	ND	67
		Intervertebral disk disease	ND	136
		Lens luxation	ND	158
		Oligodontia	ND	41
		Patellar luxation	ND	127
		Portosystemic shunting	ND	78
		Prognathism	ND	42
		Progressive retinal atrophy	ND	163
		Ulcerative keratitis	ND	151
Doberman pinscher	22			
		Acral lick dermatitis	ND	45
		Atrial septal defect	ND	30
		Brachygnathism	ND	39
		Bullous pemphigoid	ND	97
		Cardiomyopathy	ND	30
		Cataracts	AID?	147
		Cervical vertebral instability	AR	130
		Chromosomal intersex	ND	174
		Chronic inflammatory hepatic disease	ND	73
		Ciliary dyskinesia	ND	98
		Color dilution alopecia	AR?	48
		Dancing Doberman disease	ND	142
		Deafness	ND	132

Breed	AKC Rank* (1998)	Disorder†	Inheritance‡	Page
		Demodicosis	ND	50
		Diabetes mellitus	ND	65
		Familial benign pemphigus	ND	181
		Familial nephropathy	ND	53
		Fanconi syndrome	ND	180
		Flank sucking	ND	132
		Gastric dilatation-volvulus	ND	76
		Hemivertebra	ND	135
		Histiocytosis	ND	58
		Hypertrophic osteodystrophy	ND	120
		Hypothyroidism	ND	69
		Ichthyosis	ND	56
		Lupoid onychopathy	ND	57
		Malignant hyperthermia	ND	107
		Microphthalmia	ND	158
		Mucinosis	ND	58
		Narcolepsy	ND	144
		Neutrophil bactericidal defect	ND	96
		OCD–stifle	ND	124
		Oligodontia	ND	41
		Panosteitis	ND	126
		Pemphigus foliaceus	ND	97
		Peripheral vestibular disease	ND	132
		Persistent primary vitreous	ND	161
		Persistent pupillary membranes	ND	162
		Prognathism	ND	42
		Progressive retinal atrophy	ND	163
		Renal agenesis	Familial	179
		Retinal dysplasia	ND	168
		Seasonal flank alopecia	ND	71
		Sebaceous adenitis	ND	60
		Supernumerary teeth	ND	42
		Vertebral stenosis	ND	146
		Vestibular disease	ND	132
		Vitiligo	ND	62
		von Willebrand disease	AR?	89
		Wry mouth	ND	41
		Zinc-responsive dermatosis	ND	63
Dutch Kooiker dog				
		Degenerative myelopathy	AR	133
		von Willebrand disease	AID?	89
English bulldog	23			
		Anasarca	ND	47
		Brachycephalic syndrome	ND	177
		Cataracts	ND	147
		Cryptorchidism	ND	173
		Cystinuria	ND	185
		Deafness	ND	132
		Demodicosis	ND	50
		Distichiasis	ND	151
		Elbow dysplasia	ND	113
		Elongated soft palate	ND	177
		Entropion	Polygenic	154
		Factor VII deficiency	AR	82
		Factor VIII deficiency	XR	82
		Fold dermatitis	ND	53
		Hemivertebra	ND	135
		Hip dysplasia	Polygenic	116
		Hydrocephalus	ND	135
		Hypoplastic trachea	ND	177
		Hypothyroidism	ND	69
		Laryngeal paralysis	ND	177
		Lymphedema	ND	85

Breed	AKC Rank* (1998)	Disorder†	Inheritance‡	Page
		Myelodysplasia	ND	140
		Patellar luxation	ND	127
		Prolapsed gland of nictitans	ND	168
		Pulmonic stenosis	Polygenic	34
		Retinal dysplasia	ND	168
		Sacrocaudal dysgenesis	ND	142
		Seasonal flank alopecia	ND	71
		Spina bifida	ND	145
		Subaortic stenosis	ND	29
		Supernumerary teeth	ND	42
		Tetralogy of Fallot	ND	36
		Urate urolithiasis	ND	184
		Ventricular septal defect	AD, VE	37
		von Willebrand disease	AID?	89
		Wry mouth	ND	41
English setter	91			
		Allergic inhalant dermatitis	ND	93
		Brachygnathism	ND	39
		Cataracts	ND	147
		Central PRA	ND	162
		Ceroid lipofuscinosis	AR	102
		Cutaneous asthenia	ND	49
		Deafness	AID?	132
		Ectropion	ND	153
		Exocrine pancreatic insufficiency	ND	75
		Factor VIII deficiency	XR	82
		Familial benign pemphigus	AD, VE	53
		GM2-Gangliosidosis	ND	106
		Hip dysplasia	Polygenic	116
		Hypothyroidism	N	69
		Keratoconjunctivitis sicca	ND	156
		Malassezia dermatitis	ND	58
		Methemoglobin reductase deficiency	ND	85
		Patellar luxation	ND	127
		Prognathism	ND	42
		Progressive retinal atrophy	ND	163
		von Willebrand disease	AID?	89
		Wry mouth	ND	41
English toy spaniel	120			
		Cataracts	ND	147
		Cleft palate	ND	73
		Corneal dystrophy	ND	150
		Microphthalmia	AR	158
		Patellar luxation	ND	127
		Patent ductus arteriosus	ND	34
		Persistent primary vitreous	ND	161
		Retinal dysplasia	ND	168
Entlebucher mountain dog (Sennehund)				
		Cataracts	AR	147
		Fragmented coronoid process	ND	114
		Glaucoma	ND	154
		Hip dysplasia	ND	116
Field spaniel	127			
		Cataracts	ND	147
		Epilepsy	ND	143
		Hip dysplasia	Polygenic	116
		Hypothyroidism	ND	69
		Progressive retinal atrophy	ND	163
		Retinal dysplasia	ND	168
		Subaortic stenosis	ND	29
Fila Brasiliero				
		Entropion	ND	154
		Fragmented coronoid process	ND	114

Breed	AKC Rank* (1998)	Disorder†	Inheritance‡	Page
		Gastric dilatation-volvulus	ND	76
		Hip dysplasia	Polygenic	116
		Hypothyroidism	ND	69
Finnish harrier				
		Cerebellar abiotrophy	Familial	129
		Hound ataxia	ND	138
Finnish spitz	142			
		Cataracts	ND	147
		Cleft lip/palate	ND	73
		Diabetes mellitus	ND	65
		Epilepsy	ND	143
		Glaucoma	ND	154
		Hip dysplasia	Polygenic	116
		Lupus erythematosus	ND	95
		Pemphigus foliaceus	ND	97
		Pituitary dwarfism	ND	70
		Pulmonic stenosis	ND	34
		Shaker syndrome	ND	144
		Thrombopathia	ND	87
Flat-coated retriever	97			
		Cataracts	ND	147
		Corneal dystrophy	ND	150
		Distichiasis	ND	151
		Ectropion	ND	153
		Elbow dysplasia	ND	113
		Entropion	Polygenic	154
		Fragmented coronoid process	ND	114
		Hip dysplasia	ND	116
		Histiocytosis	ND	58
		Hypothyroidism	ND	69
		Optic nerve hypoplasia	ND	159
		Patellar luxation	ND	127
		Progressive retinal atrophy	ND	163
Fox terrier, smooth	86			
		Brachygnathism	ND	39
		Cervical vertebral instability	ND	130
		Deafness	ND	132
		Epilepsy	ND	143
		Legg-Calvé-Perthes disease	ND	120
		Lens luxation	N	158
		Mitral valve disease	ND	33
		Myasthenia gravis	AR	139
		Oligodontia	ND	41
		Prognathism	ND	42
		Progressive ataxia	AR	137
		Progressive retinal atrophy	ND	163
		Pulmonic stenosis	ND	34
		von Willebrand disease	AID?	89
Fox terrier, wire	62			
		Allergic inhalant dermatitis	ND	93
		Brachygnathism	ND	39
		Cataracts	AR?	147
		Cerebellar hypoplasia	ND	130
		Deafness	ND	132
		Epilepsy	ND	143
		Glaucoma	ND	154
		Legg-Calvé-Perthes disease	ND	120
		Lens luxation	ND	158
		Lissencephaly	ND	138
		Megaesophagus	AR	75
		Mitral valve disease	ND	33
		Oligodontia	ND	41
		Prognathism	ND	42
		Pulmonic stenosis	ND	34

Breed	AKC Rank* (1998)	Disorder†	Inheritance‡	Page
		Retinal pigmented epithelium dystrophy	AR?	163
		Tetralogy of Fallot	ND	36
		von Willebrand disease	AID?	89
Foxhound, American	141			
		Cricopharyngeal dysphagia	ND	75
		Cryptorchidism	ND	173
		Deafness	ND	132
		Hound ataxia	ND	138
		Hypothyroidism	ND	69
		Pelger-Huet anomaly	AID?	85
		Thrombopathia	ND	87
Foxhound, English	145			
		Brachygnathism	ND	39
		Deafness	ND	132
		Hip dysplasia	ND	116
		Hound ataxia	ND	138
		Pelger-Huet anomaly	ND	85
		Prognathism	ND	42
		Renal amyloidosis	ND	101
		Thrombopathia	ND	87
Gammel Dansk honsehund				
		Myasthenia gravis	AR	139
Garafiano shepherd dog				
		Cutaneous asthenia	ND	49
German shepherd dog	3			
		Acral lick dermatitis	ND	45
		Allergic inhalant dermatitis	ND	93
		Base-narrow canine	ND	41
		Brachygnathism	ND	39
		Calcinosis circumscripta	ND	47
		Cataracts	AD/AR	147
		Cauda equina syndrome	ND	146
		Central PRA	ND	162
		Cerebellar abiotrophy	ND	129
		Cervical vertebral instability	ND	130
		Cleft lip/palate	ND	73
		Corneal dystrophy	ND	150
		Cutaneous asthenia	ND	49
		Deafness	ND	132
		Degenerative myelopathy	Familial	133
		Demodicosis	ND	50
		Dermatomyositis	AID?	51
		Dermoid	ND	151
		Diabetes mellitus	ND	65
		Ectodermal dysplasia	XR	52
		Epilepsy	Familial	143
		Exocrine pancreatic insufficiency	Familial	75
		Factor VIII deficiency	XR	82
		Factor IX deficiency	XR	83
		Familial vasculopathy	AR?	101
		Fragmented coronoid process	ND	114
		Gastric dilatation-volvulus	ND	76
		Giant axonal neuropathy	AR	141
		Glycogen storage disease III	AR	105
		Gracilis or semitendinosus myopathy	ND	115
		GSD pyoderma	Familial	94
		Hemivertebra	AR	135
		Hip dysplasia	Polygenic	116
		Hyperparathyroidism	AR	68
		Hypertrophic osteodystrophy	ND	120
		IgA deficiency	ND	99
		Lupoid onychopathy	ND	57
		Lupus erythematosus	ND	95
		Lymphedema	ND	85

Breed	AKC Rank* (1998)	Disorder†	Inheritance‡	Page
		Masticatory myositis	ND	121
		Megaesophagus	ND	75
		Micropapilla	ND	159
		Mitral valve disease	ND	33
		Nodular dermatofibrosis	AID?	59
		OCD–stifle	ND	124
		Oligodontia	ND	41
		Optic nerve hypoplasia	ND	159
		Osteochondrodysplasia	ND	126
		Pannus	ND	159
		Panosteitis	ND	126
		Pedal panniculitis	ND	59
		Pelger-Huet anomaly	AID?	85
		Pemphigus erythematosus	ND	97
		Perianal fistulae	ND	59
		Peripheral vestibular disease	ND	132
		Pituitary dwarfism	AR	70
		Progressive retinal atrophy	ND	163
		Retinal dysplasia	ND	168
		Sebaceous adenitis	ND	60
		Silica urolithiasis	ND	185
		Small intestinal bacterial overgrowth	ND	80
		Subaortic stenosis	ND	29
		Tricuspid valve dysplasia	ND	36
		Ununited anconeal process	ND	115
		Uveodermatological syndrome	ND	99
		Vascular ring anomaly	ND	36
		Ventricular ectopy	ND	36
		Vertebral stenosis	ND	146
		Vitiligo	ND	62
		von Willebrand disease	AID?	89
		Wry mouth	ND	41
German shorthaired pointer	24			
		Acral mutilation syndrome	ND	46
		Brachygnathism	ND	39
		Cataracts	ND	147
		Cryptorchidism	ND	173
		Cutaneous lupus erythematosus	ND	96
		Entropion	Polygenic	154
		Epidermolysis bullosa	AR?	52
		Factor VIII deficiency	XR	82
		Factor IX deficiency	XR	83
		Factor XII deficiency	ND	84
		Gastric dilatation-volvulus	ND	76
		GM-2 gangliosidosis	AR	106
		Hemivertebra	AR	135
		Hip dysplasia	Polygenic	116
		Hypoadrenocorticism	ND	69
		Lupoid dermatosis	ND	57
		Lymphedema	ND	85
		Muscular dystrophy	ND	121
		Prognathism	ND	42
		Seasonal flank alopecia	ND	71
		Subaortic stenosis	ND	29
		von Willebrand disease	AR	89
		XX sex reversal	ND	174
German wirehaired pointer	75			
		Brachygnathism	ND	39
		Cataracts	ND	147
		Entropion	Polygenic	154
		Factor IX deficiency	XR	83
		Fragmented coronoid process	ND	114
		Hip dysplasia	Polygenic	116

Breed	AKC Rank* (1998)	Disorder†	Inheritance‡	Page
		Hypothyroidism	ND	69
		OCD–shoulder	ND	124
		Prognathism	ND	42
		Retinal dysplasia	ND	168
		von Willebrand disease	AR	89
Glen of Imaal terrier				
		Entropion	ND	154
		Hip dysplasia	ND	116
		Hypothyroidism	ND	69
		Seasonal flank alopecia	ND	71
Golden retriever	2			
		Acral lick dermatitis	ND	45
		Allergic inhalant dermatitis	ND	93
		Anasarca	ND	47
		Cardiomyopathy	ND	30
		Cataracts	AID?	147
		Central PRA	AR	162
		Cerebellar abiotrophy	ND	129
		Cervical vertebral instability	ND	130
		Ciliary dyskinesia	ND	98
		Corneal dystrophy	ND	150
		Degenerative myelopathy	ND	133
		Diabetes mellitus	AR?	65
		Distichiasis	ND	151
		Entropion	Polygenic	154
		Epilepsy	Familial	143
		Factor VIII deficiency	XR	82
		Fragmented coronoid process	ND	114
		Gastric dilatation-volvulus	ND	76
		Hip dysplasia	Polygenic	116
		Histiocytosis	ND	58
		Hypoadrenocorticism	ND	69
		Hypomyelinating neuropathy	ND	141
		Hypothyroidism	ND	69
		Ichthyosis	ND	56
		Juvenile cellulitis	ND	56
		Micropapilla	ND	159
		Nodular dermatofibrosis	ND	59
		OCD–shoulder	ND	124
		OCD–stifle	ND	124
		Oligodontia	ND	41
		Optic nerve hypoplasia	ND	159
		Progressive retinal atrophy	ND	163
		Proliferative episcleritis	ND	151
		Renal dysplasia	ND	179
		Retinal dysplasia	ND	168
		Seasonal flank alopecia	ND	71
		Sebaceous adenitis	ND	60
		Silica urolithiasis	ND	185
		Subaortic stenosis	ND	29
		Supernumerary teeth	ND	42
		Tetralogy of Fallot	ND	36
		von Willebrand disease	AID?	89
Gordon setter	79			
		Black hair follicular dysplasia	ND	53
		Cataracts	ND	147
		Cerebellar abiotrophy	AR	129
		Entropion	Polygenic	154
		Epilepsy	ND	143
		Fragmented coronoid process	ND	114
		Gastric dilatation-volvulus	ND	76
		Hip dysplasia	Polygenic	116
		Hypertrophic osteodystrophy	ND	120
		Juvenile cellulitis	ND	56

Breed	AKC Rank* (1998)	Disorder†	Inheritance‡	Page
		Keratoconjunctivitis sicca	ND	156
		Micropapilla	ND	159
		Progressive retinal atrophy	ND	163
		Retinal dysplasia	ND	168
Great Dane	28			
		Acral lick dermatitis	ND	45
		Brachygnathism	ND	39
		Cardiomyopathy	ND	30
		Cataracts	ND	147
		Cervical vertebral instability	AR	130
		Color dilution alopecia	AR?	48
		Cystinuria	XR?	185
		Deafness	ND	132
		Demodicosis	ND	50
		Entropion	Polygenic	154
		Epidermolysis bullosa	ND	52
		Gastric dilatation-volvulus	ND	76
		Glaucoma	ND	154
		Hemeralopia	ND	154
		Hip dysplasia	Polygenic	116
		Hypertrophic osteodystrophy	ND	120
		Hypoadrenocorticism	ND	69
		Hypothyroidism	ND	69
		Lateral patellar luxation	ND	127
		Lymphedema	ND	85
		Megaesophagus	ND	75
		Microphthalmia	ND	158
		Mitral valve disease	ND	33
		OCD–stifle	ND	124
		Oligodontia	ND	41
		Panosteitis	ND	126
		Prognathism	ND	42
		Progressive retinal atrophy	ND	163
		Retinal dysplasia	ND	168
		Spinal muscular atrophy	ND	145
		Subaortic stenosis	ND	29
		Tricuspid valve dysplasia	ND	36
		Ununited anconeal process	ND	115
		Uveal hypopigmentation	ND	171
		Vascular ring anomaly	ND	36
		von Willebrand disease	AID?	89
		Wry mouth	ND	41
		Zinc-responsive dermatosis	ND	63
Great Pyrenees	45			
		Brachygnathism	ND	39
		Cervical vertebral instability	ND	130
		Craniomandibular osteopathy	ND	112
		Deafness	ND	132
		Elbow dysplasia	ND	113
		Entropion	Polygenic	154
		Factor XI deficiency	AID?	84
		Glanzmann's thrombasthenia	ND	88
		Hip dysplasia	Polygenic	116
		OCD–shoulder	ND	124
		Optic nerve hypoplasia	ND	159
		Osteochondrodysplasia	ND	126
		Patellar luxation	ND	127
		Prognathism	ND	42
		Progressive axonopathy	ND	141
		Thrombopathia	ND	87
		Tricuspid valve dysplasia	ND	36
		Ununited anconeal process	ND	115
		von Willebrand disease	AID?	89

Breed	AKC Rank* (1998)	Disorder†	Inheritance‡	Page
Greater Swiss mountain dog	108			
		Fragmented coronoid process	ND	114
		Gastric dilatation-volvulus	ND	76
		Hip dysplasia	Polygenic	116
		OCD–shoulder	ND	124
		Panosteitis	ND	126
		von Willebrand disease	AID?	89
Greyhound	119			
		Brachygnathism	ND	39
		Cryptorchidism	ND	173
		Cutaneous and renal glomerular vasculopathy	ND	81
		Cutaneous asthenia	ND	49
		Deafness	ND	132
		Factor VIII deficiency	XR	82
		Gastric dilatation-volvulus	ND	76
		Greyhound alopecia	ND	55
		Hypothyroidism	ND	69
		Lupoid onychopathy	ND	57
		Malignant hyperthermia	ND	107
		Megaesophagus	ND	75
		OCD–shoulder	ND	124
		OCD–stifle	ND	124
		Optic nerve hypoplasia	ND	159
		Pannus	ND	159
		Persistent pupillary membranes	ND	162
		Polydontia	ND	42
		Retinal degeneration	ND	162
		Spina bifida	ND	145
		von Willebrand disease	AID?	89
Greyhound, Italian	49			
		Brachygnathism	ND	39
		Cataracts	ND	147
		Color dilution alopecia	AR?	48
		Corneal dystrophy	ND	150
		Cryptorchidism	ND	173
		Deafness	ND	132
		Pattern baldness	ND	52
		Persistent right aortic arch	ND	36
		Prognathism	ND	42
		Progressive retinal atrophy	ND	163
		Retained primary teeth	ND	42
		von Willebrand disease	AID?	89
Harrier	143			
		Cerebellar abiotrophy	ND	129
		Epilepsy	ND	143
		Hip dysplasia	ND	116
		Inguinal hernia	ND	111
Havanese	98			
		Cataracts	ND	147
		Hypothyroidism	ND	69
		Oligodontia	ND	41
		Patellar luxation	ND	127
		Portosystemic shunting	ND	78
		Progressive retinal atrophy	ND	163
		Retinal dysplasia	ND	168
Hovawart				
		Cryptorchidism	ND	173
		Hip dysplasia	ND	116
		Portosystemic shunting	ND	78
		Sebaceous adenitis	ND	60
		Subaortic stenosis	ND	29

Breed	AKC Rank* (1998)	Disorder†	Inheritance‡	Page
Ibizan hound	137			
		Brachygnathism	ND	39
		Cardiomyopathy	ND	30
		Cataracts	ND	147
		Deafness	ND	132
		Elongated soft palate	ND	177
		Epilepsy	ND	143
		Nervous system degeneration	AR	138
		Oligodontia	ND	41
		Polydontia	ND	42
		Prognathism	ND	42
Irish setter	60			
		Acral lick dermatitis	ND	45
		Allergic inhalant dermatitis	ND	93
		Brachygnathism	ND	39
		Cataracts	ND	147
		Central PRA	AR	162
		Cerebellar abiotrophy	ND	129
		Cervical vertebral instability	ND	130
		Color dilution alopecia	AR?	48
		Cutaneous asthenia	ND	49
		Degenerative myelopathy	ND	133
		Ectropion	ND	153
		Entropion	Polygenic	154
		Epilepsy	ND	143
		Factor VIII deficiency	XR	82
		Gastric dilatation-volvulus	ND	76
		Gluten-sensitive enteropathy	Familial	77
		Hip dysplasia	Polygenic	116
		Hypertrophic osteodystrophy	ND	120
		Hypothyroidism	ND	69
		Leukocyte adhesion deficiency	AR	95
		Lissencephaly	ND	138
		Lupoid onychopathy	ND	57
		Megaesophagus	ND	75
		Narcolepsy	ND	144
		Optic nerve hypoplasia	ND	159
		Osteochondrodysplasia	ND	126
		Perianal fistulae	ND	59
		Prognathism	ND	42
		Progressive retinal atrophy	AR/XR?	163
		Retained primary teeth	ND	42
		Sebaceous adenitis	ND	60
		Tricuspid valve dysplasia	ND	36
		Vascular ring anomaly	ND	36
		von Willebrand disease	AID?	89
Irish terrier	113			
		Cryptorchidism	ND	173
		Cystinuria	AR?	185
		Degenerative myelopathy	ND	133
		Microphthalmia	ND	158
		Muscular dystrophy	XR	121
		Progressive retinal atrophy	ND	163
		Uveodermatological syndrome	ND	99
Irish water spaniel	131			
		Cataracts	ND	147
		Coat dilution alopecia	ND	48
		Follicular dysplasia	ND	53
		Fragmented coronoid process	ND	114
		Hip dysplasia	Polygenic	116
		Hypothyroidism	ND	69
		Persistent pupillary membranes	ND	162
		Progressive retinal atrophy	ND	163

Breed	AKC Rank* (1998)	Disorder†	Inheritance‡	Page
Irish wolfhound	82			
		Cardiomyopathy	ND	30
		Cataracts	ND	147
		Cervical vertebral instability	ND	130
		Elbow dysplasia	ND	113
		Entropion	Polygenic	154
		Gastric dilatation-volvulus	ND	76
		Hip dysplasia	Polygenic	116
		Hypertrophic osteodystrophy	ND	120
		Hypothyroidism	ND	69
		Lateral patellar luxation	ND	127
		Micropapilla	ND	159
		OCD–stifle	ND	124
		Portosystemic shunting	ND	78
		Progressive retinal atrophy	ND	163
		Retinal dysplasia	ND	168
		Ununited anconeal process	ND	115
		von Willebrand disease	AID?	89
Jack Russell terrier	78			
		Black hair follicular dysplasia	ND	53
		Brachygnathism	ND	39
		Cataracts	ND	147
		Compulsive tail chasing	ND	131
		Deafness	ND	132
		Epilepsy	ND	143
		Factor X deficiency	AD, VE	84
		Glaucoma	ND	154
		Ichthyosis	ND	56
		Legg-Calvé-Perthes disease	ND	120
		Lens luxation	ND	158
		Mitochondrial myopathy	ND	121
		Myasthenia gravis	AR	139
		Neuroaxonal dystrophy	AR?	140
		Oligodontia	ND	41
		Prognathism	ND	42
		Progressive ataxia	AR?	137
		Progressive retinal atrophy	ND	163
		Vasculitis	ND	88
Japanese chin	73			
		Cataracts	ND	147
		Cryptorchidism	ND	173
		Elbow luxation	ND	113
		Entropion	Polygenic	154
		Hemivertebra	ND	135
		Mitral valve disease	ND	33
		Patellar luxation	ND	127
		Progressive retinal atrophy	ND	163
		Ulcerative keratitis	ND	151
Japanese retriever				
		Ceroid lipofuscinosis	AR?	102
Japanese spaniel				
		Elbow luxation	ND	113
		GM-2 Gangliosidosis	AR	106
		Patellar luxation	ND	127
Karelian bear dog				
		Cataracts	ND	147
		Deafness	ND	132
		Hip dysplasia	ND	116
		Persistent primary vitreous	ND	161
		Pituitary dwarfism	AR	70
		Progressive retinal atrophy	ND	163
		Retinal dysplasia	ND	168
Keeshond	66			
		Adrenal sex hormone imbalance	ND	65

Breed	AKC Rank* (1998)	Disorder†	Inheritance‡	Page
		Cataracts	ND	147
		Central PRA	ND	162
		Cutaneous asthenia	ND	49
		Diabetes mellitus	AR	65
		Epilepsy	Familial	143
		Glaucoma	ND	154
		Hip dysplasia	Polygenic	116
		Hypothyroidism	ND	69
		Oligodontia	ND	41
		Optic nerve hypoplasia	ND	159
		Patellar luxation	ND	127
		Patent ductus arteriosus	Polygenic	34
		Progressive retinal atrophy	ND	163
		Renal dysplasia	ND	179
		Tetralogy of Fallot	AR	36
		Ventricular septal defect	AR	37
		von Willebrand disease	AID?	89
Kerry blue terrier	107			
		Cataracts	ND	147
		Cerebellar abiotrophy	ND	129
		Craniomandibular osteopathy	ND	112
		Degenerative myelopathy	ND	133
		Dermoid sinus	ND	52
		Entropion	Polygenic	154
		Factor XI deficiency	AID?	84
		Hip dysplasia	Polygenic	116
		Hypothyroidism	ND	69
		Keratoconjunctivitis sicca	ND	156
		Oligodontia	ND	41
		Patellar luxation	ND	127
		Patent ductus arteriosus	Polygenic	34
		Progressive retinal atrophy	ND	163
		Spiculosis	ND	62
		XX sex reversal	ND	174
Komondor	134			
		Cataracts	ND	147
		Fragmented coronoid process	ND	114
		Gastric dilatation-volvulus	ND	76
		Hip dysplasia	Polygenic	116
		Hypothyroidism	ND	69
		Oligodontia	ND	41
		Prognathism	ND	42
		Retained primary teeth	ND	42
Kuvasz	114			
		Allergic inhalant dermatitis	ND	93
		Cataracts	ND	147
		Cruciate ligament rupture	ND	112
		Deafness	ND	132
		Dermatomyositis	AID?	51
		Gastric dilatation-volvulus	ND	76
		Hip dysplasia	Polygenic	116
		OCD–shoulder	ND	124
		Prognathism	ND	42
		von Willebrand disease	AID?	89
Labrador retriever	1			
		Acral lick dermatitis	ND	45
		Allergic inhalant dermatitis	ND	93
		Cataracts	AID?	147
		Central axonopathy	AR	138
		Central PRA	AD, VE	162
		Cerebellar abiotrophy	Familial	129
		Cervical vertebral instability	ND	130

Breed	AKC Rank* (1998)	Disorder†	Inheritance‡	Page
		Chronic inflammatory hepatic disease	ND	73
		Cleft lip/palate	ND	75
		Degenerative myelopathy	ND	133
		Diabetes mellitus	ND	65
		Ectropion	ND	153
		Entropion	Polygenic	154
		Epilepsy	Familial	143
		Factor VIII deficiency	XR	82
		Factor IX deficiency	XR	83
		Fanconi syndrome	ND	181
		Fibrinoid leukodystrophy	ND	138
		Follicular dysplasia	ND	53
		Fragmented coronoid process	Polygenic	114
		Gastric dilatation-volvulus	ND	76
		Hereditary myopathy	AR	115
		Hip dysplasia	Polygenic	116
		Hypertrophic osteodystrophy	ND	120
		Hypotrichosis	ND	48
		Juvenile cellulitis	ND	56
		Lymphedema	ND	85
		Malignant hyperthermia	AD	107
		Megaesophagus	ND	75
		Micropapilla	ND	159
		Microphthalmia	ND	158
		Mucinosis	ND	58
		Myelodysplasia	ND	140
		Myoclonus		122
		Narcolepsy	AR	144
		Neuroaxonal dystrophy	ND	140
		OCD–hock	ND	124
		OCD–shoulder	ND	124
		OCD–stifle	ND	124
		Oligodontia	ND	41
		Optic nerve colobomas	ND	159
		Optic nerve hypoplasia	ND	159
		Osteochondrodysplasia	AR	126
		Panosteitis	ND	126
		Persistent pupillary membranes	ND	162
		Progressive retinal atrophy	AR	163
		Retinal dysplasia	AR	168
		Seasonal flank alopecia	ND	71
		Sebaceous adenitis	ND	60
		Silica urolithiasis	ND	18
		Spongiform leukodystrophy	ND	137
		Supernumerary teeth	ND	42
		Tetralogy of Fallot	ND	36
		Tricuspid valve dysplasia	Familial	36
		Ununited anconeal process	ND	115
		Vitamin A-responsive dermatosis	ND	62
		Vitiligo	ND	62
		von Willebrand disease	AID?	89
Lakeland terrier	123			
		Cataracts	AR	147
		Cryptorchidism	ND	173
		Glaucoma	ND	154
		Legg-Calvé-Perthes disease	ND	120
		Lens luxation	ND	158
		Microphthalmia	AR?	158
		Prognathism	ND	42
		Progressive retinal atrophy	ND	163
		von Willebrand disease	AID?	89
Leonberger				
		Fragmented coronoid process	ND	114

Breed	AKC Rank* (1998)	Disorder†	Inheritance‡	Page
		Hip dysplasia	Polygenic	116
		Hypoadrenocorticism	Familial	69
		Hypothyroidism		69
		OCD–shoulder	ND	124
		Panosteitis	ND	126
Lhasa apso	29			
		Allergic inhalant dermatitis	ND	93
		Brachycephalic syndrome	ND	177
		Calcium oxalate urolithiasis	ND	184
		Cataracts	ND	147
		Corneal dystrophy	ND	150
		Demodicosis	ND	50
		Distichiasis	ND	151
		Ectodermal defect	ND	52
		Entropion	Polygenic	154
		Epilepsy	ND	143
		Factor IX deficiency	XR	83
		Hip dysplasia	Polygenic	116
		Hydrocephalus	ND	135
		Hypotrichosis	ND	48
		Intervertebral disk disease	ND	136
		Juvenile cellulitis	ND	56
		Keratoconjunctivitis sicca	ND	156
		Lissencephaly	ND	138
		Oligodontia	ND	41
		Pancreatitis	ND	78
		Progressive retinal atrophy	ND	163
		Prolapsed gland of nictitans	ND	168
		Renal dysplasia	Familial	179
		Seasonal flank alopecia	ND	71
		Sebaceous adenitis	ND	60
		Ulcerative keratitis	ND	151
		Urolithiasis	ND	182
		Vertebral stenosis	ND	146
		von Willebrand disease	AID?	89
Lowchen	140			
		Cataracts	ND	147
		Hypothyroidism	ND	69
		Legg-Calvé-Perthes disease	ND	120
		Patellar luxation	ND	127
		Progressive retinal atrophy	ND	163
Lurcher				
		Dysmyelinogenesis	ND	134
Maltese	21			
		Brachygnathism	ND	39
		Cleft lip/palate	ND	73
		Cryptorchidism	ND	173
		Deafness	ND	132
		Glaucoma	ND	154
		Glycogen storage disease	AR	104
		Hydrocephalus	ND	135
		Mitral valve disease	ND	33
		Necrotizing meningoencephalitis	ND	139
		Oligodontia	ND	41
		Patent ductus arteriosus	Polygenic	34
		Portosystemic shunting	ND	78
		Prognathism	ND	42
		Progressive retinal atrophy	ND	163
		Retained primary teeth	ND	42
		Retinal dysplasia	ND	168
		Sebaceous adenitis	ND	60
		Shaker syndrome	ND	144
		Tracheal collapse	ND	178
		Wry mouth	ND	41

Breed	AKC Rank* (1998)	Disorder†	Inheritance‡	Page
Manchester terrier	102			
		Cataracts	ND	147
		Cleft lip/palate	ND	73
		Cutaneous asthenia	ND	49
		Diabetes mellitus	ND	65
		Hydrocephalus	ND	135
		Legg-Calvé-Perthes disease	ND	120
		Lens luxation	ND	158
		Oligodontia	ND	41
		Progressive retinal atrophy	ND	163
		Retained primary teeth	ND	42
		von Willebrand disease	AR	89
Mastiff	41			
		Cruciate ligament rupture	ND	112
		Cystinuria	ND	185
		Elbow dysplasia	ND	113
		Entropion	Polygenic	154
		Gastric dilatation-volvulus	ND	76
		Hip dysplasia	Polygenic	116
		Hypothyroidism	ND	69
		Microphthalmia	AR?	158
		OCD–hock	ND	124
		OCD–shoulder	ND	124
		OCD–stifle	ND	124
		Persistent pupillary membranes	ND	162
		Prognathism	ND	42
		Progressive retinal atrophy	AR?	163
		Pulmonic stenosis	ND	34
		Retinal dysplasia	ND	168
		Subaortic stenosis	ND	29
Mexican hairless (Xoloitzcuintli)				
		Hairlessness	AD	48
		Oligodontia	ND	41
		Thymic atrophy	ND	99
Miniature pinscher	16			
		Cataracts	ND	147
		Color dilution alopecia	AR?	48
		Cystinuria	ND	185
		Deafness	ND	132
		Diabetes mellitus	ND	65
		Elbow luxation	ND	113
		Glaucoma	ND	154
		Legg-Calvé-Perthes disease	ND	120
		Mucopolysaccharidosis VI	AR	108
		Pannus	ND	159
		Progressive retinal atrophy	ND	163
		Sebaceous adenitis	ND	60
Munsterlander				
		Cataracts	ND	147
		Cystinuria	ND	185
		Hip dysplasia	Polygenic	116
		Oligodontia	ND	41
Neopolitan mastiff				
		Cataracts	ND	147
		Fragmented coronoid process	ND	114
		Hip dysplasia	ND	116
		Hypothyroidism	ND	69
		Patent ductus arteriosus	ND	34
		Progressive retinal atrophy	ND	163
		Prolapsed gland of nictitans	ND	168
Newfoundland	53			
		Cardiomyopathy	ND	30
		Cruciate ligament rupture	ND	112
		Cystinuria	AR	185

Breed	AKC Rank* (1998)	Disorder†	Inheritance‡	Page
		Entropion	Polygenic	154
		Fragmented coronoid process	ND	114
		Gastric dilatation-volvulus	ND	76
		Glomerulosclerosis/glomerulofibrosis	ND	180
		Hip dysplasia	Polygenic	116
		Hypothyroidism	ND	69
		OCD–shoulder	ND	124
		OCD–stifle	ND	124
		Pemphigus foliaceus	ND	97
		Prognathism	ND	42
		Retinal dysplasia	ND	168
		Subaortic stenosis	AD, VE	29
		Tricuspid valve dysplasia	ND	36
		Ununited anconeal process	ND	115
		Ventricular septal defect	ND	37
Norfolk terrier	112			
		Allergic inhalant dermatitis	ND	93
		Brachygnathism	ND	39
		Cataracts	ND	147
		Glaucoma	ND	154
		Inguinal hernia	ND	111
		Lens luxation	ND	158
		Micropapilla	ND	159
		Optic nerve hypoplasia	ND	159
		Patellar luxation	ND	127
		Prognathism	ND	42
Norwegian Buhund				
		Cataracts	AD	147
		Hip dysplasia	ND	116
		Hypothyroidism	ND	69
Norwegian Dunkerhound				
		Deafness	ND	132
		Heterochromia iridis	ND	171
Norwegian Elkhound	74			
		Brachygnathism	ND	39
		Cataracts	ND	147
		Ciliary dyskinesia	ND	98
		Entropion	Polygenic	154
		Fanconi syndrome	ND	181
		Glaucoma	Familial	154
		Hip dysplasia	Polygenic	116
		Hypothyroidism	ND	69
		Oligodontia	ND	41
		Osteochondrodysplasia	ND	126
		Osteogenesis imperfecta	ND	126
		Prognathism	ND	42
		Progressive retinal atrophy	AR	163
		Renal glucosuria	Familial	182
		Retinal dysplasia	ND	168
		XX sex reversal	ND	174
Norwegian Lundehund				
		Intestinal lymphangectasia		79
Norwich terrier	104			
		Allergic inhalant dermatitis	ND	93
		Brachygnathism	ND	39
		Cataracts	AR	147
		Corneal dystrophy	ND	150
		Lens luxation	ND	158
		Patellar luxation	ND	127
		Prognathism	ND	42
Nova Scotia duck tolling retriever				
		Cataracts	ND	147
		Cryptorchidism	ND	173

Breed	AKC Rank* (1998)	Disorder†	Inheritance‡	Page
		Hip dysplasia	Polygenic	116
		Hypoadrenocorticism	Familial	69
		Patellar luxation	ND	127
		Persistent pupillary membranes	ND	162
		Progressive retinal atrophy	ND	163
Old English sheepdog	65			
		Anasarca	ND	47
		Atrial septal defect	ND	30
		Brachygnathism	ND	39
		Cardiomyopathy	ND	30
		Cataracts	Familial	147
		Cervical vertebral instability	ND	130
		Ciliary dyskinesia	ND	98
		Cryptorchidism	ND	173
		Deafness	ND	132
		Degenerative myelopathy	ND	133
		Demodicosis	ND	50
		Diabetes mellitus	ND	65
		Entropion	Polygenic	154
		Factor IX deficiency	XR	83
		Gastric dilatation-volvulus	ND	76
		Hip dysplasia	Polygenic	116
		Hypoadrenocorticism	ND	69
		Hypothyroidism	ND	69
		Lymphedema	ND	85
		Micropapilla	ND	159
		Microphthalmia	ND	158
		Mitochondrial myopathy	ND	121
		Optic nerve hypoplasia	ND	159
		Persistent pupillary membranes	ND	162
		Prognathism	ND	42
		Progressive retinal atrophy	ND	163
		Retinal dysplasia	ND	168
		Sebaceous adenitis	ND	60
		Silica urolithiasis	ND	185
		Tricuspid valve dysplasia	ND	36
		von Willebrand disease	AID?	89
Otterhound	144			
		Brachygnathism	ND	39
		Epilepsy	ND	143
		Factor II deficiency	ND	81
		Fragmented coronoid process	ND	114
		Gastric dilatation-volvulus	ND	76
		Hip dysplasia	Polygenic	116
		Prognathism	ND	42
		Thrombopathia	AID?	87
Papillon	47			
		Black hair follicular dysplasia	ND	53
		Cataracts	ND	147
		Cleft lip/palate	ND	73
		Cryptorchidism	ND	173
		Deafness	ND	132
		Inguinal hernia	ND	111
		Neuroaxonal dystrophy	ND	140
		Patellar luxation	ND	127
		Progressive retinal atrophy	AR	163
		Retained primary teeth	ND	42
		von Willebrand disease	AID?	89
Pekingese	26			
		Brachycephalic syndrome	ND	177
		Cleft lip/palate	ND	73
		Cryptorchidism	ND	173
		Distichiasis	ND	151
		Elongated soft palate	ND	177

Breed	AKC Rank* (1998)	Disorder†	Inheritance‡	Page
		Entropion	Polygenic	154
		Fold dermatitis	ND	53
		Hydrocephalus	ND	135
		Keratoconjunctivitis sicca	ND	156
		Legg-Calvé-Perthes disease	ND	120
		Medial patellar luxation	ND	127
		Microphthalmia	ND	158
		Prognathism	ND	42
		Progressive retinal atrophy	ND	163
		Pseudohermaphrodism	ND	174
		Renal dysplasia	ND	179
		Tracheal hypoplasia	ND	177
		Ulcerative keratitis	ND	151
		Wry mouth	ND	41
Peruvian inca orchid				
		Hairlessness	AD	48
		Umbilical hernia	ND	111
Petit Basset Griffon Vendeen	111			
		Corneal dystrophy	ND	150
		Epilepsy	ND	143
		Fragmented coronoid process	ND	114
		Hip dysplasia	Polygenic	116
		Patellar luxation	ND	127
		Retinal dysplasia	ND	168
Pharaoh hound	132			
		Demodicosis	ND	50
		Epilepsy	ND	143
		Hypothyroidism	ND	69
		Shoulder luxation	ND	124
Plott hound	146			
		Mucopolysaccharidosis I	AR	107
Pointer (English pointer)	93			
		Acral mutilation syndrome	AR?	46
		Black hair follicular dysplasia	ND	53
		Cataracts	AID?	147
		Central PRA	ND	162
		Cerebellar ataxia	XR	130
		Ciliary dyskinesia	ND	98
		Cleft lip/palate	ND	73
		Corneal dystrophy	ND	150
		Deafness	AR	132
		Demodicosis	ND	50
		Entropion	Polygenic	154
		Gastric dilatation-volvulus	ND	76
		Hip dysplasia	Polygenic	116
		Hypoadrenocorticism	ND	69
		Juvenile cellulitis	ND	56
		Malignant hyperthermia	ND	107
		Pannus	ND	159
		Prognathism	ND	42
		Progressive retinal atrophy	ND	163
		Spinal muscular atrophy	AR	145
		Subaortic stenosis	ND	29
		Ununited anconeal process	ND	115
Polish Owczarek Nizinny dog				
		Ceroid lipofuscinosis	AR?	102
		Entropion	ND	154
		Fragmented coronoid process	ND	114
		Hip dysplasia	ND	116
		Hypothyroidism	ND	69
		Patent ductus arteriosus	ND	34
Pomeranian	10			
		Adrenal sex hormone imbalance	ND	65

Breed	AKC Rank* (1998)	Disorder†	Inheritance‡	Page
		Cataracts	ND	147
		Cryptorchidism	ND	173
		Cyclic hematopoiesis	ND	94
		Deafness	ND	132
		Entropion	Polygenic	154
		Globoid cell leukodystrophy	AR?	103
		Growth hormone-responsive dermatosis	ND	67
		Hydrocephalus	ND	135
		Hypothyroidism	ND	69
		Intervertebral disk disease	ND	136
		Legg-Calvé-Perthes disease	ND	120
		Medial patellar luxation	ND	127
		Methemoglobin reductase deficiency	ND	85
		Oligodontia	ND	41
		Patent ductus arteriosus	Polygenic	34
		Prognathism	ND	42
		Progressive retinal atrophy	ND	163
		Sebaceous adenitis	ND	60
		Tracheal collapse	ND	178
Poodle	7*			
		Adrenal sex hormone imbalance	ND	65
		Allergic inhalant dermatitis	ND	93
		Anterior crossbite	ND	41
		Base-narrow canines	ND	41
		Calcium oxalate urolithiasis	ND	184
		Cataracts	AR	147
		Cerebellar abiotrophy	Familial	129
		Ceroid lipofuscinosis	AR?	102
		Corneal dystrophy	ND	150
		Cryptorchidism	ND	173
		Cystinuria	ND	185
		Deafness	ND	132
		Diabetes mellitus	ND	65
		Distichiasis	ND	151
		Ectodermal defect	ND	52
		Entropion	Polygenic	154
		Epilepsy	ND	143
		Factor VIII deficiency	XR	82
		Factor XII deficiency	AD/AR?	84
		Fibrinoid leukodystrophy	ND	138
		Glaucoma	ND	154
		Globoid cell leukodystrophy	AR?	103
		Growth hormone-responsive dermatosis	ND	67
		Hemeralopia	AR?	154
		Hip dysplasia	Polygenic	116
		Hydrocephalus	ND	135
		Hyperadrenocorticism	ND	67
		Hypothyroidism	ND	69
		Hypotrichosis	ND	48
		Intervertebral disk disease	ND	136
		Keratoconjunctivitis sicca	ND	156
		Lafora body disease	ND	106
		Legg-Calvé-Perthes disease	ND	120
		Leukodystrophy	ND	137
		Lymphedema	ND	85
		Macrocytosis/dyshematopoiesis	ND	85
		MAP urolithiasis	ND	183
		Medial patellar luxation	ND	127
		Methemoglobin reductase deficiency	ND	85
		Micropapilla	ND	159
		Mitral valve disease	ND	33
		Narcolepsy	AR	144
		Nodular panniculitis	ND	59
		Non-spherocytic hemolytic anemia	ND	85

Breed	AKC Rank* (1998)	Disorder†	Inheritance‡	Page
		OCD–shoulder	ND	124
		Oligodontia	ND	41
		Optic nerve aplasia	ND	159
		Optic nerve hypoplasia	AR	159
		Osteogenesis imperfecta	ND	126
		Pancreatitis	ND	78
		Patent ductus arteriosus	Polygenic	34
		Prekallikrein deficiency	AR	86
		Progressive retinal atrophy	AR	163
		Prolapsed gland of nictitans	ND	168
		Proliferative episcleritis	ND	151
		Pseudohermaphrodism	ND	174
		Retinal dysplasia	ND	168
		Sebaceous adenitis	AR?	60
		Sphingomyelinosis	AR?	109
		Systemic lupus erythematosus	ND	95
		Tracheal collapse	ND	178
		von Willebrand disease	AR	89
		Wry mouth	ND	41
Poodle, standard	7*			
		Brachygnathism	ND	39
		Cardiomyopathy	ND	30
		Cataracts	AR	147
		Color dilution alopecia	AR?	48
		Factor XII deficiency	ND	84
		Gastric dilatation-volvulus	ND	76
		Glaucoma	ND	154
		Hemeralopia	ND	154
		Hypoadrenocorticism	Familial	69
		Ichthyosis	ND	56
		Microphthalmia	ND	158
		OCD–stifle	ND	124
		Oligodontia	ND	41
		Optic nerve hypoplasia	ND	159
		Persistent pupillary membranes	ND	162
		Prognathism	ND	42
		Progressive retinal atrophy	AR?	163
		Renal dysplasia	ND	179
		Retinal dysplasia	ND	168
		Sebaceous adenitis	AR?	60
		Stationary night blindness	AR?	171
		von Willebrand disease	AR	89
		Wry mouth	ND	41
Poodle, toy	7*			
		Corneal dystrophy	ND	150
		Cryptorchidism	ND	173
		Deafness	ND	132
		Distichiasis	ND	151
		Glaucoma	ND	154
		Growth hormone-responsive dermatosis	ND	67
		Medial patellar luxation	ND	127
		Micropapilla	ND	159
		Optic nerve hypoplasia	ND	159
		Patent ductus arteriosus	Polygenic	34
		Retinal dysplasia	ND	168
		Sebaceous adenitis	AR?	60
		Tetralogy of Fallot	ND	36
		Vertebral stenosis	ND	146
Portuguese water dog	83			
		Cataracts	ND	147
		Coat dilution alopecia	ND	48
		Familial renal disease	NR	179
		Follicular dysplasia	ND	53
		GM-1 gangliodisosis	AR	105

Breed	AKC Rank* (1998)	Disorder†	Inheritance‡	Page
		Hip dysplasia	Polygenic	116
		Hypoadrenocorticism	Familial	69
		Hypothyroidism	ND	69
		Juvenile cardiomyopathy	AR?	30
		Microphthalmia	ND	158
		Progressive retinal atrophy	AR	163
Pudel Pointer				
		Hip dysplasia	Polygenic	116
Pug	17			
		Allergic inhalant dermatitis	ND	93
		Brachycephalic syndrome	ND	177
		Brachygnathism	ND	39
		Cataracts	ND	147
		Cleft palate	ND	73
		Cryptorchidism	ND	173
		Degenerative myelopathy	ND	133
		Demodicosis	ND	50
		Distichiasis	ND	151
		Elongated soft palate	ND	177
		Entropion	Polygenic	154
		Fold dermatitis	ND	53
		Hemivertebra	ND	135
		Hypothyroidism	ND	69
		Keratoconjunctivitis sicca	ND	156
		Legg-Calvé-Perthes disease	ND	120
		Lentigo	ND	56
		Necrotizing meningoencephalitis	ND	139
		Oligodontia	ND	41
		Patellar luxation	ND	127
		Progressive retinal atrophy	ND	163
		Sacrocaudal dysgenesis	ND	142
		Spina bifida	ND	145
		Ulcerative keratitis	ND	151
		Urolithiasis	ND	182
		XX sex reversal	ND	174
Puli	129			
		Cataracts	ND	147
		Hip dysplasia	Polygenic	116
		Hypothyroidism	ND	69
		Micropapilla	ND	159
		Oligodontia	ND	41
		Progressive retinal atrophy	ND	163
		Retinal dysplasia	ND	168
Redbone coonhound				
		Central PRA	ND	162
		Ectropion	ND	153
		Entropion	ND	154
		Hip dysplasia	ND	116
		Hypothyroidism	ND	69
		Pelger-Huet anomaly	AID?	85
Rhodesian ridgeback	57			
		Cataracts	ND	147
		Cervical vertebral instability	ND	130
		Deafness	ND	132
		Degenerative myelopathy	ND	133
		Dermoid sinus	AR?	52
		Entropion	Polygenic	154
		Hemivertebra	ND	135
		Hip Dysplasia	Polygenic	116
		Myotonia	ND	122
		Renal dysplasia	ND	179

Breed	AKC Rank* (1998)	Disorder†	Inheritance‡	Page
Rottweiler	4			
		Atrophic membranous glomerulopathy	ND	181
		Brachygnathism	ND	39
		Cataracts	Familial	147
		Cervical vertebral instability	ND	130
		Ciliary dyskinesia	ND	98
		Corneal dystrophy	ND	150
		Cruciate ligament rupture	ND	112
		Deafness	ND	132
		Demodicosis	ND	50
		Entropion	Polygenic	154
		Fragmented coronoid process	Familial	114
		Gastric dilatation-volvulus	ND	76
		Hemivertebra	ND	135
		Hip dysplasia	Polygenic	116
		Histiocytosis	ND	58
		Hypertrophic osteodystrophy	ND	120
		Hypoadrenocorticism	ND	69
		Hypothyroidism	ND	69
		Incomplete ossification of humeral condyle	ND	114
		Leukodystrophy	AR	137
		Lymphedema	ND	85
		Microphthalmia	ND	158
		Muscular dystrophy	XR	121
		Myelodysplasia	ND	140
		Narcolepsy	ND	144
		Neuroaxonal dystrophy	AR	140
		OCD–hock	ND	124
		OCD–shoulder	ND	124
		OCD–stifle	ND	124
		Oligodontia	ND	41
		Panosteitis	ND	126
		Polyneuropathy	AR	141
		Prognathism	ND	42
		Progressive retinal atrophy	ND	163
		Retinal dysplasia	ND	168
		Seasonal flank alopecia	ND	71
		Spinal muscular atrophy	ND	145
		Subaortic stenosis	ND	29
		Ulcerative keratitis	ND	151
		Vasculitis	ND	88
		Vitiligo	ND	62
		von Willebrand disease	AID?	89
		Wry mouth	ND	41
Russian Terrier				
		Cataracts	ND	147
		Microphthalmia	ND	158
St. Bernard	38			
		Cataracts	ND	147
		Cutaneous asthenia	ND	49
		Deafness	ND	132
		Dermoid sinus	ND	52
		Distichiasis	ND	151
		Entropion	Polygenic	154
		Epilepsy	ND	143
		Factor IX deficiency	XR	83
		Gastric dilatation-volvulus	ND	76
		Hip dysplasia	Polygenic	116
		Hypofibrinogenemia	ND	81
		Hypothyroidism	ND	69
		Lateral patellar luxation	ND	127
		Malignant hyperthermia	ND	107
		Microphthalmia	ND	158

Breed	AKC Rank* (1998)	Disorder†	Inheritance‡	Page
		Narcolepsy	ND	144
		Optic nerve hypoplasia	ND	159
		Panosteitis	ND	126
		Prolapsed gland of nictitans	ND	168
		Retinal dysplasia	ND	168
		Sebaceous adenitis	ND	60
Saluki	109			
		Black hair follicular dysplasia	ND	53
		Brachygnathism	ND	39
		Ceroid lipofuscinosis	AR?	102
		Color dilution alopecia	AR?	48
		Glaucoma	ND	154
		Prognathism	ND	42
		Progressive retinal atrophy	ND	163
Samoyed	54			
		Adrenal sex hormone imbalance	ND	65
		Atrial septal defect	ND	30
		Cataracts	AR	147
		Cerebellar abiotrophy	ND	129
		Corneal dystrophy	AR	150
		Deafness	ND	132
		Dysmyelinogenesis	Familial	134
		Factor VIII deficiency	XR	82
		Gastric dilatation-volvulus	ND	76
		Glaucoma	Familial	154
		Glomerulonephropathy	XR?	180
		Growth hormone-responsive dermatosis	ND	67
		Hip dysplasia	Polygenic	116
		Microphthalmia	Familial	158
		Muscular dystrophy	XR	121
		Myasthenia gravis	AR	139
		Myelodysplasia	ND	140
		OCD–stifle	ND	124
		Oligodontia	ND	41
		Osteochondrodysplasia	AR	126
		Pelger-Huet anomaly	AID?	85
		Persistent pupillary membranes	ND	162
		Progressive retinal atrophy	AR?	163
		Pulmonic stenosis	ND	34
		Retinal dysplasia	ND	168
		Sebaceous adenitis	ND	60
		Shaker syndrome	ND	144
		Spina bifida	ND	145
		Spongiform leukodystrophy	ND	137
		Subaortic stenosis	ND	29
		Ulcerative keratitis	ND	151
		Uveodermatological syndrome	ND	99
		Ventricular septal defect	ND	37
		von Willebrand disease	AID?	89
		Zinc-responsive dermatosis	ND	63
Schipperke	55			
		Black hair follicular dysplasia	ND	53
		Cataracts	ND	147
		Color dilution alopecia	AR?	48
		Diabetes mellitus	ND	65
		Galactosialidosis		103
		Hip dysplasia	ND	116
		Legg-Calvé-Perthes disease	ND	120
		Pancreatitis	ND	78
		Pemphigus foliaceus	ND	97
		Prognathism	ND	42
		Progressive retinal atrophy	Familial	163
Schnauzer, giant	80			
		Brachygnathism	ND	39

Breed	AKC Rank* (1998)	Disorder†	Inheritance‡	Page
		Cataracts	ND	147
		Cobalamin malabsorption	AR	109
		Cryptorchidism	ND	173
		Epilepsy	ND	143
		Fragmented coronoid process	ND	114
		Glaucoma	ND	154
		Hip dysplasia	Polygenic	116
		Hypothyroidism	ND	69
		Narcolepsy	ND	144
		Prognathism	ND	42
		Progressive retinal atrophy	ND	163
		Retinal dysplasia	ND	168
		Tricuspid valve dysplasia	ND	36
		von Willebrand disease	ND	89
Schnauzer, miniature	14			
		Acquired aurotrichia	ND	45
		Allergic inhalant dermatitis	ND	93
		Anterior crossbite	ND	41
		Base-narrow canines	ND	41
		Brachygnathism	ND	39
		Calcium oxalate urolithiasis	ND	184
		Cataracts	AR	147
		Ceroid lipofuscinosis	AR?	102
		Cleft lip/palate	ND	73
		Comedo syndrome	ND	60
		Cryptorchidism	ND	173
		Cutaneous asthenia	ND	49
		Deafness	ND	132
		Diabetes mellitus	ND	65
		Factor VII deficiency	AR	82
		Fanconi syndrome	ND	181
		Glaucoma	ND	154
		Hyperlipidemia	ND	106
		Hypothyroidism	ND	69
		IgA deficiency	ND	99
		Keratoconjunctivitis sicca	ND	156
		Macrocytosis/Stomatocytosis	ND	85
		MAP urolithiasis	ND	183
		Megaesophagus	AD	75
		Microphthalmia	AR	158
		Mitral valve disease	ND	33
		Muscular dystrophy	XR	121
		Mycobacterial susceptibility	ND	96
		OCD–stifle	ND	124
		Optic nerve hypoplasia	ND	159
		Pancreatitis	ND	78
		Persistent Mullerian duct syndrome	AR	175
		Portosystemic shunting	ND	78
		Prognathism	ND	42
		Progressive retinal atrophy	AR/ND	163
		Pulmonic stenosis	ND	34
		Renal dysplasia	ND	179
		Retinal dysplasia	ND	168
		Seasonal flank alopecia	ND	71
		Sick sinus syndrome	ND	35
		von Willebrand disease	AID?	89
		Wry mouth	ND	41
Schnauzer, standard	103			
		Anterior crossbite	ND	41
		Base-narrow canines	ND	41
		Cataracts	AR	147
		Hip dysplasia	Polygenic	116
		Persistent primary vitreous	ND	161
		Prognathism	ND	42

Breed	AKC Rank* (1998)	Disorder†	Inheritance‡	Page
		Pulmonic stenosis	ND	34
		Retinal dysplasia	ND	168
		Urolithiasis	ND	182
		Wry mouth	ND	41
Scottish deerhound	125			
		Cardiomyopathy	ND	30
		Cataracts	ND	147
		Cystinuria	ND	185
		Exocrine pancreatic insufficiency	ND	75
		Fragmented coronoid process	ND	114
		Gastric dilatation-volvulus	ND	76
		Hypothyroidism	ND	69
Scottish terrier	42			
		Allergic inhalant dermatitis	ND	93
		Brachygnathism	ND	39
		Cataracts	ND	147
		Copper toxicosis	ND	74
		Craniomandibular osteopathy	AR	112
		Cystinuria	AR?	185
		Deafness	ND	132
		Factor IX deficiency	XR	83
		Fibrinoid leukodystrophy	ND	137
		Lens luxation	ND	158
		MAP urolithiasis	ND	183
		Persistent pupillary membranes	ND	162
		Progressive retinal atrophy	ND	163
		Renal glucosuria	ND	182
		Scotty cramp	AR?	142
		Seasonal flank alopecia	ND	71
		Sebaceous adenitis	ND	60
		von Willebrand disease	AR	89
Sealyham terrier	139			
		Brachygnathism	ND	39
		Cataracts	AR?	147
		Deafness	ND	132
		Glaucoma	ND	154
		Keratoconjunctivitis sicca	ND	156
		Lens luxation	ND	158
		Prognathism	ND	42
		Progressive retinal atrophy	ND	103
		Retinal dysplasia	AR	168
Shetland sheepdog	15			
		Brachygnathism	ND	39
		Bullous pemphigoid	ND	97
		Central PRA	AD, VE	162
		Collie eye anomaly	AR?	147
		Color dilution alopecia	AR?	48
		Corneal dystrophy	ND	150
		Cryptorchidism	ND	173
		Deafness	ND	132
		Dermatomyositis	AID?	51
		Distichiasis	ND	151
		Epilepsy	ND	143
		Factor VIII deficiency	XR	82
		Factor IX deficiency	XR	83
		Fanconi syndrome	ND	181
		Hip dysplasia	Polygenic	116
		Hypothyroidism	ND	69
		Lupus erythematosus	ND	95
		Mucinosis	ND	58
		Muscular dystrophy	ND	121
		Oligodontia	ND	41
		Optic nerve hypoplasia	ND	159
		Patent ductus arteriosus	Polygenic	34

Breed	AKC Rank* (1998)	Disorder†	Inheritance‡	Page
		Pemphigus erythematosus	ND	97
		Peripheral vestibular disease	ND	132
		Posterior crossbite	ND	41
		Progressive retinal atrophy	ND	163
		Renal agenesis	Familial	179
		Retinal dysplasia	ND	168
		Rostrally displaced maxillary canine	ND	41
		Stationary night blindness	AR	171
		Ulcerative dermatosis	ND	62
		Uveal hypopigmentation	ND	171
		Uveodermatological syndrome	ND	99
		von Willebrand disease	AR	89
Shiba Inu	58			
		Base-narrow canines	ND	41
		Hip dysplasia	Polygenic	116
		Hypothyroidism	ND	69
		Microcytosis	ND	85
		Oligodontia	ND	41
		Patellar luxation	ND	127
		Rostrally displaced maxillary canine	ND	41
		Uveodermatological syndrome	ND	99
		von Willebrand disease	ND	89
		Wry mouth	ND	41
Shih tzu	11			
		Allergic inhalant dermatitis	ND	93
		Brachycephalic syndrome	ND	177
		Calcium oxalate urolithiasis	ND	184
		Cleft lip/palate	Familial	73
		Dermoid sinus	ND	52
		Distichiasis	ND	151
		Entropion	Polygenic	154
		Glaucoma	ND	154
		Hip dysplasia	Polygenic	116
		Hydrocephalus	ND	135
		Intervertebral disk disease	ND	136
		Keratoconjunctivitis sicca	ND	156
		Malassezia dermatitis	ND	58
		Oligodontia	ND	41
		Prognathism	ND	42
		Progressive retinal atrophy	ND	163
		Prolapsed gland of nictitans	ND	168
		Renal dysplasia	Familial	179
		Retinal dysplasia	ND	168
		Sebaceous adenitis	ND	60
		Tricuspid valve dysplasia	ND	36
		Ulcerative keratitis	ND	151
		Urolithiasis (calcium oxalate)	ND	184
		von Willebrand disease	AID?	89
Shropshire terrier				
		Deafness	ND	132
Siberian husky	18			
		Cataracts	AR	147
		Corneal dystrophy	AR?	150
		Cryptorchidism	ND	173
		Cutaneous lupus erythematosus	ND	96
		Deafness	ND	132
		Degenerative myelopathy	ND	133
		Demodicosis	ND	50
		Entropion	Polygenic	154
		Eosinophilic granuloma	ND	47
		Epilepsy	ND	143
		Factor VIII deficiency	XR	82
		Follicular dysplasia	ND	53
		Glaucoma	AR?	154

Breed	AKC Rank* (1998)	Disorder†	Inheritance‡	Page
		Hypertension	ND	34
		Hypothyroidism	ND	69
		Laryngeal paralysis	ND	177
		Microphthalmia	ND	158
		Myelodysplasia	ND	140
		Pannus	ND	159
		Persistent primary vitreous	ND	161
		Progressive retinal atrophy	XR	163
		Retinal dysplasia	ND	168
		Tetralogy of Fallot	ND	36
		Uveal hypopigmentation	ND	171
		Uveodermatological syndrome	ND	99
		Ventricular septal defect	ND	37
		von Willebrand disease	AID?	89
		Wooly syndrome	ND	54
		Zinc-responsive dermatosis	ND	63
Silky terrier	61			
		Brachygnathism	ND	39
		Cataracts	ND	147
		Color dilution alopecia	ND	48
		Cryptorchidism	ND	173
		Cystinuria	ND	185
		Diabetes mellitus	ND	65
		Glucocerebrosidosis	AR?	104
		Hydrocephalus	ND	135
		Legg-Calvé-Perthes disease	ND	120
		Patellar luxation	ND	127
		Prognathism	ND	42
		Progressive retinal atrophy	ND	163
		Spongiform leukodystrophy	ND	137
Skye terrier	130			
		Allergic inhalant dermatitis	ND	93
		Chronic inflammatory hepatic disease	ND	73
		Copper hepatopathy	ND	74
		Lens luxation	ND	158
		Oligodontia	ND	41
		Tracheal collapse	ND	178
		von Willebrand disease	AID?	89
Soft-coated wheaten terrier	59			
		Anterior crossbite	ND	41
		Brachygnathism	ND	39
		Cutaneous asthenia	ND	49
		Glomerulonephritis	Familial	181
		Hypoadrenocorticism	ND	69
		Ichthyosis	ND	56
		Intestinal lymphangiectasia	ND	79
		Microphthalmia	ND	158
		Optic nerve hypoplasia	ND	159
		Prognathism	ND	42
		Progressive retinal atrophy	ND	163
		Protein-losing enteropathy/nephropathy	Familial	79
		Renal dysplasia	AR?	179
		Retinal dysplasia	ND	168
		von Willebrand disease	AID?	89
Spinoni Italiani				
		Fragmented coronoid process	ND	114
		Hip Dysplasia	Polygenic	116
		Portosystemic shunting	ND	78
Springer spaniel, English	27			
		Cataracts	Familial	147
		Central PRA	AR	162
		Cerebellar abiotrophy	ND	129
		Ciliary dyskinesia	ND	98
		Cutaneous asthenia	AD	49

Breed	AKC Rank* (1998)	Disorder†	Inheritance‡	Page
		Deafness	ND	132
		Diabetes mellitus	ND	65
		Ectropion	ND	153
		Entropion	Polygenic	154
		Epilepsy	ND	143
		Factor XI deficiency	AID?	84
		Fucosidosis	AR	103
		Glaucoma	ND	154
		GM-1 gangliodisosis	AR	105
		Hip dysplasia	Polygenic	116
		Lichenoid-psoriasiform dermatitis	ND	57
		Microphthalmia	ND	158
		Myasthenia gravis	AR	139
		Narcolepsy	ND	144
		Patent ductus arteriosus	Polygenic	34
		Persistent atrial standstill	ND	35
		Phosphofructokinase deficiency	AR	108
		Progressive retinal atrophy	ND	163
		Protein-losing enteropathy	ND	79
		Rage syndrome	ND	142
		Retinal dysplasia	AR	168
		Ventricular septal defect	AID?	37
		von Willebrand disease	AID?	89
		Wooly syndrome	ND	54
Springer spaniel, Welsh	118			
		Cataracts	AR	147
		Dysmyelinogenesis	XR	134
		Glaucoma	Familial	154
		Hip dysplasia	Polygenic	116
		Hypothyroidism	ND	69
		Prognathism	ND	42
		Progressive retinal atrophy	N	163
		Retinal dysplasia	ND	168
Sussex spaniel	136			
		Cataracts	ND	147
		Distichiasis	ND	151
		Hip dysplasia	ND	116
		Mitochondrial myopathy	Mitochondrial	121
		Prognathism	ND	42
		Pulmonic stenosis	ND	34
		Retinal dysplasia	N	168
Swedish Lapland dog				
		Cerebellar abiotrophy	ND	129
		Glycogen storage disease II	AR?	105
		Spinal muscular atrophy	ND	145
Swiss hound				
		Progressive retinal atrophy	N	163
Swiss sheepdog				
		Cleft lip/palate	ND	73
Tibetan mastiff				
		Demodicosis	ND	50
		Factor VIII deficiency	XR	82
		Hip dysplasia	Polygenic	116
		Hypertrophic neuropathy	AR	142
		Hypothyroidism	N	69
Tibetan spaniel	105			
		Brachygnathism	ND	39
		Entropion	Polygenic	154
		Epilepsy	ND	143
		Micropapilla	ND	159
		Microphthalmia	Familial	158
		Optic nerve hypoplasia	ND	159
		Patent ductus arteriosus	ND	34

Breed	AKC Rank* (1998)	Disorder†	Inheritance‡	Page
		Prognathism	ND	42
		Progressive retinal atrophy	AR	163
		Retinal dysplasia	ND	168
Tibetan terrier	94			
		Brachygnathism	ND	39
		Cataracts	ND	147
		Ceroid lipofuscinosis	AR	102
		Glaucoma	ND	154
		Hip dysplasia	Polygenic	116
		Lens luxation	ND	158
		Night blindness	ND	171
		Polydontia	ND	42
		Prognathism	ND	42
		Progressive retinal atrophy	AR	163
		Retinal dysplasia	Familial	168
		von Willebrand disease	AID?	89
Toy pinscher				
		Pituitary dwarfism	ND	70
Turkish naked dog				
		Hairlessness	AD	48
Vizsla	48			
		Entropion	Polygenic	154
		Factor I deficiency	ND	81
		Factor VIII deficiency	XR	82
		Hip dysplasia	Polygenic	116
		OCD–shoulder	ND	124
		Progressive retinal atrophy	ND	163
		Sebaceous adenitis	ND	60
		von Willebrand disease	AID?	89
Walker American foxhound				
		Deafness	ND	132
		Hip dysplasia	ND	116
		Hound ataxia	ND	138
		Hypothyroidism	ND	69
Weimaraner	37			
		Corneal dystrophy	ND	150
		Dysmyelinogenesis	Familial	134
		Factor VIII deficiency	XR	82
		Factor XI deficiency	AID?	84
		Familial glomerulonephropathy	ND	181
		Gastric dilatation-volvulus	ND	76
		Hip dysplasia	Polygenic	116
		Hypertrophic osteodystrophy	ND	120
		Hypothyroidism	ND	69
		Immunodeficiency	ND	100
		Lupoid onychopathy	ND	57
		Muscular dystrophy	ND	121
		Myelodysplasia	Codominant	140
		Pituitary dwarfism	ND	70
		Prognathism	ND	42
		Renal dysplasia	ND	179
		Sebaceous adenitis	ND	60
		Tricuspid valve dysplasia	ND	36
		Ununited anconeal process	ND	115
		XX sex reversal	ND	179
Welsh Corgi, Cardigan	89			
		Cataracts	ND	147
		Central PRA	ND	162
		Ceroid lipofuscinosis	ND	102
		Combined Immunodeficiency	XR	100
		Cystinuria	ND	185
		Hip dysplasia	Polygenic	116
		Intervertebral disk disease	ND	136
		Methemoglobin reductase deficiency	ND	85

Breed	AKC Rank* (1998)	Disorder†	Inheritance‡	Page
		Patellar luxation	ND	127
		Persistent pupillary membranes	ND	162
		Progressive retinal atrophy	AR	163
		Retinal dysplasia	N	168
Welsh Corgi, Pembroke	34			
		Brachygnathism	ND	39
		Cataracts	ND	147
		Corneal dystrophy	ND	150
		Cryptorchidism	ND	173
		Cutaneous asthenia	ND	49
		Cystinuria	ND	185
		Degenerative myelopathy	ND	133
		Dermatomyositis	ND	51
		Epilepsy	ND	143
		Hip dysplasia	Polygenic	116
		Intervertebral disk disease	ND	136
		MAP urolithiasis	ND	183
		Methemoglobin reductase deficiency	ND	85
		Narcolepsy	ND	144
		Persistent pupillary membranes	ND	162
		Prognathism	ND	42
		Progressive retinal atrophy	ND	163
		Renal telangiectasia	ND	179
		Retinal dysplasia	N	168
		von Willebrand disease	AID?	89
Welsh terrier	99			
		Cataracts	ND	147
		Glaucoma	AR?	154
		Lens luxation	ND	158
		Patellar luxation	ND	127
		Progressive retinal atrophy	ND	163
		von Willebrand disease	ND	89
West Highland white terrier	33			
		Allergic inhalant dermatitis	ND	93
		Cataracts	AR/ND	147
		Chronic inflammatory hepatic disease	ND	73
		Copper hepatopathy	ND	74
		Craniomandibular osteopathy	AR	112
		Deafness	ND	132
		Diabetes mellitus	ND	65
		Epidermal dysplasia	ND	52
		Glaucoma	ND	154
		Globoid cell leukodystrophy	AR	103
		Hypoadrenocorticism	ND	69
		Ichthyosis	ND	56
		IgA deficiency	ND	99
		Keratoconjunctivitis sicca	ND	156
		Legg-Calvé-Perthes disease	ND	120
		Malassezia dermatitis	ND	58
		Microphthalmia	AR	158
		Oligodontia	ND	41
		Persistent pupillary membranes	ND	162
		Prognathism	ND	42
		Pulmonic stenosis	ND	34
		Pyruvate kinase deficiency	AR	86
		Retained primary teeth	ND	42
		Retinal dysplasia	N	168
		Shaker syndrome	ND	144
Whippet	64			
		Brachygnathism	ND	39
		Cataracts	Familial	147
		Color dilution alopecia	AR?	48
		Corneal dystrophy	ND	150
		Cryptorchidism	ND	173

Breed	AKC Rank* (1998)	Disorder†	Inheritance‡	Page
		Ectodermal defect	ND	52
		Gastric dilatation-volvulus	ND	76
		Micropapilla	ND	159
		OCD–shoulder	ND	124
		Progressive retinal atrophy	ND	163
		Prognathism	ND	42
		von Willebrand disease	AID?	89
Wirehaired pointing griffon	122			
		Hip dysplasia	Polygenic	116
		Narcolepsy	ND	144
Xoloitzcuintli				
		Cryptorchidism	N	173
		Hairlessness	AD	48
Yorkshire terrier	9			
		Calcium oxalate urolithiasis	ND	184
		Cataracts	AR	147
		Color dilution alopecia	AR?	48
		Corneal dystrophy	ND	150
		Cryptorchidism	ND	173
		Dermoid sinus	ND	52
		Hyperadrenocorticism	ND	67
		Hypotrichosis	ND	48
		Keratoconjunctivitis sicca	ND	156
		Legg-Calvé-Perthes disease	ND	120
		Medial patellar luxation	ND	127
		Mitral valve disease	ND	33
		Necrotizing meningoencephalitis	ND	139
		Patent ductus arteriosus	Polygenic	34
		Portosystemic shunting	ND	78
		Progressive retinal atrophy	ND	163
		Retained primary teeth	ND	42
		Retinal dysplasia	AR?	168
		Shaker syndrome	ND	144
		Tracheal collapse	ND	178
		von Willebrand disease	AID?	89
Yugoslavian sheepdog				
		Ceroid lipofuscinosis	AR?	102

*AKC number reflects registration rank for 1998, e.g., an AKC number of 1 means that it was the most commonly registered breed in that year. A space is left blank for breeds not recognized by the AKC.

†Italic indicates that the condition is reported in the breed, but not from peer reviewed sources.

‡AR = autosomal recessive; AD = autosomal dominant; AID = autosomal dominant, incomplete penetrance; XR = x-linked recessive; ND = not determined; ? = the relationship is suspected but not proven.

References

A

1. Ackerman LJ. Canine nodular panniculitis. Compend Contin Educ Pract Vet 1984; 6:818–24.
2. Ackerman LJ. Pemphigus and pemphigoid in the dog and cat. Part I. Pemphigus. Compend Contin Educ Pract Vet 1985; 7:89–97.
3. Ackerman LJ. Pemphigus and pemphigoid in the dog and cat. Part II. Pemphigoid. Compend Contin Educ Pract Vet 1985; 7: 281–6.
4. Ackerman L. Lichenoid-psoriasiform dermatosis in a springer spaniel. Mod Vet Prac 1988; 69: 32–3.
5. Acland G, Aguirre, G. PRA today: current research in progressive retinal atrophy. http://mendel.berkeley.edu/dogs/disease/pra/classes. html. May 10, 1998.
6. Acland GM, Blanton SH, Hershfield B, Aguirre GD. Xlpr—a canine retinal degeneration inherited as an X-linked trait. Am J Med Genet 1994; 52(1):27–33.
7. Acland GM, Fletcher RT, Gentlman S, et al. Non-allelism of three genes (rcd1, rcd2, erd) for early-onset hereditary retinal degeneration. Experim Eye Res 1989; 49:983–98.
8. Acland GM, Ray K, Mellersh CS, et al. Linkage analysis and comparative mapping of canine progressive rod-cone degeneration (prcd) establishes potential locus homology with retinitis pigmentosa (Rp17) in humans. Proceedings of Nat Acad Sciences of US 1998; 95(6):3048–53.
9. Adams WM, Dueland RT, Meinen J, et al. Early detection of canine hip dysplasia: Comparison of two palpation and five radiographic methods. J Am Anim Hosp Assoc 1998; 34(4):339–47.
10. Aguirre GD, Baldwin V, Pearce-Kelling S, et al. Congenital stationary night blindness in the dog: Common mutation in the RPE65 gene indicates founder effect. Molecular Vision 1998; 4: 23–6.
11. Alexander JW. The pathogenesis of canine hip dysplasia. Vet Clin N Am, Sm Anim Pract 1992; 22(3):503–11.
12. Alhaidari Z, Olivry T, Ortonne, J-P. Melanocytogenesis and melanogenesis: genetic regulation and comparative clinical diseases. Vet Derm 1999; 10(1):3–16.
13. Allan FJ, Thompson, KG, Jones, BR, et al. Neutropenia with a probable hereditary basis in border collies. New Zealand Vet J 1996; 44:67–72.
14. Allen L, Stobie D, Mauldin N, Baer KE. Clinicopathologic features of dogs with hepatic microvascular dysplasia with and without portosystemic shunts: 42 cases (1991–1996). JAVMA 1999; 214(2): 218–20.
15. Allen WM, Pocock PI, Dalton PM, et al. Cyclic neutropenia in collies. Vet Rec 1996; 138(15): 371–2.
16. Alroy J, Knowles K, Schelling SH, et al. Retarded bone formation in GM1 gangliosidosis: a study of the infantile form and comparison with two canine models. Virchows Archiv—an International Journal of Path 1995; 426:141–8.
17. Alroy J, Orgad U, DeGasperi, R et al. Canine GM1-gangliosidosis: a clinical morphological, histochemical and biochemical comparison of two different models. Am J Path 1992; 140:657–63.
18. Amann JF, Laughlin H, Korthuis RJ. Muscle hemodynamics in hereditary myopathy of Labrador retrievers. Am J Vet Res 1988; 49(7):1127–30.
19. Ameratunga R, Winkelstein JA, Brody L, et al. Molecular analysis of the third component of canine complement (C3) and identification of the mutation responsible for hereditary canine C3 deficiency. J Immunol, 1998; 160(6): 2824–30.
20. Anderson JG, Harvey CE: Masticatory muscle myositis. J Vet Dent 1993; 10(1):6–8.
21. Anderson RK. Canine acanthosis nigricans. Compend Contin Educ Pract Vet 1979; 1:466–71.
22. Angeles JM, Feldman EC, Nelson RW, Feldman, MS. Use of urine cortisol-creatinine ratio versus adrenocorticotropic hormone stimulation testing for monitoring mitotane treatment of pituitary-dependent hyperadrenocorticism in dogs. JAVMA 1997; 211(8):1002–8.
23. Araujo RB, Rezende CMF, Neto JMF, Muzzi LAL. Hip dysplasia frequency in fila Brasiliero dogs. Arquivo Brasiliero de Medicina Veterinaria E Zootecnia 1997; 49(3):379–83.
24. Arnold S, Muller A, Binder H, et al. Plasma von Willebrand factor concentrations in Bernese mountain dogs. Schweizer Archiv für Tierheilkunde 1997; 139(4):177–82.
25. Autran de Morais HS, DiBartola SP, Chew DJ. Juvenile renal disease in golden retrievers: 12 cases (1984–1994). JAVMA 1996; 209(4):792–7.

B

26. Bailey CS, Morgan JP. Congenital spinal malformations. Vet Clin N Am, Sm Anim Pract 1992; 22(4):985–1015.
27. Barclay KB, Haines DM. Immunohistochemical evidence for immunoglobulin and complement deposition in spinal cord lesions in degenerative myelopathy in German shepherd dogs. Can J Vet Res 1994; 58(1):20–4.
28. Bardet JF. Arthroscopy of the elbow in dogs. 2. The cranial portals in the diagnosis and treatment of the lesions of the coronoid process. Vet Compar Orthopaedics and Traumatol 1997; 10(2): 60–6.
29. Bardet JF, Bureau S. Fragmentation of the coronoid process in dogs—a case control study of 83 elbows treated by shortening osteotomy of the proximal ulna. Pratique Medicale et Chirurgicale de L'Animal de Compagnie 1996; 31(5):451–463.
30. Barker CG, Herrtage ME, Shanahan F, Winchester BG. Fucosidosis in English springer spaniels: results of a trial screening programme. J Sm Anim Pract 1988; 29(10):623–30.
31. Barnett KC: Hereditary cataract in the miniature schnauzer. J Sm Anim Pract 1985; 26(11):635–43.
32. Barnett KC. Hereditary cataract in the Welsh springer spaniel. J Sm Anim Pract 1980; 21:621–5.
33. Barnett KC. Hereditary cataract in the German shepherd dog. J Sm Anim Pract 1986; 27(6):387–95.
34. Barnett, KC. Inherited eye disease in the dog and cat. J Sm Anim Pract 1988; 29(7):462–75.
35. Barnett KC, Startup FG. Hereditary cataract in the standard poodle. Vet Rec 1985; 117:15–6.

36. Barrie J, Watson TDG. Hyperlipidemia. In: Kirk's current veterinary therapy XII, Small animal practice. Philadelphia: WB Saunders, 1995:430–4.
37. Bartges JW, Osborne CA, Lulich JP, et al. Canine urate urolithiasis—etiopathogenesis, diagnosis, and management. Vet Clin N Am, Sm Anim Prac 1999; 29(1):161–174.
38. Bartges JW, Osborne CA, Lulich JP, et al. Prevalence of cystine and urate uroliths in bulldogs and urate uroliths in dalmatians. JAVMA 1994; 204(12): 1914–18.
39. Bartlett RJ, Winand, NJ, Secore SL, et al. Mutation segregation and rapid carrier detection of X-linked muscular dystrophy in dogs. Am J Vet Res 1996; 57:650–4.
40. Batt RM. Exocrine pancreatic insufficiency. Vet Clin N Am, Sm Anim Pract 1993; 23(3):595–608.
41. Bauer JE. Evaluation and dietary considerations in idiopathic hyperlipidemia in dogs. JAVMA 1995; 206(11):1684–8.
42. Beco L, Fontaine J, Gross TL. Charlier G. Color dilution alopecia in 7 dachshunds—a clinical study and the hereditary, microscopic and ultrastructural aspect of the disease. Vet Derm 1996; 7(2):91–7.
43. Bedford PGC. Collie eye anomaly in the Lancashire heeler. Vet Rec 1998; 143(13): 354–6.
44. Behrend EN, Kemppainen RJ. Medical therapy of canine Cushing's syndrome. Compend Contin Educ Pract Vet 1998; 20(6):679–86.
45. Behrend EN, Kemppainen RJ, Young DW. Effect of storage conditions on cortisol, total thyroxine, and free thyroxine concentrations in serum and plasma of dogs. JAVMA 1998; 212(10):1564–8.
46. Bell J. Sex-related genetic disorders: Did mama cause them? AKC Gazette 1994 (Feb):74–8.
47. Bennett PF, Clarke RE. Laryngeal paralysis in a rottweiler with neuroaxonal dystrophy. Austral Vet J 1997; 75(11):784–6.
48. Bensignor E. A case of dermatomyositis in a Beauce shepherd dog. Recueil de Medecine Veterinaire 1997; 173(4–6):125–31.
49. Bensignor E, Pin D, Carlotti DN. Pemphigus foliaceus in dogs and cats—a review. Annales de Medecine Veterinaire 1998; 142(1):5–13.
50. Berendt M, Gram L. Epilepsy and seizure classiciation in 63 dogs: a reappraisal of veterinary epilepsy terminology. J Vet Intern Med 1999; 13(1):14–20.
51. Bergeaud P. Repositioning of the parotid duct. Point Veterinaire 1996; 27(174):83–5.
52. Bergvall K. Treatment of symmetrical onychomadesis and onychodystrophy in five dogs with omega–3 and omega–6 fatty acids. Vet Derm 1998; 9: 263–8.
53. Besso JG, Penninnck DG, Gliatto JM. Retrospective ultrasonographic evaluation of adrenal lesions in 26 dogs. Vet Radiology & Ultrasound 1997; 38(6):448–55.
54. Biefelt SW, Redman HC, McClellan RO. Sire and sex related differences in rates of epileptiform seizures in a purebred beagle colony. Am J Vet Res 1971; 32: 2039–48.
55. Bingel SA, Sande RD. Chondrodyysplasia in five Great Pyrenees. JAVMA 1994; 205:845–48.
56. Bingel SA, Sande RD. Chondrodysplasia in the Norwegian elkhound. Am J Path 1982; 107:219–29.
57. Binns MM, Holmes NG, Marti E, Bowen N. Dog parentage testing using canine microsatellites. J Sm Anim Pract 1995; 36(11):493–7.
58. Bissett SA, Guilford WG, Spohr A. Breath hydrogen testing in small animal practice. Compend Contin Educ Pract Vet 1997; 19(8):916–26.
59. Bjerkas E, Haaland MB. Pulverulent nuclear cataract in the Norwegian buhund. J Sm Anim Pract 1995; 36(11):471–4.
60. Bjerkas E, Narfstrom K. Progressive retinal atrophy in the Tibetan spaniel in Norway and Sweden. Vet Rec 1994; 134(15):377–9.
61. Bjerkas I. Hereditary "cavitating" leucodystrophy in Dalmatian dogs: light and electron microscopic studies 1977; Acta Neuropathol (Berl) 40:163–8.
62. Bjorling DE. Laryngeal paralysis. In: Kirk's current veterinary therapy XII, small animal practice. Philadelphia: WB Saunders, 1995:901–5.
63. Blakemore JC. Gastrointestinal allergy. Vet Clin N Am, Sm Anim Pract 1994; 24(4):655–95.
64. Boari A, Williams DA, Famiglibergamini, P. Observations on exocrine pancreatic insufficiency in a family of English setter dogs. J Sm Anim Pract 1994; 35:247–50.
65. Bolognia J, Pawelek JM. Biology of hypopigmentation. J Am Acad Derm 1988; 19:217–55.
66. Bond R, Lloyd DH. Skin and mucosal populations of Malassezia pachydermatis in healthy and seborrheic basset hounds. Vet Derm 1997; 8(2):101–6.
67. Boord MJ, Griffin CE, Rosenkrantz WS. Onychectomy as a therapy for symmetic claw and claw fold disease in the dog. J Am Anim Hosp Assoc 1997; 33:131–8.
68. Booth MJ. Atypical dermoid sinus in a chow chow dog. J S African Vet Assoc 1998; 69(3): 102–4.
69. Boroffka SAEB, Verbruggen AMJ, Boeve MH, Stades FC. Ultrasonographic diagnosis of persistent hyperplastic tunica vasculosa lentis, persistent hyperplastic primary vitreous in 2 dogs. Vet Radiol & Ultrasound 1998; 39(5): 440–4.
70. Boudreaux MK. Platelet and coagulation disorders. In: Morgan RV, ed. Handbook of small animal medicine, 3d ed. Philadelphia: WB Saunders, 1997: 698–718.
71. Boudreaux MK. Platelets and coagulation, an update. Vet Clin N Am, Sm Anim Pract 1996; 26(5): 1065–87.
72. Boudreaux MK, Crager C, Dillon AR, et al. Identification of an intrinsic platelet function defect in Spitz dogs. J Vet Intern Med 1994; 8: 93–6.
73. Boudreaux MK, Kvam K, Dillon AR, et al. Type I Glanzmann's thrombasthenia in a Great Pyrenees dog. Vet Path 1996; 33:505–6.
74. Boulay JP. Fragmented medial coronoid process of the ulna in the dog. Vet Clin N Am, Sm Anim Pract 1998; 28(1):51–74.
75. Bounous DI, Boudreaux MK, Hoskins JD. The hematopoietic and lymphoid systems. In: Hoskins JD, ed. Veterinary pediatrics. Philadelphia: WB Saunders, 1995:337–76.
76. Bounous DI, Carmichael KP, Kaswan RL, et al. Effects of ophthalmic cyclosporine on lacrimal gland pathology and function in dogs with keratoconjunctivitis sicca. Veterinary & Comparative Ophthal 1995; 5(1):5–12.
77. Bourdin M. Canine acral lick dermatits—a model of obsessive-compulsive disorder. Sciences et Techniques de L'Animal de Laboratoire 1994; 19(4):265–73.
78. Bovée KC, McGuire T. Qualitative and quantitative analysis of uroliths in dogs: definitive determination of chemical type. JAVMA 1984; 185:983–7.
79. Bovée KC, Littman MP, Crabtree BJ, et al. Essential hypertension in a dog. JAVMA 1989; 195: 81–3.
80. Bowles MH, Mosier DA. Renal amyloidosis in a family of beagles. JAVMA 1992; 201(4):569–74.
81. Braun JP, Medaille C. Diagnosis and monitoring of diabetes mellitus in dogs and cats use of fructosamine measurement: a review. Revue de Medecine Veterinaire 1997; 148(12):945–50.
82. Braund KG. Degenerative causes of myopathies in dogs and cats. Vet Med 1997; 92(7):608–17.
83. Braund KG. Degenerative causes of neuropathies in dogs and cats. Vet Med 1996; 91(8): 722–39.
84. Braund KG. Endogenous causes of myopathies in dogs and cats. Vet Med 1997; 92(7):618–28.
85. Braund KG. Endogenous causes of neuropathies in dogs and cats. Vet Med 1996; 91(8): 740–54.
86. Braund KG. Hereditary myopathy in Labrador retrievers. Calif Vet 1985; 39(2):18–24.
87. Braund KG. Identifying degenerative peripheral neuropathies in pets. Vet Med 1987; 82(4):352–80.
88. Braund KG. Idiopathic and exogenous causes of myopathies in dogs and cats. Vet Med 1997; 92(7):629–34.
89. Braund KG. Idiopathic and exogenous causes of neuropathies in dogs and cats. Vet Med 1996; 91(8): 755–69.
90. Braund KG. Laryngeal paralysis-polyneuropathy complex in young Dalmatian dogs. In: Kirk's current veterinary therapy XII, Small animal practice. Philadelphia: WB Saunders, 1995:1136–40.

91. Braund KG, Mehta JR, Toivio-Kinnucan M, et al. Congenital hypomyelinating polyneuropathy in two golden retriever littermates. Vet Path 1989; 26(3):202–8.
92. Braund KG, Shores A, Lowrie CT, et al. Idiopathic polyneuropathy in Alaskan malamutes. J Vet Intern Med 1997; 11(4):243–9.
93. Braund KG, Steinberg S, Shores A, et al. Laryngeal paralysis in immature and mature dogs as one sign of a more diffuse polyneuropathy. JAVMA 1989; 194(12): 1735–40.
94. Braund KG, Toiviokinnucan M, Vallat JM, et al. Distal sensorimotor polyneuropathy in mature rottweiler dogs. Vet Path 1994; 31(3):316–26.
95. Bray JP, Burbidge HM. The canine intervertebral disk. Part II: degenerative changes—nonchondrodystrophoid versus chondrodystrophoid disks. J Am Anim Hosp Assoc 1998; 34(2):135–44.
96. Breathnach SM. Amyloid and amyloidosis. J Am Acad Derm 1988; 18(1):1–16.
97. Brechue WF, Gropp KE, Ameredes BT, et al. Metabolic and work capacity of skeletal muscle of PFK-deficient dogs studied in situ. J Appl Physiol 1994; 77(5):2456–467.
98. Breen M, Langford CF, Dickens HF, et al. Canine FISH cytogenetics. Canine Pract 1998; 23(1):37–8.
99. Breitschwerdt EB, Hirakawa DA, Hurlbert SA, et al. Effects of dietary protein source on basenjis with immunoproliferative enteropathy. Am J Vet Res 1992; 5(2):234–8.
100. Breitschwerdt EB, Kornegay JN, Wheeler SJ, et al. Episodic weakness associated with exertional lactic acidosis and myopathy in Old English sheepdog littermates. JAVMA 1992; 201(5):731–6.
101. Brenner O, DeLahunta A, Summers BA, et al. Hereditary polioencephalomyelopathy of the Australian cattle dog. Acta Neuropathol 1997; 94(1):54–66.
102. Breur GJ, Zerebe CA, Slocombe RF, et al. Clinical, radiographic, pathologic, and genetic features of osteochondrodysplasia in Scottish deerhounds. JAVMA 1989; 195(5):606–12.
103. Brewer GJ. Wilson disease and canine copper toxicosis. Am J Clin Nutr 1998; 67(suppl):1087S–1090S.
104. Briggs OM. Lentiginosis profusa in the pug: Three case reports. J Sm Anim Pract 1985; 26:675–80.
105. Briggs OM, Botha WS. Color mutant alopecia in a blue Italian greyhound. J Am Anim Hosp Assoc 1986; 22(5):611–4.
106. Bright JM. The cardiovascular system. In: Hoskins JD, ed. Veterinary pediatrics. Philadelphia: WB Saunders, 1995: 95–123.
107. Brinkhous K, Landen C, Monroe D, et al. F-IX pathophysiology and gene therapy of canine hemophilia. B. Dynamics of fIX distribution from extravascular sites (subcutaneous, intramuscular, and intraperitoneal). FASEB Journal 1993; 7(3-Part I): A117.
108. Brix AE, Howerth EW, McConkierrosell A, et al. Glycogen storage disease type Ia in two littermate Maltese puppies. Vet Path 1995; 32(5):460–5.
109. Brockman DJ, Washabau RJ, Drobatz KJ. Canine gastric dilatation/volvulus syndrome in a veterinary critical care unit—295 cases (1986–1992). JAVMA 1995; 207(4):460–4.
110. Brooks, DE. Canine and feline glaucomas. Current veterinary therapy IX. Philadelphia: WB Saunders, 1986: 656–9.
111. Brooks DE, Dziezyc J. The canine glaucomas: pathogenesis, diagnosis, and treatment. Compend Contin Educ Pract Vet 1983; 5(4):292–8.
112. Brooks M. Hereditary bleeding disorders. Proceedings of the 16th ACVIM Forum, San Diego, 1998; 424–6.
113. Brooks M, Dodds J, Raymond, SL. Epidemiologic features of von Willebrand's disease in Doberman pinschers, Scottish terriers and Shetland sheepdogs: 260 cases (1984–1988). JAVMA 1992; 200(8):1123–7.
114. Brooks M, Raymond S, Catalfamo J. Severe, recessive von Willebrand's disease in German wirehaired pointers. JAVMA 1996; 209(5):926–9.
115. Brooks MB, Gu W, Ray K. Complete deletion of factor IX gene and inhibition of factor IX activity in a Labrador retriever with hemophilia. Brit J Am Vet Med Assoc 1997; 211(11):1418–21.
116. Brooks PN. Necrotizing vasculitis in a group of beagles. Lab Anim 1984; 18:285–90.
117. Brourman JD, Schertel ER, Allen DA, et al. Factors associated with perioperative mortality in dogs with surgically managed gastric dilatation-volvulus: 137 cases (1988–1993). JAVMA 1996; 208(11):1855–8.
118. Brown CA, Crowell WA, Brown SA, et al. Suspected familial renal disease in chow chows. JAVMA 1990; 196:1279–84.
119. Brown SA. Fanconi's syndrome. In: Kirk RW, ed. Current veterinary therapy X, Small animal practice. Philadelphia: WB Saunders, 1989:1163–5.
120. Brown SA. Glomerulonephritis. Proceedings of the 16th ACVIM Forum, San Diego, 1998, 20–1.
121. Brown SA, Henik RA. Diagnosis and treatment of systemic hypertension. Vet Clin N Am, Sm Anim Pract 1998; 28(6): 1481–94.
122. Brown WA. Ventricular septal defect in the English springer spaniel. In: Kirk's current veterinary therapy XII, Small animal practice. Philadelphia: WB Saunders, 1995:827–30.
123. Brunson DB, Hogan K, Powers P, et al: Investigation of the causal mutation for malignant hyperthermia in black Labrador retrievers. Canine Pract 1998; 23(1):48.
124. Bruyette DS, Ruehl WW, Entriken TL, et al. Treating canine pituitary-dependent hyperadrenocorticism with L-Deprenyl. Vet Med 1997; 92(8): 710–8.
125. Buback JL, Boothe HW, Hobson HP. Surgical treatment of tracheal collapse in dogs: 90 cases (1983–1993). JAVMA 1996; 208(3):380–4.
126. Buchanan JW. Causes and prevalence of cardiovascular disease. In: Current veterinary therapy XI, Small animal practice. Philadelphia:WB Saunders, 1992:647–55.
127. Buchanan JW. Changing breed predispositions in canine heart disease. Canine Pract 1993; 18(6):12–4.
128. Buchanan JW, Beardow AW, Sammarco, CD: Femoral artery occlusion in Cavalier King Charles spaniels. JAVMA 1997; 211(7):872–4.
129. Budsberg SC, Spurgeon TL, Liggitt HD. Anatomic predisposition to perianal fistulae formation in the German shepherd dog. Am J Vet Res 1985; 46(7):1468–72.
130. Bunch, SE. Diseases of the large intestine. In: Morgan RV, ed. Handbook of small animal practice. 3d. Philadelphia: WB Saunders, 1997:371–82.
131. Bundza A, Lowden JA, Charlton KM. Niemann-Pick disease in a poodle dog. Vet Path 1979; 16:530–8.
132. Burbidge HM. A review of Wobbler syndrome in the Doberman pinscher. Austral Vet Practitioner 1995; 25(3):147–56.
133. Burrows CF, Ignaszewski LA. Canine gastric dilatation-volvulus. J Sm Anim Pract 1990; 10:21–6.
134. Burton S, DeLay J, Holmes A, et al. Hypoadrenocorticism in young related Nova Scotia duck tolling retrievers. Can Vet J 1997; 38:231–4.
135. Buskirk RV. The lens epithelium of American cocker spaniels with inherited and non-inherited lens cataracts. Res Vet Sci 1977; 22:237–42.

C

136. Calderwood Mays MB, Bergeron J. Cutaneous histiocytosis in dogs. JAVMA 1986; 188(4): 377–81.
137. Callan MB, Bennett, JS, Phillips DK et al. Inherited platelet ë-storage pool disease in dogs causing severe bleeding: an animal model for a specific ADP deficiency. Thrombosis and Haemostasis 1995; 74(3):949–53.
138. Calvert CA. Diagnosis and management of ventricular tachyarrhythmias in Doberman pinschers with cardiomyopathy. In: Kirk's current veterinary therapy XII, Small animal practice. Philadelphia: WB Saunders, 1995:799–806.
139. Calvert CA. Dilated congestive cardiomyopathy in Doberman pinschers. Compend Contin Educ Pract Vet 1986; 8(6):417–22.
140. Calvert CA, Hall G, Jacobs G, Pickus C. Clinical and pathological findings in Doberman pinschers with occult cardiomyopathy that died suddenly or developed congestive heart failure—54 cases (1984–1991). JAVMA 1997; 210(4):505–13.

141. Calvert CA, Jacobs GJ, Kraus M. Possible ventricular late potentials in Dobermann pinschers with occult cardiomyopathy. JAVMA 1998; 213(2):235–9.
142. Calvert CA, Jacobs GJ, Medleau L, et al. Thyroid-stimulating hormone stimulation tests in cardiomyopathic Doberman pinschers—A retrospective study. J Vet Intern Med 1998; 12(5): 343–8.
143. Calvert CA, Pickus CW, Jaccobs GJ, Brown J. Signalment, survival, and prognostic factors in Doberman pinschers with end-stage cardiomyopathy. J Vet Intern Med 1997; 11(6):323–6.
144. Cameron C, Notley C, Hoyle S, et al. The canine factor VIII cDNA and 5' flanking sequence. Thrombosis & Haemostasis 1998; 79:317–22.
145. Campbell BG, Wootton JAM, Krook L, et al. Clinical signs and diagnosis of osteogenesis imperfecta in 3 dogs. JAVMA 1997; 211(2):183–6.
146. Campbell KL. Canine cyclic hematopoiesis. Compend Contin Educ Pract Vet 1985; 7(1):57–62.
147. Campbell KL. Growth hormone-related disorders in dogs. Compend Contin Educ Pract Vet 1988; 10(4):484–92.
148. Cantile C, Buonaccorsi A, Pepe V, Arispici M. Juvenile neuronal ceroid lipofuscinosis (Batten disease) in a poodle dog. Prog in Vet Neurol 1996; 7:82–7.
149. Cardinet III GH, Kass PH, Walace LJ, Guffy MM. Association between pelvic muscle mass and canine hip dysplasia. JAVMA 1997; 210(10):1466–73.
150. Carmichael S, Griffiths IR, Harvey MJA. Familial cerebellar ataxia with hydrocephalus in bullmastiffs. Vet Rec 1983; 112:354–8.
151. Carothers MA, Kwochka KW, Rojko JL. Cyclosporine-responsive granulomatous sebaceous adenitis in a dog. JAVMA 1991; 198(9):1645–8.
152. Carpenter JL, Andelman NCC, Moore FM, King Jr. NW, Idiopathic cutaneous and renal glomerular vasculopathy of greyhounds. Vet Path 1988; 25:401–7.
153. Carpenter L. Legg-Calvé-Perthes disease. In: Tilley LP, Smith FWK Jr., eds. The 5 minute veterinary consult. Baltimore: Williams & Wilkins, 1997:762–3.
154. Carrig CB, MacMillan A, Brundage S, et al. Retinal dysplasia associated with skeletal abnormalities in Labrador retrievers. JAVMA 1977; 170:49–57.
155. Carrig CB, Sponenberg DP, Schmidt GM, Tvedten HW. Inheritance of associated ocular and skeletal dysplasia in Labrador retrievers. JAVMA 1988; 193(10):1269–72.
156. Casal ML, Giger U, Bovée KC, Patterson DF. Inheritance of cystinuria and renal defect in Newfoundlands. JAVMA 1995; 207(12): 1585–9.
157. Casal ML, Jezyk PF, Greek JM, et al. X-linked ectodermal dysplasia in the dog. J Hered 1997; 88(6):513–7.
158. Case LC, Ling GV, Franti CE, et al. Cystine-containing urinary calculi in dogs: 102 cases (1981–1989). JAVMA 1992; 201(1): 129–33.
159. Caswell J, Yager JA, Parker WM, Moore PF. A prospective study of the immunophenotype and temporal changes in the histologic lesions of canine demodicosis. Vet Path 1997; 34(4):279–87.
160. Caswell JL, Yager JA, Ferrer L, Weir JAM. Canine demodicosis—a reexamination of the histopathologic lesions and description of the immunophenotype of infiltrating cells. Vet Derm 1995; 6(1):9–19.
161. Catalfamo JL, Dodds WJ. Hereditary and acquired thrombopathias. Vet Clin N Am 1988; 18(1):185–93.
162. Center SA, Smith CA, Wilkinson E, et al. Clinicopathologic, renal immunofluorescent, and light microscopic features of glomerulonephritis in the dog: 41 cases (1975–1985). JAVMA 1987; 190(1):81–90.
163. Cederberg R, Nishino S, Dement WC, Mignot E. Breeding history of the Stanford colony of narcoleptic dogs. Vet Rec 1998; 142:31–6.
164. Cerundolo R, Lloyd DH, Pidduck HG. Studies on the inheritance of hair loss in the Irish water spaniel. 14th Proceedings of AAVD/ACVD meeting, Concurrent Session Notes. San Antonio, 1998: 95–6.
165. Chabanne L, Fournel C, Monestier M, et al. Canine systemic lupus erythematosus. Part I. Clinical and biological aspects. Compen Contin Edu Prac Vet 1999; 21(2):135–141.
166. Chabanne L, Marchal T, Denerolle P. Lymphocyte subset abnormalities in German shepherd dog pyoderma (GSP). Vet Immunology and Immunopathology 1995, 49(3):189–98.
167. Chalmers SA, Medleau L. An update on atopic dermatitis in dogs. Vet Med 1994: 89(4):3–12.
168. Chapmann BL, Giger U. Inherited erythrocyte pyruvate kinase deficiency in the West Highland white terrier. J Sm Anim Pract 1990; 31: 610–3.
169. Chaudieu G. Cases of inherited retinal pigmented epithelium dystrophy in wire-haired fox terriers—an original clinical study and a review of the literature. Revue de Medecine Veterinaire 1997; 148(6):537–46.
170. Chaudieu G. Dysplasia of the pectinate ligament in the Siberian husky. A clinical, biometrical and anatomical pathological study. Pratique Medicale et Chirurgicale de L'Animal de Compagnie 1997; 32(5):393–402.
171. Chaudieu G. Study of inherited focal degeneration (retinopathy) in the borzoi. A report on 160 dogs. Pratique Medicale et Chirurgicale de L' Animal de Compagnie 1995; 30(4):461–72.
172. Chaudieu G, Molonnoblot S. Corneal dystrophy and degeneration. Pratique Medicale et Chirurgicale de L'Animal de Compagnie 1997; 32(4):103–11.
173. Chaudieu G, Molonnoblot S, Duprat P. Rod dysplasia and early retinal degeneration in a briard shepherd pup. Clinical, histological, and ultrastructural study. A case report and literature review. Revue de Medecine Veterinaire 1994; 145(11):825–7.
174. Chastain CB. Pediatric cytogenetics. Compend Contin Educ Pract Vet 1992; 14(3):333–40.
175. Chastain CB. The endocrine and metabolic systems. In: Hoskins JD, ed. Veterinary Pediatrics. Philadelphia: WB Saunders, 1995:377–97.
176. Chastain CB, Swayne DE. Congenital hypotrichosis in male basset hound littermates. JAVMA 1985; 187:845–6.
177. Chinn DR, Dodds WJ, Selcer BA. Prekallikrein deficiency in a dog. JAVMA 1986; 188(1):69–71.
178. Chouinard L, Martineau D, Forget C, Girard C. Use of polymerase chain reaction and immunohistochemistry for detection of canine adenovirus type 1 in formalin-fixed, paraffin-embedded liver of dogs with chronic hepatitis or cirrhosis. J Vet Diag Investig 1998; 10(4):320–5.
179. Chrisman, CL. Neuroaxonal dystrophy and leukoencephalomyelopathy of rottweiler dogs. In: Kirk RW, ed. Current veterinary therapy IX, Small animal practice. Philadelphia: WB Saunders, 1986:805–6.
180. Clark P, Bowden DK, Parry BW. Studies to detect carriers of hemophilia A in German shepherd dogs using diagnostic DNA polymorphisms in the human factor VIII gene. V J 1997; 153(1):71–4.
181. Clark RD, Stainer JR. Medical & genetic aspects of purebred dogs. Fairway, KS: Forum Publications, 1994. 687 p.
182. Clements PJM, Sargan DR, Gould DJ, Petersen-Jones SM. Recent advances in understanding the spectrum of canine generalized progressive retinal atrophy. J Sm Anim Pract 1996; 37:155–62.
183. Clemmons RM. Degenerative myelopathy. Vet Clin N Am 1992; 22(4):965–71.
184. Clemmons RM. Degenerative myelopathy of german shepherd dogs. http://neuro.vetmed.ufl.edu/neuro/DM_Web/DmofGS.htm, accessed August 23, 1998.
185. Clerc B. Chronic superficial keratitis in German shepherd dogs and other breeds. Canine Pract 1996; 21(6):6–12.
186. Clerc B, Jegou JP, Dehaas V, et al. The treatment of canine keratoconjunctivitis sicca. Pratique Medicale et Chirurgicale de L'Animal de Compagnie 1996; 31(4):331–8.
187. Coates JR, Kline KL. Congenital and inherited neurologic disorders in dogs and cats. In: Kirk's current veterinary therapy XII, Small animal practice. Philadelphia: WB Saunders, 1995: 1111–20.

188. Collins RL, Birchard SJ, Chew DJ, Heuter KJ. Surgical treatment of urate calculi in dalmatians—38 cases (1980–1995). JAVMA 1998; 213(6): 833–5.
189. Comegliani L, Ghibaudo G. A dermoid sinus in a Siberian husky. Vet Derm 1999; 10(1):47–49.
190. Conroy JD. Alopecia of dogs and cats. J Am Anim Hosp Assoc 1968; 4:200–69.
191. Conroy JD, Rasmusen, BA. Small E. hypotrichosis in miniature poodle siblings. JAVMA 1975; 166:697–9.
192. Cook AK, Breitschwerdt EB, Levine, JF, et al. Risk factors associated with acute pancreatitis in dogs: 101 cases (1985–1990). JAVMA 1993; 203(5):673–9.
193. Cook CS. Diseases of the orbit. In: Morgan RV, ed. Handbook of small animal practice. 3d ed. Philadelphia: WB Saunders, 1997:1076–84.
194. Cook CS. Surgery for glaucoma. Vet Clin N Am, Sm Anim Pract 1997; 27(5):1109–26.
195. Cook JL, Tomlinson JL, Constantinescu G. Pathophysiology, diagnosis, and treatment of canine hip dysplasia. Compend Contin Educ Pract Vet 1996; 18(8):853–9.
196. Cook SM, Dean DF, Golden DL, et al. Renal failure attributable to atrophic glomerulopathy in four related rottweilers. JAVMA 1993; 202(1):107–9.
197. Cooley PL, Dice PF. Corneal dystrophy in the dog and cat. Vet Clin N Am, Sm Anim Pract 1990; 20:681–92.
198. Cooper HK, Mattern GW. Genetic studies of cleft lip and palate in dogs. Carnivore Genet Newsletter 1970; 9:204–9.
199. Cooper Jr. RC, Weber WJ, Goodwin, J-K. The surgical treatment of common congenital heart defects. Vet Med 1992; 87(7):676–88.
200. Corcoran KA, Koch S, Peiffer RL. Primary glaucoma in the chow chow. Vet & Comp Ophthalmol 1994; 4(4):193–7.
201. Cordy DR, Holliday TA. A necrotizing meningoencephalitis in pug dogs. Vet Path 1989; 26(3):191–4.
202. Cork LC. Canine ventral horn cell diseases. In: Kirk's current veterinary therapy XI, Small animal practice. Philadelphia: WB Saunders, 1992:1031–4.
203. Cork LC, Green SL, Pinter MJ. Hereditary canine spinal muscular atrophy—genetics, neurophysiology, and pathology. J Neurol Sci 1997; 152(Suppl 1):S74.
204. Cork LC, Morris JM, Olson JL, et al. Membranoproliferative glomerulonephritis in dogs with a genetically determined deficiency of the third component of complement. Clinical Immunology and Immunopathology 1991; 60:455–70.
205. Corley EA. Role of the Orthopedic Foundation for Animals in the control of canine hip dysplasia. Vet Clin N Am, Sm Anim Pract 1992; 22(3):579–93.
206. Corley EA, Keller G, Lattimer JC, Ellersieck MR. Reliability of early radiographic evaluations for canine hip dysplasia obtained from standard ventrodorsal radiographic projection. JAVMA 1997; 211(9):1142–6.
207. Cottrell BO, Barnett KC. Primary glaucoma in the Welsh springer spaniel. J Sm Anim Prac 1988; 29:185–99.
208. Cowan LA, Hertzke DM, Fenwick BW, et al. Clinical and clinicopathologic abnormalities in greyhounds with cutaneous and renal glomerular vasculopathy: 18 cases (1992–1994). JAVMA 1997; 210(6):789–93.
209. Coward TG. Persistent right aortic arch in two Great Dane litter mates. J Sm Anim Pract 1964; 5:245–7.
210. Cox NR, Kwapien RP, Sorjonen, DC. Myeloencephalopathy resembling Alexander's disease in a Scottish terrier dog. Acta Neuropathol 1986; 71:163–7.
211. Cox VS, Wallace LF, Jessen CR. An anatomic and genetic study of canine cryptorchidism. Teratology 1978; 18:233–7.
212. Cozzi F, Vite CH, Wenger DA, et al. MRI and electrophysiological abnormalities in a case of canine globoid cell leukodystrophy. J Sm Anim Pract 1998; 39(8): 401–5.
213. Crawford MA, Foil CS. Vasculitis: clinical syndromes in small animals. Compend Contin Educ Pract Vet 1989; 11(4):400–15.
214. Crawford MA, Schall WD, Jensen RK, Tasker, JB. Chronic active hepatitis in 26 Doberman pinschers. JAVMA 1985; 187(12):1343–50.
215. Cross AR, Chambers JN. Ununited anconeal process of the canine elbow. Compend Contin Educ Pract Vet 1997; 19(3):349–57.
216. Crystal MA. Epistaxis. In: Tilley L, Smith F, eds. The 5 minute veterinary consult. Baltimore: Williams & Wilkins, 1997:64–5.
217. Cummings JF, DeLahunta A. Canine neurodegenerative diseases involving motor neurons. In Kirk's current veterinary therapy XII, Small animal practice. Philadelphia: WB Saunders, 1995:1132–6.
218. Cummings JF, George C, Delahunta, A, et al. Focal spinal muscular atrophy in 2 German shepherd pups. Acta Neuropathol 1989; 79:113–6.
219. Cummings JF, Wood PA, Walkley SU, et al. GM2 gangliosidosis in a Japanese spaniel. Acta Neuropathol (Berl) 1985; 67:247–53.
220. Cunningham JC, Farnbach GC. Inheritance and idiopathic canine epilepsy. J Am Anim Hosp Assoc 1988; 24:421–9.
221. Curtis CF, Evans H, Lloyd DH. Investigation of the reproductive and growth-hormone status of dogs affected by idiopathic recurrent flank alopecia. J Sm Anim Pract 1996; 37(9):417–22.
222. Curtis R. Retinal diseases in the dog a cat: an overview and update. J Sm Anim Pract 1988; 29(7):3 -415.
223. Curtis R, Barnett KC. A survey of catar ts in golden and Labrador retrievers. J Sm Anim Pract 1 39; 30:277–86.
224. Curtis R, Barnett KC. Progressive retinal atrophy in miniature longhaired dachshund dogs. Br Vet J 1993; 149(1):71–85.

D

225. Dale DC, Rodger E, Cebon J, et al. Long-term treatment of canine cyclic hematopoiesis with recombinant canine stem cell factor. Blood 1995; 85(1):74–9.
226. Dambach DM, Lannon A, Sleeper MM, Buchanan J. Familial dilated cardiomyopathy of young Portuguese water dogs. J Vet Intern Med 1999; 13(1):65–71.
227. Daminet, SC. Gluten-sensitive enteropathy in a family of Irish setters. Can Vet J 1996; 37:745–6.
228. Darke PGG. Mitral valve disease in Cavalier King Charles spaniels. In: Kirk's current veterinary therapy XII, Small animal practice. Philadelphia: WB Saunders, 1995:837–41.
229. Davidson MG. Diseases of the anterior uveal tract. In: Handbook of small animal practice. 3d ed. In: Morgan RV, ed. Philadelphia: WB Saunders, 1997:1020–9.
230. Davidson MG, Geoly FJ, Gilger BC, et al. Retinal degeneration associated with vitamin E deficiency in hunting dogs. JAVMA 1998; 213(5): 645–8.
231. Davies C. Medical treatment of canine perianal fistulas. Vet Med 1997; 92(12):1056–60.
232. Davies AP, Hardy R, Larsen R, et al. Primary lymphedema in three dogs. JAVMA 1979; 174(12):1316–20.
233. Davis KE, Finnie JW, Hooper PT. Lafora's disease in a dog. Australian Vet J 1990; 67:192–3.
234. Day MJ. An immunohistochemical study of the lesions of demodicosis in the dog. J Comp Pathol 1997; 116(2):203–16.
235. Day MJ. Immunopathology of anal furunculosis in the dog. J Sm Anim Pract 1993; 34:381–9.
236. Day MJ. Inheritance of serum autoantibody, reduced serum IgA and autoimmune disease in a canine breeding colony. Vet Immunology and Immunopathology 1996; 53(3–4):207–19.
237. Day MJ. Low IgA concentration in the tears of German shepherd dogs. Australian Vet J 1996; 74(6):433–4.
238. Day MJ, Power C, Oleshko J, Rose M. Low serum immunoglobulin concentrations in related Weimaraner dogs. J Sm Anim Pract 1997; 38(7):311–5.
239. DeBosschere H, Watzeels F, Ducatelle R. Juvenile nephropathy in a Newfoundlander. Vlaams Diergeneeskundig Tijdschrift 1998; 67(6):347–351.
240. DeBowes LJ. Dental disease and care. In: Hoskins JD, ed. Veterinary pediatrics. Philadelphia: WB Saunders, 1995: 125–32.
241. Degen M. Pseudohyperkalemia in Akitas. JAVMA 1987; 190(5): 541–3.

242. Degopegui RR, Feldman BF. Acquired and inherited platelet dysfunction in small animals. Compend Contin Educ Pract Vet 1998; 20(9): 1039–47.
243. Degopegui RR, Felman BF. Von Willebrand's disease. Comparative Haematology International 1997; 7(4):187–96.
244. Dehaan JJ, Goring RL, Beale BS. Evaluation of polysulfated glycosaminoglycan for the treatment of hip dysplasia in dogs. Vet Surg 199; 23:177–81.
245. Delahunta A, Averill DR. Hereditary cerebellar cortical and extrapyramidal nuclear abiotrophy in Kerry blue terriers. JAVMA 1976; 168:1119–22.
246. Delahunta A, Ingram JT, Cummings JF, Bell JSS. Labrador retriever central axonopathy. Prog in Vet Neurol 1994; 5(3):117–22.
247. Delellis LA, Thomas WP, Pion PD. Balloon dilatation of congenital subaortic stenosis in the dog. J Vet Intern Med 1993; 7:153–62.
248. Delles EK, Willard MD, Simpson RB, et al. Comparison of species and numbers of bacteria in concurrently cultured samples of proximal small intestinal fluid and endoscopically obtained duodenal mucosa in dogs with intestinal bacterial overgrowth. Am J Vet Res 1994; 55(7):957–64.
249. Delverdier M, Seltensperger T, Amardeilh MF, Magnol JP. Cutaneous mucinosis in dogs and cat—a histological and histochemical study of 106 cases. Revue de Medecine Veterinaire 1995; 146(5):333–9.
250. Demarco J, Center S, Dykes N, et al. A syndrome resembling idiopathic noncirrhotic portal hypertension in 4 young Doberman pinschers. J Vet Intern Med 1998; 12(3):147–56.
251. Demorais HAS, Dibartola SP, Chew DJ. Juvenile renal disease in golden retrievers—12 cases (1984–1994). JAVMA 1996; 209(4):792–7.
252. Denerolle P, Bourdoiseau G, Magnol J-P, et al. German shepherd dog pyoderma: a prospective study of 23 cases. Vet Derm 1998; 9: 243–8.
253. Denhertog E, Braakman JCA, Teske E, et al. Treatment of pituitary-dependent hyperadrenocorticism in the dog by nonselective adrenocorticolysis with O,P'-DDD. Vet Quarterly 1997; 19(1):S17-S19.
254. Derooster H, Vanryssen B, Vanbree H. Diagnosis of cranial cruciate ligament injury in dogs by tibial compression radiography. Vet Rec 1998; 142(14):366–8.
255. Deykin AR, Guandalini A, Rato A. A retrospective histopathologic study of primary episcleral and scleral inflammatory disease in dogs. Vet & Compar Ophthalmol 1997; 7(4):245–8.
256. DiBartola SP. Renal amyloidosis. Proceedings of the 16th ACVIM Forum, San Diego, 1998, 23–4.
257. DiBartola SP, Chew DJ, Boyce, JT. Juvenile renal disease in related standard poodles. JAVMA 1983; 183:693–6.
258. DiBartola SP, Tarr MJ, Webb DM, Giger U. Familial renal amyloidosis in Chinese shar pei dogs. JAVMA 1990; 197:483–7.
259. DiBartola SP, Tarr MJ, Parker AT, et al. Clinicopathologic findings in dogs with renal amyloidosis: 59 cases (1976–1986). JAVMA 1989; 195(3):358–64.
260. Dillberger JE, Altman NH. Focal mucinosis in dogs: Seven cases and review of cutaneous mucinoses of man and animals. Vet Path 1986; 23:132–9.
261. Dimski DS. Chronic active hepatitis. In: Tilley LP, Smith FWK Jr., eds. The 5 minute veterinary consult. Baltimore: Williams & Wilkins, 1997: 656–7.
262. Dimski DS, Hawkins EC. Canine systemic hypertension. Compend Contin Educ Pract Vet 1988; 10(10):1152–8.
263. Dodds WJ. Bleeding disorders. In: Morgan RV, ed. Handbook of small animal medicine. 2d ed. New York: Churchill Livingstone, 765–7.
264. Dodds WJ. Von Willebrand's disease. UDC Focus 1997; 2:6.
265. Dodds WJ, Raymond SL, Brooks MB. Inherited and acquired von Willebrand's disease. Vet Pract Staff 1993; 5(4/5):1,14–7, 21–3.
266. Dodman NH, Knowles KE, Shuster L, et al. Behavioral changes associated with suspected complex partial seizures in bull terriers. JAVMA 1996; 208(5):688–91.
267. Dodman NH, Shuster L, White SD, et al. Use of narcotic antagonists to modify stereotypic self-licking, self-chewing, and scratching behavior in dogs. JAVMA 1988; 194: 815–9.
268. Dole RS, Spurgeon TL. Frequency of supernumerary teeth in a dolicocephalic canine breed, the greyhound. Am J Vet Res 1998; 59(1):16–7.
269. Duclos DD, Jeffers, JG, Shanley KJ. Prognosis for treatment of adult-onset demodicosis in dogs: 34 cases (1979–1990). JAVMA 1994; 204(4):616–9.
270. Dugan SJ, Ketring KL, Severin GA, Render JA. Variant nodular granulomatous episclerokeratitis in 4 dogs. J Am Anim Hosp Assoc 1993; 29(5):403–9.
271. Duncan ID. Abnormalities of myelination of the central nervous system associated with congenital tremor. J Vet Intern Med 1987; 1(1):10–23.
272. Duncan ID, Cuddon PA. Sensory neuropathy. In: Kirk RW, ed. Current veterinary therapy X, Small animal practice. Philadelphia: WB Saunders, 1989:822–7.
273. Duncan ID, Griffiths IR, Carmichael S, Henderson S. Inherited canine giant axonal neuropathy. Muscle Nerve 1981; 4:223–7.
274. Dunn KJ, Herrtage ME, Dunn JK. Use of ACTH stimulation tests to monitor the treatment of canine hyperadrenocorticism. Vet Rec 1995; 137(7):161–5.
275. Dunstan RW, Credille KM, Walder EJ. The light and the skin. Advances in Vet Derm 1998; 3:3–35.
276. Dunstan RW, et al. A disease resembling junctional epidermolysis bullosa in a toy poodle. Am J Dermatopathol 1988; 10:442–7.
277. Dunstan RW, Hargis AM. The diagnosis of sebaceous adenitis in standard poodle dogs. In: Kirk's current veterinary therapy XII, Small animal practice. Philadelphia: WB Saunders, 1995:619–22.
278. DuPont G. Personal communication 1998.
279. Dupuis J, Harari J. Cruciate ligament and meniscal injuries in dogs. Compend Contin Educ Pract Vet 1993; 15(2):215–32.

E

280. Eckstein RA, Hart BL. Treatment of canine acral lick dermatitis by behavior modification using electronic stimulation. J Am Anim Hosp Assoc 1996; 32(3):225–30.
281. Eger CE, Huxtable CRR, Chester ZC, Summers BA. Progressive tetraparesis and laryngeal paralysis in a young Rottweiler with neuronal vacuolation and axonal degeneration: an Australian case. Australian Vet J 1998; 76(11): 733–7.
282. Eggers JS, Parker GA, Braaf HA, Mense MG. Disseminated mycobacterium avium infection in 3 miniature schnauzer littermates. J Vet Diag Invest 1997; 9(4):424–7.
283. Eigenmann JE. Diagnosis and treatment of dwarfism in a German shepherd dog. J Am Anim Hosp Assoc 1981; 17(5):798–804.
284. Ekesten B, Bjerkas E, Kongsengen K, Narfstrom K. Primary glaucoma in the Norwegian elkhound. Vet & Compar Ophthalmol 1997; 7(1):14–18.
285. Ekesten B, Torrang I. Heritability of the depth of the opening of the ciliary cleft in Samoyeds. Am J Vet Res 1995; 56(9):1138–43.
286. Ekman S, Carlson CS. The pathophysiology of osteochondrosis. Vet Clin N Am, Sm Anim Pract 1998; 28(1):17–32.
287. Eksell P, Haggstrom J, Kvart C, Karlsson A. Thrombocytopenia in the Cavalier King Charles spaniel. J Sm Anim Pract 1994; 35(3):153–5.
288. Elliott DA, Nelson RW, Feldman EC, Neal, LA. Glycosylated hemoglobin concentrations in the blood of healthy dogs and dogs with naturally developing diabetes mellitus, pancreatic beta-cell neoplasia, hyperadrenocorticism, and anemia. JAVMA 1997; 211(6):723–9.
289. Ellison GW. Treatment of perianal fistulas in dogs. JAVMA 1995; 206(11):1680–2.
290. Ellison GW, Bellah J, Stubbs WP, Vangilder J. Treatment of perianal fistulas with Nd-YAG laser—results in 20 cases. Vet Surg 1995; 24(2):140–7.

291. Elmwood CM. Risk factors for gastric dilatation in Irish setter dogs. J Sm Anim Pract 1998; 39(4):185–90.
292. Elwood JM, Colquhoun TA. Observations on the prevention of cleft palate in dogs by folic acid and potential relevance to humans. New Zealand Vet J 1997; 45:254–6.
293. English RV. Diseases of the lens and vitreous. In: Morgan RV, ed. Handbook of small animal practice. 3d ed. Philadelphia: WB Saunders, 1997:1036–46.
294. Evers P, Kramek BA, Wallace, LJ, et al. Clinical and radiographic evaluation of intertrochanteric osteotomy in dogs—a retrospective study of 18 dogs. Vet Surg 1997; 26(3):217–22.

F

295. Falco MJ, Barker J, Wallace ME. The genetics of epilepsy in the British Alsatian. J Sm Anim Pract 1974; 15:685–92.
296. Famula TR, Oberbauer AM. Reducing the incidence of epileptic seizures in the Belgian Tervuren through selection. Prevent Vet Med 1998; 33(1–4):251–9.
297. Famula TR, Oberbauer AM, Brown KN. Heritability of epileptic seizures in the Belgian Tervuren. J Sm Anim Pract 1997; 38(8):349–52.
298. Famula TR, Oberbauer AM, Sousa CA. A threshold model analysis of deafness in dalmatians. Mammalian Genome 1996; 7(9):650–3.
299. Farber DB, Danciger JS, Aguirre G. The beta subunit of cyclic GMP phosphodiesterase messenger RNA is deficient in canine rod-cone dysplasia–1. Neuron 1992; 9:349–56.
300. Farnbach G. Seizures in the dog. Part I. Basis, classification, and predilection. Compend Contin Educ Pract Vet 1984; 6(6):569–74.
301. Farrow BRH, Hartley WJ, Pollard AC, et al. Gaucher disease in the dog. In: Gaucher disease: a century of delineation and research. New York: Alan R. Liss, Inc., 1985:645–53.
302. Farrow BRH, Malik R. Hereditary myotonia in the chow chow. J Sm Anim Pract 1981; 22:451–65.
303. Fatone G, Brunetti A, Lamagna F, Potena A. Dermoid sinus and spinal malformations in a Yorkshire terrier: diagnosis and follow-up. J Sm Anim Pract 1995; 36(4):178–80.
304. Feldman DG, Brooks MB, Dodds WJ. Hemophilia B (factor IX deficiency) in a family of German shepherd dogs. JAVMA 1995; 206:1901–5.
305. Feldman EC, Nelson RW, Feldman MS. Use of low-dose and high-dose dexamethasone tests for distinguishing pituitary-dependent from adrenal tumor hyperadrenocorticism in dogs. JAVMA 1996; 209(4):772–7.
306. Felkai C, Voros K, Vrabely T, et al. Ultrasonographic findings of renal dysplasia in cocker spaniels—8 cases. Acta Veterinaria Hungaricaa 1997; 45(4):397–408.
307. Fellows CG, Lerche P, King G, Tometzki A. Treatment of patent ductus arteriosus by placement of 2 intravascular embolization coils in a puppy. J Sm Anim Pract 1998; 39(4):196–9.
308. Felsburg PJ. Overview of the immune system and immunodeficiency diseases. Vet Clin N Am, Sm Anim Pract 1994; 24(4):629–53.
309. Felsburg PJ. Primary immunodeficiencies. In: Current veterinary therapy XI, Small animal practice. Philadelphia: WB Saunders 1992: 448–53.
310. Felsburg PJ, Somberg, RL, Hartnett, BJ et al. Canine X-linked severe combined immunodeficiency. Immunol Res 1998; 17(1–2):63–73.
311. Fenner WR. Neurology of the geriatric patient. Vet Clin N Am, Sm Anim Pract 1988; 18(3):711–24.
312. Ferguson J. Patellar luxation in the dog and cat. Practice 1997; 19(4):174–81.
313. Ferrara ML, Occhiodoro T, Muler M, et al. Canine fucosidosis—a model for retroviral gene transfer into hematopoietic stem cells. Neuromuscular Disorders 1997; 7(5):361–6.
314. Finco DR. Familial renal disease in Norwegian elkhound dogs: morphologic examinations. Am J Vet Res 1977; 38:941–7.
315. Fine DM, Eyster GE, Anderson LK, Smitley A. Cyanosis and congenital methemoglobinemia in a puppy. J Am Anim Hosp Assoc 1999, 35(1):33–35.
316. Fingland RB, Bonagura JD, Myer, CW. Pulmonic stenosis in the dog: 29 cases (1975–1984). JAVMA 1986; 189(2):218–26.
317. Fischer A, Carmichael KP, Munnell JF, et al. Mucopolysaccharidosis IIIA (Sanfilippo A) in dachshunds. Proceedings of the 14th ACVIM Forum 1996:678–9.
318. Fitch RB, Beale BS. Osteochondrosis of the canine tibiotarsal joint. Vet Clin N Am, Sm Anim Prac 1998; 28(1):95–113.
319. Fogh JM. A study of hemophilia A in German shepherd dogs in Denmark. Vet Clin N Am 1988; 18(1):245–54.
320. Fogh JM, Fogh IT. Inherited coagulation disorders. Vet Clin N Am 1988; 18(1):231–43.
321. Foil CS. The skin. In: Hoskins JD, ed. Veterinary pediatrics. Philadelphia: WB Saunders, 1995:227–96.
322. Foley CW, Lasley JF, Osweiler GD. Abnormalities of companion animals: analysis of heritability. Ames: Iowa State University Press, 1979. 270 p.
323. Fontaine J, Beco L, Paradis M. Recurrent flank alopecia—A study carried out on 12 cases of Griffon Korthals. Point Veterinaire 1998; 29(192): 67–71.
324. Fontaine J, Gilbert S, Pypendop B, Verstegen J. Use of medetomidine as stimulating agent in the GH test in the dog and interest of the induced hyperglycemic response in dermatology. Annales de Medecine Veterinaire 1996; 140(2):65–70.
325. Ford L. Hereditary aspects of human and canine cyclic neutropenia. J Hered 1969; 60:293–9.
326. Ford RB. Clinical management of lipemic patients. Compend Contin Educ Pract Vet 1996; 18(10):1053–60.
327. Ford RB. Idiopathic hyperchylomicroanemia in miniature schnauzers. J Sm Anim Pract 1993; 34:488–92.
328. Fossum TW (Ed.). Small animal surgery. St. Louis: Mosby Year Book 1997.
329. Foster SJ, Curtis R, Barnett KC. Primary lens luxation in the Border collie. J Sm Anim Pract 1986; 27: 1–4.
330. Franch J, Cesari JR, Font J. Craniomandibular osteopathy in 2 Pyrenean mountain dogs. Vet Rec 1998; 142(17):455–9.
331. Franklin RJM, Jeffery ND, Ramsey, IK. Neuroaxonal dystrophy in a litter of papillon pups. J Sm Anim Pract 1995; 36(10):441–4.
332. Freeman LJ. Ehlers-Danlos syndrome in dogs and cats. Sem Vet Med Surg 1987; 2(3):221–7.
333. Freeman LM, Michel KE, Brown DJ, et al. Idiopathic dilated cardiomyopathy in dalmatians—9 cases (1990–1995). JAVMA 1996; 209(9):1592–6.
334. Freshman JL. Diseases of the testes and epididymides. In: Morgan RV, ed. Handbook of small animal practice. 3d ed. Philadelphia: WB Saunders, 1997:588–93.
335. Fries CL, Remedios AM. The pathogenesis and diagnosis of canine hip dysplasia—review. Can Vet J 1995; 36(8):494–502.
336. Fry TR, Clark DM. Canine hip dysplasia: clinical signs and physical diagnosis. Vet Clin N Am, Sm Anim Pract 1992; 22(3):551–8.
337. Fuentealba C, Guest S, Haywood S, Horney B. Chronic hepatitis—a retrospective study in 34 dogs. Can Vet J 1997; 38(6):365–73.
338. Fyfe JC, Jezyk PF, Giger U, Patterson DF. Inherited selective malabsorption of vitamin B12 in giant schnauzers. J Am Anim Hosp Assoc 1989; 25(5):533–9.

G

339. Gaiddon J, Lallement PE, Peiffer RL. Positive correlation between coat color and electroretinographically diagnosed progressive retinal atrophy in miniature poodles in Southern France. Vet & Compar Ophthal 1995; 5(2):74–7.
340. Gaiddon J, Lallement PE, Peiffer RL. Study and statistics of 207 electroretinograms performed on miniature poodles suspected of progressive retinal atrophy. Pratique Medicale et Chirurgicale de L'Animal de Compagnie 1997; 32(1):77–81.
341. Gamble DA, Chrisman CL. A leukoencephalomyelopathy of rottweiler dogs. Vet Path 1984:274–8.
342. Garden OA, Manners HK, Sorensen SH, et al. Intestinal permeability of Irish setter puppies challenged with a controlled oral dose of gluten. Res in Vet Sci 1998; 65(1): 23–8.

343. Gavaghan BJ, Kittleson MD. Dilated cardiomyopathy in an American cocker spaniel with taurine deficiency. Australian Vet J 1997; 75: 862–8.
344. Gelatt KN. Corneal diseases in the dog. In: Glaze MB, ed. Ophthalmology in small animal practice. Trenton, NJ: Veterinary Learning Systems, 1996:31–8.
345. Gelatt KN. Lens and cataract formation in the dog. In: Glaze MB, ed. Ophthalmology in small animal practice. Trenton, NJ: Veterinary Learning Systems, 1996: 25–30.
346. Gelatt KN, Brooks DE, Samuelson DA. Comparative glaucomatology I. The spontaneous glaucomas. J Glaucoma 1998; 7(3):187–201.
347. Gelatt KN, Gum G. Inheritance of primary glaucoma in the beagle. Am J Vet Res 1981; 42:1691–3.
348. Gelatt KN, Powell G, Huston K. Inheritance of microphthalmia with coloboma in the Australian sheep dog. Am J Vet Res 1981; 42:1686–90.
349. Gelatt KN, Whitley RD, Lavach, JD, et al.Cataracts in Chesapeake Bay retrievers. JAVMA 1979; 175:1176–8.
350. Genetics Committee of the American College of Veterinary Ophthalmologists. Ocular disorders presumed to be inherited in purebred dogs. 2d ed.: Genetics Committee 1996.
351. Gerard VA, Conarck CN. Identifying the cause of early onset of seizures in puppies with epileptic parents. Vet Med 1991; 86: 1060–1.
352. Gerhardt A, Risse R, Meyerlindenberg A. Necrotizing vasculitis of the spinal and cerebral leptomeninges in a Bernese mountain dog. Deutsche Tierarztliche Wochenschrift 1998; 105(4): 139–41.
353. Gerlach KF, Skrodzki M, Trautvetter E. Balloon valvuloplasty for the treatment of pulmonic stenosis in the dog. Tierarztliche Praxis Ausgabe Kleintiere Heimtiere 1997; 25(6):643–65.
354. Gibbs C. The BVA/KC scoring scheme for control of hip dysplasia. Interpretation of criteria. Vet Rec 1997; 141:275–84.
355. Gibson TE, Roberts SM, Severin GA, et al. Comparison of gonioscopy and ultrasound biomicroscopy for evaluating the iridocorneal angle in dogs. JAVMA 1998; 213(5): 635–7.
356. Giger U. Primary immunodeficiency in small animals. Kleintierpraxis 1994; 39(6):433–8.
357. Giger U, Felsburg PJ. Immunodeficiency disorders. In: Morgan RV, ed. Handbook of small animal medicine. 3d ed. Philadelphia: WB Saunders, 1997:779–85.
358. Giger U, Harvey JW. Hemolysis caused by phosphofructokinase deficiency in English springer spaniels: Seven cases (1983–1986). JAVMA 1987; 191: 453–7.
359. Giger U, Mason GD, Wang P. Inherited erythrocyte pyruvate kinase deficiency in a beagle dog. Vet Clin Path 1991; 20: 83–5.
360. Giger U, Noble NA. Determination of erythrocyte pyruvate kinase deficiency in basenjis with chronic hemolytic anemia. JAVMA 1991; 198:1755–8.
361. Giger U, Smith BF, Woods CB, et al. Inherited phosphofructokinase deficiency in an American cocker spaniel. JAVMA 1992; 201: 1569–771.
362. Ginel PJ, Novales M, Lozano MD, et al: Local secretory IgA in dogs with low systemic IgA levels. Vet Rec 1993; 132(13):321–3.
363. Gionfriddo J. Corneal dystrophy in dogs. http://www.vet.purdue.edu/ ~yshen/dx2.html, May 10, 1998.
364. Gionfriddo JR. Recognizing and managing acute and chronic cases of glaucoma. Vet Med 1995; 90(3):265–74.
365. Glaze MB, Carter, JD. The eye. In: Hoskins JD, ed. Veterinary Pediatrics. Philadelphia: WB Saunders, 1995: 297–336.
366. Gleadhill A. Juvenile nephropathies in dogs and cats. Practice 1997; 19(5):270–6.
367. Glickman L, Emerick T, Glickman N, et al. Radiological assessment of the relationship between thoracic conformation and the risk of gastric dilatation-volvulus in dogs. Vet Radiol & Ultrasound 1996; 37(3):174–80.
368. Glickman LT, Glickman NW, Perez CM, et al. Analysis of risk factors for gastric dilatation and dilatation-volvulus in dogs. JAVMA 1994; 204(9):1465–71.
369. Glickman LT, Lantz GC, Schellenberg DB, Glickman NW. A prospective study of survival and recurrence following the acute gastric dilatation-volvulus syndrome in 136 dogs. J Am Anim Hosp Assoc 1998; 34(3):253–9.
370. Glover TD, Constantinescu GM. Surgery for cataracts. Vet Clin N Am, Sm Anim Pract 1997; 27(5):1143–59.
371. Goldberger E, Rapoport, JL. Canine acral lick dermatitis: Response to the antiobsessional drug clomipramine. J Am Anim Hosp Assoc 1991; 27(2):179–82.
372. Goldsmith LA, Thorpe JM, Mash RF. Tyrosine aminotransferase deficiency in mink (Mustela vison): A model for human tyrosinemia II. Biochem Genet 1981; 19:687–93.
373. Goldstein GS. The diagnosis and treatment of orthodontic problems. Problems in Vet Med 1990; 2(1):195–19.
374. Goodwin J-K. Familial distribution of cardiomyopathy in boxers. Canine Pract 1998; 23(1):49.
375. Goodwin J-K. Atrial septal defect. In: Tilley LP, Smith FWK Jr., eds. The 5 minute veterinary consult. Baltimore: Williams & Wilkins, 1997:378.
376. Goodwin J-K. Atrioventricular valve dysplasia. In: Tilley LP, Smith FWK Jr., eds. The 5 minute veterinary consult. Baltimore: Williams & Wilkins, 1997: 380–1.
377. Goodwin, J-K, Cooper RC Jr. Understanding the pathophysiology of congenital heart defects. Vet Med 1992; 87(7):650–68.
378. Goodwin J-K, Cooper RC Jr., Weber WJ. The medical management of pets with congenital heart defects. Vet Med 1992; 87(7):670–5.
379. Goodwin J-K, Lombard CW: Patent ductus arteriosus in adult dogs: clinical features of 14 cases. J Am Anim Hosp Assoc 1992; 28(4):349–54.
380. Gookin JL, Bunch SE, Rush LJ, Grindem, CB. Evaluation of microcytosis in 18 Shibas. JAVMA 1998; 212(8):1258–9.
381. Goossens MMC, Feldman EC, Theon AP, Koblik PD. Efficacy of cobalt–60 radiotherapy in dogs with pituitary-dependent hyperadrenocorticism. JAVMA, 1998; 212(3):374–8.
382. Gorospe J, Hoffman E, McQuarrier P, et al. Duchenne muscular dystrophy in a wire-haired fox terrier: A new dog model with no somatic reversion. VIIIth International Congress on Human Genetics, 1991, p. 97.
383. Greco DS. Congenital canine hypothyroidism. Canine Pract 1997; 22(1):23–4.
384. Greco DS. Pediatric endocrinology. In: Kirk's current veterinary therapy XII, Small animal practice. Philadelphia: WB Saunders, 1995:347–51.
385. Greenfield CL. Canine laryngeal paralysis. Compend Contin Educ Pract Vet 1987; 9(10):1011–7.
386. Greibrokk T. Hereditary deafness in the Dalmatian—relationship to eye and coat color. J Am Anim Hosp Assoc 1994; 30(2):170–6.
387. Grieshaber TL, Blakemore JC, Yaskulski, S: Congenital alopecia in a bichon frisé. JAVMA 1986; 188:1053–4.
388. Griffiths IR. Progressive axonopathy: an inherited neuropathy of boxer dogs. I. Further studies of the clinical and electrophysiological features. J Sm Anim Pract 1985; 26(7):381–92.
389. Griffiths IR. Progressive axonopathy of boxer dogs. In: Kirk RW, ed. Current veterinary therapy X, Small animal practice. Philadelphia: WB Saunders,1989:828–30.
390. Griffiths IR, Duncan ID, McCulloch M, Carmichael S. Hereditary hypomyelination of the CNS in springer spaniel pups. Neuropathol and Appl Neurobiol 1981; 7:80–6.
391. Grifka, RG, Miller, MW, Frischmeyer KJ, Mullins CE: Transcatheter occlusion of a patent ductus arteriosus in a Newfoundland puppy using the Gianturco-Grifka vascular occlusion device. J Vet Intern Med 1996; 10:42–44.
392. Grodecki KM, Gains MJ, Baumal R, et al. Treatment of x-linked hereditary nephritis in Samoyed dogs with angiotensin-converting enzyme (ACE) inhibitor. J Compar Path 1997; 117(3):209–25.
393. Grondalen J. Arthrosis in the elbow joint of young rapidly growing dogs. Nord Vet Med 1982; 34:65–75.
394. Gross TL. Calcinosis circumscripta and renal dysplasia in a dog. Vet Derm 1997; 8:27–32.
395. Gross TL, Halliwell RE, McDougal BJ, Rosencrantz S. Psoriasiform lichenoid dermatitis in the springer spaniel. Vet Path 1986; 23(1):76–8.
396. Gross TL, Pascaltenorio A, Munn RJ, et al. Follicular lipidosis in 3 rottweilers. Vet Derm 1997; 8(1):33–9.

397. Gu W, Acland GM, Langston, AA, et al. Identification of a RAPD marker linked to inherited progressive rod-cone degeneration (prcd) in dogs. Mammalian Genome 1998. In press.
398. Gu W, Ray K, Acland GM, Aguirre GD. RAPD analysis identifies canine genomic DNA polymorphisms, and a marker linked to progressive rod-cone degeneration. Canine Pract 1998; 23(1):41–2.
399. Gu WK, Ray K. A polymorphic (Ttta), tandem repeat in an intron of the canine factor IX gene. Anim Genet 1997; 28(5):370–1.
400. Guaguere E, Magnol JP, Cauzinille L, et al. Familial canine dermatomyositis in 8 Beauceron shepherds. In: Kwochka KW, Willemse T, von Tscharner C, eds. Advances in veterinary dermatology. Vol 3. Oxford, England: Butterworth-Heinemann, 1998: 527–8.
401. Guaguere E, Olivry T, Poujadedelverdier A, Magnol JP. Junctional epidermolysis bullosa associated with an absent expression of collagen XVII (Bpage (2), Bp180) in German shorthaired pointers. A report of 2 cases. Pratique Medicale et Chirurgicale de L'Animal de Compagnie 1997; 32(6):471–80.
402. Guenther LC. Inherited disorders of complement. J Am Acad Derm 1983; 9:815–39.
403. Guevara-Fujita ML, Loechel R, Venta PJ, et al. Chromosomal assignment of seven genes on canine chromosomes by fluorescence in situ hybridization. Mammalian Genome 1996; 7(4):268–70.
404. Guilford, WG: Breed-associated gastrointestinal disease. In: Kirk's Current veterinary therapy XII, Small animal practice. Philadelphia: WB Saunders, 1995:695–7.
405. Gupthhill L, Scottmoncrieff JC, Widmer WR. Diagnosis of canine hyperadrenocorticism. Vet Clin N Am, Sm Anim Pract 1997; 27(2):215–28.
406. Gwim RM, Wyman M, Lim DJ, et al. Multiple ocular defects associated with partial albinism and deafness in the dog. J Am Anim Hosp Assoc 1981; 17(3):401–8.

H

407. Hackner SG. Approach to the diagnosis of bleeding disorders. Compend Contin Educ Pract Vet 1995; 17(3):331–49.
408. Hakanson N, Narfstrom K. Progressive retinal atrophy in papillon dogs in Sweden. A clinical survey. Vet & Compar Ophthal 1995; 5(2):83–7.
409. Hall, JA. Diseases of the exocrine pancreas. In: Morgan RV, ed. Handbook of small animal practice. 3d ed. Philadelphia: WB Saunders, 1997: 403–16.
410. Hall SJG, Wallace ME. Canine epilepsy—a genetic counselling programme for keeshonds. Vet Rec 1996; 138:358–60.
411. Hamann F, Wedell H, Bauer J. Canine demodicosis. Kleintierpraxis 1997; 42(9):745–8.
412. Hanichen T, Brem G, Spiess C, Hermanns W. Canine lipid storage disease. Eur J Vet Path 1995; 1:37–44.
413. Hannigan MM. A refractory case of schnauzer comedo syndrome. Can Vet J 1997; 38:238–9.
414. Hansen P, Clercx C, Henroteaux M, et al. Neutrophil phagocyte dysfunction in a Weimaraner with recurrent infections. J Sm Anim Pract, 1995; 36(3):128–31.
415. Hanson SM, Smith MO, Walker TL, Shelton GD. Juvenile-onset distal myopathy in rottweiler dogs. J Vet Intern Med 1998; 12(2):103–8.
416. Hanssen I, Falck G, Grammeltvedt AT, Haug E, Isaksen CV. Hypochondroplastic dwarfism in the Irish setter. J Sm Anim Pract 1998; 39(1):10–4.
417. Harari J. Osteochondrosis of the femur. Vet Clin N Am, Sm Anim Pract 1998; 28(1):87–94.
418. Hargis AM, Haupt KH, Hebreberg GA, et al. Familial canine dermatomyositis: initial characterization of the cutaneous and muscular lesions. Am J Path 1984; 116:234–44.
419. Hargis AM, Haupt KH, Prieur DJ, et al. A skin disorder in three Shetland sheepdogs: comparison with familial canine dermatomyositis of collies. Compend Contin Educ Pract Vet 1985; 7:306–15.
420. Hargis AM, Haupt KH, Prieur DJ, Moore MP. Familial canine dermatomyositis: animal model of human disease. Am J Path 1985; 120(2):323–5.
421. Hargis AM, Mundell AC. Familial canine dermatomyositis. Compend Contin Educ Pract Vet 1995; 14:55–64.
422. Harkin KR, Walshaw R, Mullaney TP. Association of perianal fistula and colitis in the German shepherd dog. Response to high dose prednisone and dietary therapy. J Am Anim Hosp Assoc 1996; 32(6):515–20.
423. Harrington ML, Bagley RS, Moore MP. Hydrocephalus. Vet Clin N Am, Sm Anim Pract 1996; 26(4):843–56.
424. Harvey CE. Inherited and congenital airway conditions. J Sm Anim Pract 1989; 30(3):184–7.
425. Harvey, CE. Palate defects in dogs and cats. Compend Contin Educ Pract Vet 1987; 9(4):404–16.
426. Harvey JW. Congenital erythrocyte enzyme deficiencies. Vet Clin N Am, Sm Anim Pract 1996; 26(5): 1003–16.
427. Harvey JW. Methemoglobinemia and Heinz-body hemolytic anemia. In: Kirk's current veterinary therapy XII, Small animal practice, 3rd ed. Philadelphia: WB Saunders, 1995:443–46.
428. Harvey JW, Kaneko JJ, Hudson EB. Erythrocyte pyruvate kinase deficiency in a beagle dog. Vet Clin Path 1977; 6: 13–6.
429. Harvey JW, Smith JE. Hematology and clinical chemistry of English springer spaniel dogs with phosphofructokinase deficiency. Comparative Haematology International 1994; 4(2):70–5.
430. Haskins M, Giger U. Lysosomal storage diseases. In: Clinical biochemistry of domestic animals. 5th ed. 1997; 741–60.
431. Haskins ME, Aguirre GD, Jezyk PF et al. Mucopolysaccharidosis type VII (Sly syndrome)—Beta glucuronidase-deficient mucopolysaccharidosis in the dog. Am J Pathol 1991; 138:1553–5.
432. Haskins ME, Otis EJ, Hayden JE, et al. Hepatic storage of glycosaminoglycans in feline and canine models of Mucopolysaccharidose I, Mucopolysaccharidose VI, and Mucopolysaccharidose VII. Vet Path 1992; 29:112–9.
433. Haupt KH, Prieur DJ, Moore, MP, et al. Familial canine dermatomyositis: clinical, electrodiagnostic, and genetic studies. Am J Vet Res 1985; 46(9):1861–75.
434. Hay CW, Dueland RT, Dubielzig RR, Bjorenson JE. Idiopathic mutifocal osteopathy in four Scottish terriers (1991–1996). J Am Anim Hosp Assoc 1999; 35(1):62–67.
435. Hayes HM. Congenital umbilical and inguinal hernias in cattle, horses, swine, dogs and cats: Risk by breed and sex among hospital patients. Am J Vet Res 1974; 35: 839–42.
436. Haywood S, Rutgers HC, Christian MK. Hepatitis and copper accumulation in Skye terriers. Vet Path 1988; 25:408–14.
437. Hegreberg GA, Padgett GA. Inherited progressive epilepsy of the dog with comparisons to Lafora's disease of man. Federation Proceedings, 1976; 35:1202–5.
438. Held J-P, Prater, PE. Diseases of the external genitalia. In: Morgan RV, ed. Handbook of small animal practice. 3d ed. Philadelphia: WB Saunders, 1997:607–14.
439. Helman RG, Rames DS, Chester DK. Ichthyosiform dermatosis in a soft-coated wheaten terrier. Vet Derm 1997; 8(1):53–8.
440. Hendricks JC. Recognition and treatment of congenital respiratory tract defects in brachycephalics. In: Kirk's current veterinary therapy XII, Small animal practice. Philadelphia: WB Saunders, 1995:892–4.
441. Hendricks MJ, Dunagan CA. Focal necrotizing granulomatous panniculitis associated with subcutaneous injection of rabies vaccine in cats and dogs: 10 cases (1988–1989) JAVMA, 1991; 198(2): 304–305.
442. Henthorn PS, Somberg RL, Fimiani VM, et al. IL–2R gamma gene microdeletion demonstrates that canine X-linked severe combined immunodeficiency is a homologue of the human disease. Genomics 1994; 23:69–74.
443. Herrtage ME, Seymour CA, White RAS, Small GM, Wight DGD. Inherited copper toxicosis in the Bedlington terrier: the prevalence in asymptomatic dogs. J Sm Anim Pract 1988; 28(12):1141–51.
444. Hertzke DM, Cowan LA, Schoning,P, Fenwick BW. Glomerular ultrastructural lesions of idiopathic cutaneous and renal glomerular vasculopathy of greyhounds. Vet Path 1995; 32(5):451–9.
445. Hess RS, Kass PH, Shofer FS, et al. Evaluation of risk factors for fatal acute pancreatitis in dogs. JAVMA 1999; 214(1): 46–51.

446. Hess RS, Kass PH, Ward CR. Association between hyperadrenocorticism and development of calcium-containing uroliths in dogs with urolithiasis. JAVMA 1998; 212(12):1889–91.
447. Hewson CJ, Luescher UA, Parent JM, et al. Efficacy of clomipramine in the treatment of canine compulsive disorder. JAVMA 1998; 213(12): 1760–66.
448. Heynold Y, Faissler D, Steffen F, Jaggy A. Clinical, epidemiologic and treatment results of idiopathic epilepsy in 54 Labrador retrievers—a long-term study. J Sm Anim Pract 1997; 38(1):7–14.
449. Higgins RJ, Lecouteur RA, Kornegay JN, Coates JR. Late-onset progressive spinocerebellar degeneration in Brittany spaniel dogs. Acta Neuropathol 1998; 96(1):97–101.
450. Hill SL, Shelton GD, Lenehan TM. Myotonia is a cocker spaniel. J Am Anim Hosp Assoc 1995; 31(6):506–9.
451. Hoenig M. Pathophysiology of canine diabetes. Vet Clin N Am, Sm Anim Pract 1995; 25(3):553–61.
452. Hofmeyer CFB: Dermoid sinus in the ridgeback dog. J Sm Anim Pract 1963; 4:5–8.
453. Hogenesch H, Snyder PW, Scott-Montcrieff JCR, et al. Interleukin–6 activity in dogs with juvenile polyarteritis syndrome—effect of corticosteroids. Clin Immunology and Immunopathology 1995; 77(1):107–10.
454. Holliday TA, Nelson HJ, Williams DC, Willits N. Unilateral and bilateral brainstem auditory-evoked response abnormalities in 900 Dalmatian dogs. J Vet Intern Med 1990; 6:166–74.
455. Holmes NG, Herrtage ME, Ryder EJ, Binns MM. DNA marker C04107 for copper toxicosis in a population of Bedlington terriers in the United Kingdom. Vet Rec 1998; 142(14):351–2.
456. Holmstrom SE, Frost P, Gammon RL. Veterinary dental techniques for the small animal practitioner. Philadelphia: WB Saunders, 1992. 430 p.
457. Holt D, Brockman D. Diagnosis and management of laryngeal disease in the dog and cat. Vet Clin N Am, Sm Anim Pract 1994; 24(5):855–71.
458. Hood JC, Robinson WF, Huxtable CR, et al. Hereditary nephritis in the bull terrier: evidence for inheritance by an autosomal dominant gene. Vet Rec 1990; 126:456–9.
459. Hosgood G, Davidson JR. Disease of muscles and tendons. In: Morgan RV, ed. Handbook of small animal medicine. 3d ed. Philadelphia: Saunders, 1997:846–65.
460. Hoskins JD, Dimski DS. The digestive system. In: Hoskins JD, ed. Veterinary pediatrics. Philadelphia: WB Saunders, 1995:133–87.
461. Hoskins JD, Taboada J. Congenital defects of the dog. Compend Contin Educ Pract Vet 1992; 14(7):873–97.
462. Howell JM, Fletcher S, Kakulas BA, et al. Use of the dog model for Duchenne muscular dystrophy in gene therapy trials. Neuromuscular Disorders 1997; 7:325–8.
463. Hughes D, Goldschmidt MH, Washabau RJ, Kueppers F. Serum alpha–1-antitrypsin concentration in dogs with panniculitis. JAVMA 1996; 209(9):1582–4.

I

464. Ihrke PJ, Gross TL. Ulcerative dermatosis of Shetland sheepdogs and collies. In: Kirk's current veterinary therapy XII, Small animal practice. Philadelphia: WB Saunders, 1995:639–40.
465. Ihrke PJ, Mueller RS, Stannard AA. Generalized congenital hypotrichosis in a female rottweiler. Vet Derm 1993; 4(2):65–9.1
466. Inada S, Yamauchi C, Igata A, et al. Canine storage disease characterized by hereditary progressive neurogenic muscular atrophy: breeding experiments and clinical manifestations. Am J Vet Res 1986; 47(10):2294–9.
467. Inzana KD, Massicotte C. Disorders of peripheral nerves. In: Morgan RV, ed. Handbook of small animal practice. 3d ed. Philadelphia: WB Saunders, 272–91.
468. Iwasaki T, Olivry T, Lapiere JC, et al. Canine bullous pemphigoid (BP)—identification of the 180-kD canine BP antigen by circulating autoantibodies. Vet Path 1995; 32(4):387–93.
469. Iwasaki T, Okumura J, Muryama M, Saegusa S. Canine familial dermatomyositis in a family of Shetland sheepdogs. 15th Proceedsings of AAVD/ACVD meeting 1999; Maui, Hawaii, 15–16.
470. Iwasaki T, Shimizu M, Obata H, et al. Detection of canine pemphigus foliaceus autoantigen by immunoblotting. Vet Immunology and Immunopathology 1997; 59(1–2):1–10.

J

471. Jackson KF, Kuncan ID. Hypomyelination in dogs. In: Kirk RW, ed. Current veterinary therapy X, Small animal practice. Philadelphia: WB Saunders, 1989: 834–8.
472. Jaenke RS, Allen TA. Membranous nephropathy in the dog. Vet Path 1986; 23(6):718–33.
473. Jaggy A, Bernardini M. Idiopathic epilepsy in 125 dogs—a long-term study. Clinical and electroencephalographic findings. J Sm Anim Pract 1998; 39(1):23–9.
474. Jaggy A, Gaillarrd C, Lang J, Vandevelde M. Hereditary cervical spondylopathy (Wobbler syndrome) in the borzoi dog. J Am Anim Hosp Assoc 1988; 24(4):453–60.
475. Jaggy A, Heynold Y. Idiopathic epilepsy in the dog. Schweizer Archiv für Tierheilkunde 1996; 138(11):523–31.
476. Jaggy A, Vandevelde M. Multisystem neuronal degeneration in cocker spaniels. J Vet Intern Med 1988; 2(3):117–20.
477. Jansen B, Valli VEO, Thorner P, et al. Samoyed hereditary glomerulopathy: serial, clinical and laboratory (urine, serum biochemistry and hematology) studies. Can J Vet Res 1987; 51:387–93.
478. Jenkins CC, DeNovo, RC Jr. Diseases of the stomach. In Morgan RV, ed. Handbook of small animal practice. 3d ed. Philadelphia: WB Saunders 1997: 334–43.
479. Jergens AE. Diseases of the esophagus. In: Morgan RV, ed. Handbook of small animal practice, 3d ed. Philadelphia: WB Saunders, 1997: 323–33.
480. Jezyk RF, Haskins ME, MacKay-Smith WE, Patterson DF. Lethal acrodermatitis in bull terriers. JAVMA 1986; 188(8):833–9.
481. Jian ZJ, Alley MR, Cayzer J, Swinney GR. Lafora's disease in an epileptic basset hound. New Zealand Vet J 1990; 38:75–9.
482. Johnson CA, Armstrong PJ, Hauptman JG. Congenital portosystemic shunts in dogs: 46 cases (1979–1986). JAVMA 1987; 191(11):1478–85.
483. Johnson G. Progress on candidate gene research. Canine Pract 1998; 23(1):11–2.
484. Johnson GF, Sternlieb I, Tweld DC, et al. Inheritance of copper toxicosis in Bedlington terriers. Am J Vet Res 1980; 41:1865–6.
485. Johnson GS, Turrentine MA, Kraus KH. Canine von Willebrand's disease: a heterogeneous group of bleeding disorders. Vet Clin N Am 1988; 18(1):195–229.
486. Johnson JP, McLean RH, Cork LC, Winkelstein JA. Genetic analysis of an inherited deficiency of the third component of complement in Brittany spaniel dogs. Am J Med Genet 1986; 25:557–62.
487. Johnson KH, Sletten K, Hayden DW, et al. AA Amyloidosis in Chinese shar-pei dogs—immunohistochemical and amino acid sequence analyses. Amyloid—International J Exper and Clinical Investig 1995; 2(4):92–9.
488. Johnson KH, Westermark P, Sletten K, Obrien TD. Amyloid proteins and amyloidosis in domestic animals. Amyloid—International J Exper and Clinical Investig 1996; 3(4):270–89.
489. Johnson L. Diseases of the trachea. In: Morgan RV, ed. Handbook of small animal practice. 3d ed. Philadelphia: WB Saunders, 1997: 155–63.
490. Johnston SA. Conservative and medical management of hip dysplasia. Vet Clin N Am, Sm Anim Pract 1992; 22(3):595–606.
491. Johnston SA: Osteochondritis dissecans of the humeral head. Vet Clin N Am, Sm Anim Pract 1998; 28(1):33–49.
492. Johnstone IB, Lotz F. An inherited platelet function defect in Basset hounds. Can Vet J 1979; 20: 211–4.
493. Johnstone IB, Norris AM, Hirzer L. Type II von Willebrand's disease in Scottish terriers—a report of 2 cases. Can Vet J 1993; 34:679–81.

494. Jolly RD, Hartley BR, Jones AC et al. Generalized ceroid lipofuscinosis and brown bowel syndrome in cocker spaniel dogs. New Zealand Vet J 1994; 42(6):236–39.
495. Jolly RD, Palmer DN, Studdert VP, et al. Canine ceroid lipofuscinoses—a review and classification. J Sm Anim Pract 1994; 35(6):299–306.
496. Jolly RD, Sutton, RH, Smith RIE, Palmer, DN. Ceroid lipofuscinosis in miniature schnauzer dogs. Australian Vet J 1997; 75(1):67–9.
497. Jolly RD, Walkley SU. Lysosomal storage diseases of animals—an essay in comparative pathology. Vet Path 1997; 34(6): 527–48.
498. Jonen H, Nickel RF. The persistent Mullerian duct syndrome—a hereditary type of male pseudohermaphroditism in a basset hound. Kleintierpraxis 1996; 41(12):911–12.
499. Joseph SA; Brooks MB, Coccari PJ, Riback SC. Hemophilia A in a German shorthaired pointer—clinical presentations and diagnosis. J Am Anim Hosp Assoc 1996; 32(1):25–8.
500. Jull BA, Merryman JI, Thomas WB, McArthur A. Necrotizing encephalitis in a Yorkshire terrier. JAVMA 1997; 211(8):1005.

K

501. Kakkis ED, McEntee MF, Schmidtchen A, et al. Long-term and high-dose trials of enzyme replacement therapy in the canine model of mucopolysaccharidosis I. Biochem Mol Med 1996; 58(2): 156–67.
502. Kammermann B, Gmur J, Stunzi, H. Afibrinogenemia in the dog. Zentralblatt fur Veterinarmedizin 1971; 18:192–205.
503. Kaneene JB, Mostosky UV, Padgett GA. Retrospective cohort study of changes in hip joint phenotype of dogs in the United States. JAVMA 1997; 211(12):1542–4.
504. Kaswan HI, Martin CI, Dawe, DL. Rheumatoid factor determination in 50 dogs with keratoconjunctivitis sicca. JAVMA 1983; 183:1073–5.
505. Katherman, AE. A comparative review of canine and human narcolepsy. Compend Contin Educ Pract Vet 1980; 2(10):818–20.
506. Katz ML, Siakotos AN. Canine hereditary ceroid lipofuscinosis—evidence for a defect in the carnitine biosynthetic pathway. Am J Med Genetics 1995; 57(2):266–71.
507. Kawakami E, Yamada Y, Tsutsui T, et al. Changes in plasma androgen levels and testicular histology with descent of the testis in the dog. J Vet Med Sci 1993; 55(6):931–5.
508. Kay MA, Rothenberg S, Landen CN, et al. In vivo gene therapy of hemophilia B. Sustained partial correction in factor IX deficient dogs. Science 1993; 262(5130):117–9.
509. Kaye EM, Alroy J, Raghavan SS, et al. Dysmyelinogenesis in animal model of GM1 gangliosidosis. Pediat Neurol 1992; 8:255–61.
510. Kealy RD, Lawler DF, Ballam JM, et al. 5-year longitudinal study on limited food consumption and development of osteoarthritis in coxofemoral joints of dogs. JAVMA 1997; 210(2):222–7.
511. Kealy RD, Lawler DF, Monti KL, et al. Effects of dietary electrolyte balance on subluxation of the femoral head in growing dogs. Am J Vet Res 1993; 54(4):555–62.
512. Kealy RD, Olsson S, Monti KL, et al. Effects of limited food consumption on the incidence of hip dysplasia in growing dogs. JAVMA 1992; 201(6):857–63.
513. Keene BW, Kittleson MD, Rush JE. Myocardial carnitine deficiency associated with dilated cardiomyopathy in Doberman pinschers. J Vet Intern Med 1989; 3(2):126.
514. Keene BW, Panciera DP, Atkins, CE, et al. Myocardial L-carnitine deficiency in a family of dogs with dilated cardiomyopathy. JAVMA 1991; 198:647–50.
515. Kelch WJ, Smith CA, Lynn RC, New JC. Canine hypoadrenocorticism (Addison's Disease). Compend Contin Educ Pract Vet 1998; 20(8): 921–9.
516. Kellner SJ. Mesodermal goniodysplasia in the Siberian husky. Kleintierpraxis 1996; 41:19–26.
517. Kelly MJ. Myasthenia gravis—a receptor disease. Compend Contin Educ Pract Vet 1981; 3(6):544–53.
518. Kemppainen RJ, Clark TP. Etiopathogenesis of canine hypothyroidism. Vet Clin N Am 1994; 24(3):467–76.
519. Kerlin RL, van Winkle TJ. Renal dysplasia in golden retrievers. Vet Path 1995; 32:327–9.
520. Kern TJ. Disorders of the lacrimal system. In: Current veterinary therapy IX. Philadelphia: WB Saunders, 1986:634–41.
521. Kern TJ. Disorders of the lacrimal and nasolacrimal system. In: Morgan RV, ed. Handbook of Sm Anim Pract. 2d ed. Churchill-Livingstone, New York: 1992: 1053–61.
522. Kertesz P. A colour atlas of veterinary dentistry and oral surgery. Aylesbury, England: Wolfe Publishing, 1993; 312 p.
523. Kienle RD, Thomas WP, Pion PD. The natural clinical history of canine congenital subaortic stenosis. J Vet Intern Med 1994; 8:423–31.
524. Kimura T, Ohshima S, Doi K. The inheritance and breeding results of hairless descendants of Mexican hairless dogs. Lab Anim 1993; 27:55–8.
525. Kintzer PP, Peterson ME. Treatment and long-term follow-up of 205 dogs with hypoadrenocorticism. J Vet Intern Med 1997; 1192:43–9.
526. Kirberger RM, Lobetti RG. Radiographic aspects of *Pneumocystis carinii* pneumonia in the miniature Dachshund. Vet Radiol & Ultrasound 1998; 39(4): 313–7.
527. Kirschner SE. Diseases of the cornea and sclera. In: Morgan RV, ed. Handbook of small animal practice. 3d ed. Philadelphia: WB Saunders, 1997: 1007–19.
528. Kishnani PS, Bao Y, Wu JY, et al. Isolation and nucleotide sequence of canine glucose-6-phosphatase mRNA—identification of mutation in puppies with glycogen storage disease type Ia. Biochemical & Molecular Med 1997; 61:168–77.
529. Kittleson MD, Keene B, Pion PD, Loyer CG, et al. Results of the multicenter spaniel trial (Must)—taurine-responsive and carnitine-responsive dilated cardiomyopathy in American cocker spaniels with decreased plasma taurine concentration. J Vet Intern Med 1997; 11(4):204–11.
530. Knoll JS. Disorders of white blood cells. In: Morgan RV, ed. Handbook of small animal practice. 3d ed. Philadelphia: WB Saunders, 1997:673–89.
531. Knottenbelt CM, Knottenbelt MK. Black hair follicular dysplasia in a tricolor Jack Russell terrier. Vet Rec 1996; 138(19):475–6.
532. Knowler C, Giger U, Dodds WJ, Brooks M. Factor XI deficiency in Kerry blue terriers. JAVMA 1994; 205:1557–61.
533. Knowles K. Deafness. In: Morgan RV, ed. Handbook of small animal practice. Philadelphia: WB Saunders, 1997: pp. 1104–1108.
534. Knowles K, Alroy J, Castagnaro M, et al. Adult-onset lysosomal storage disease in a schipperke dog: clinical, morphological and biochemical studies. Acta Neuropathol (Berl) 1993; 86:306–12.
535. Kocabatmaz M, Keskin E, Durgun Z, Eryavuz A. Effect of garlic oil on plasma, erythrocyte and erythrocye membrane total lipids, cholesterol and phospholipid levels of hypercholesterolaemic dogs. Med Sci Res 1997; 25:265–7.
536. Koch SA. Cataracts in interrelated Old English sheepdogs. JAVMA 1972; 160:299–301.
537. Kociba GJ. Von Willebrand's disease. In: Tilley L and Smith F, eds. The 5 minute veterinary consult. Baltimore: Williams & Wilkins, 1997: 1158–9.
538. Koeman JP, Biewenga WJ, Gruys E. Proteinuria associated with glomerulosclerosis and glomerular collagen formation in three Newfoundland dog littermates. Vet Path 1994; 31: 188–93.
539. Kolb E, Nestler K, Piechotta D. Studies of copper metabolism in dogs—the development, treatment and prevention of copper storage disease in Bedlington and other terriers. Tierarztliche Umschau 1991; 46:93–7.
540. Komaromy AM, Smith PJ, Brooks DE. Electroretinography in dogs and cats. Part II. Technique, interpretation, and indications. Compend Contin Educ Pract Vet 1998; 20(3):355–63.
541. Kommonen B, Kylma T, Karhunen U, et al. Impaired retinal function in young Labrador retriever dogs heterozygous for late-onset rod-cone degeneration. Vision Research 1997; 37:365–70.

542. Kooistra HS, Voorhout G, Selman PJ, Rijnberk A. Progestin-induced growth-hormone (GH) production in the treatment of dogs with congenital GH deficiency. Domestic Animal Endocrinology 1998; 15(2):93–102.
543. Kornegay JE. Golden retriever myopathy. In: Kirk RW, ed. Current veterinary therapy IX, Small animal practice. Philadelphia: WB Saunders, 1986:792–4.
544. Kornegay JE. The X-linked muscular dystrophies. In: Kirk's current veterinary therapy XI, Small animal practice. Philadelphia: WB Saunders, 1992: 1042–47.
545. Kornegay JN. Cerebellar vermian hypoplasia in dogs. Vet Path 1986; 23(4):374–9.
546. Kornegay JN. The nervous system. In: Hoskins JD, ed. Veterinary Pediatrics. Philadelphia: WB Saunders, 1995, 451–95.
547. Kortz G. Canine myotonia. Sem Vet Med Surg 1989; 4(2):141–6.
548. Krahwinkel DJ Jr. Diseases of the anus and perineum. In: Morgan RV, ed. Handbook of small animal practice, 3d ed. Philadelphia: WB Saunders, 1997: 417–24.
549. Kramer JW, Klaasen JK, Baskin DG, et al. Inheritance of diabetes mellitus in keeshond dogs. Am J Vet Res 1988; 49:428–31.
550. Kramer JW, Schiffer WP, Sande RD, et al. Characterization of heritable thoracic hemivertebra of the German shorthaired pointer. JAVMA 1982; 15:814–5.
551. Kruger JM, Osborne CA, Lulich JP, et al. The urinary system. In: Hoskins JD, ed. Veterinary pediatrics. Philadelphia: WB Saunders, 1995:399–426.
552. Kunkle GA. A problem-oriented approach to canine pediatric dermatology. Compend Contin Educ Pract Vet 1985; 7(5):377–86.
553. Kunkle GA. Canine dermatomyositis: a disease with an infectious origin. Compend Contin Educ Pract Vet 1992; 7(5):377–86.
554. Kunkle GA. Congenital hypotrichosis in two dogs. JAVMA 1984; 185:84–5.
555. Kunkle GA, Jezyk PF, West CS, et al. Tyrosinemia in a dog. J Am Anim Hosp Assoc 1984; 20(4):615–20.
556. Kunz E, Rensing H. Castration-responsive alopecia in a male Samoyed. Kleintierpraxis 1997; 42(11):921–4.9]
557. Kural E, Lindley D, Drohne S. Canine glaucoma: clinical signs and diagnosis. In: Glaze MB, ed. Ophthalmology in small animal practice. Trenton, NJ: Veterinary Learning Systems, 1996: 38–44.
558. Kural E, Lindley D, Drohne S. Canine glaucoma. 1. Compend Contin Educ Pract Vet 1995; 17(8):1017–26.
559. Kural E, Lindley D, Drohne S. Canine glaucoma. 2. Compend Contin Educ Pract Vet 1995; 17(10):1253–62.
560. Kvart C, French AT, Fuentes VL, et al. Analysis of murmur intensity, duration and frequency components in dogs with aortic stenosis. J Sm Anim Pract 1998; 39(7): 318–24.
561. Kwochka KW, Rademakers AM. Cell proliferation kinetics of epidermis, hair follicles, and sebaceous glands of cocker spaniels with idiopathic seborrhea. Am J Vet Res 1989; 50(11):1918–22.

L

562. Ladds PW. Lethal congenital edema in bulldog pups. JAVMA 1971, 159: 881–6.
563. Lafond E, Smith GK, Gregor TP, et al. Synovial fluid cavitation during distraction radiography of the coxofemoral joint in dogs. JAVMA 1997; 210(9):1294–7.
564. Landsberg G, Hunthausen W, Ackerman L. Handbook of behaviour problems in the dog and cat. Oxford, England: Butterworth-Heinemann, 1997. 211 p.
565. Lang J, Busato A, Baumgartner D, et al. Comparison of 2 classification protocols in the evaluation of elbow dysplasia in the dog. J Sm Anim Pract 1998; 39(4):169–74.
566. Latimer KS, Kircher IM, Lindl PA, et al. Leukocyte function in Pelger-Huet anomaly of dogs. J Leukocyte Biol 1989; 45:301–10.
567. Lavach JD, Gelatt KN. Disease of the eyelids (Part II). In: Glaze MB, ed. Ophthalmology in small animal practice. Trenton, NJ: Veterinary Learning Systems, 1996:192–200.
568. Lawler DF, Keltner DG, Hoffman WE, et al. Benign familial hyperphosphatasemia in Siberian huskies. Am J Vet Res 1996; 57(5):612–7.
569. Lees GE. Canine hereditary nephritis—an update. Proc 15th ACVIM Forum, Lake Buena Vista, FL, 1997, 331–3.
570. Lees GE. Congenital renal diseases. Vet Clin N Am, Sm Anim Pract 1996; 26(6):1379–99.
571. Lees GE. Congenital renal disease in dogs and cats. Proc 16th ACVIM Forum, San Diego, 1998, 20–1.
572. Lees GE, Helman RG, Homco LD, et al. Early diagnosis of familial nephropathy in English cocker spaniels. J Am Anim Hosp Assoc 1998; 34(3):189–95.
573. Lees GE, Helman RG, Kashtan CE, et al. A model of autosomal recessive Alport syndrome in English cocker spaniel dogs. Kidney Internat 1998; 54(3): 706–19.
574. Lees GE, Wilson PD, Helman RG, et al. Glomerular ultrastructural findings similar to hereditary nephritis in 4 English cocker spaniels. J Vet Intern Med 1997; 11(2):80–5.
575. Lehmkuhl LB, Bonagura JD. Canine subvalvular aortic stenosis. In: Kirk's current veterinary therapy XII, Small animal practice. Philadelphia: WB Saunders, 1995: 822–27.
576. Lehmkuhl LB, Bonagura JD. Congenital diseases. In: Morgan RV, ed. Handbook of small animal practice. 3d ed. Philadelphia: WB Saunders, 1997:53–62.
577. Leib MS, Blass CE. Gastric dilatation-volvulus in dogs: an update. Compend Contin Educ Pract Vet 1984; 6(11):961–9.
578. Leighton EA. Genetics of canine hip dysplasia. JAVMA 1997; 210(10):1474–9.
579. Leighton RL, Suter PF. Primary lymphedema of the hindlimb in the dog. JAVMA, 1979; 175(4):369–74.
580. Lemarie SL. Canine demodicosis. Compend Contin Educ Pract Vet 1996; 18(4):353–63.
581. Lemarie SL, Horohov DW. Evaluation of interleukin–2 production and interleukin–2 receptor expression in dogs with generalized demodicosis. Vet Derm 1996; 7(4):213–9.
582. Lemarie SL, Hosgood G, Foil CS. A retrospective study of juvenile-onset and adult-onset generalized demodicosis in dogs (1986–91). Vet Derm 1996; 7(1):3–10.
583. Lemonick M. A terrible beauty: an obsessive focus on showring looks is crippling, sometimes fatally, America's purebred dogs. TIME 1994:144(24):60–64.
584. Leon A, Curtis R, Barnett KC. Hereditary persistent hyperplastic primary vitreous in the Staffordshire bull terrier. J Am Anim Hosp Assoc 1986; 22(6):765–74.
585. Leveille-Webster CR. Diseases of the hepatobiliary system. In: Morgan RV, ed. Handbook of small animal practice. 3d ed. Philadelphia: WB Saunders, 1997:383–401.
586. Leveque NW. Canine genome mapping: a dogged pursuit. Am J Vet Res 1997; 58:936–937.
587. Lewis DD, McCarthy RJ, Pechman RD. Diagnosis of common developmental orthopedic conditions in canine pediatric patients. Compend Contin Educ Pract Vet 1992; 14(3):287–301.
588. Lewis DD, Parker RB, Hager DA. Fragmented medial coronoid process of the canine elbow. Compend Contin Educ Pract Vet 1989; 11(6):703–34.
589. Lewis DD, Shelton GD, Piras A, et al. Gracilis or semitendinosus myopathy in 18 dogs. J Am Anim Hosp Assoc 1997; 33:177–88.
590. Lewis DG, Kelly DF, Sansom KJ. Congenital microphthalmia and other developmental ocular anomalies in the Doberman. J Sm Anim Pract 1986; 27(9):559–66.
591. Lewis DT, Ford MJ, Kwochka KW. Characterization and management of a Jack Russell terrier with congenital ichthyosis. Vet Derm 1998; 9(2):111–8.
592. Lewis DT, Messinger LM, Ginn PE, Ford MJ. A hereditary disorder of cornification and multiple congenital defects in five rottweiler dogs. Vet Derm 1998; 9:61–72.
593. Lewis RM. Immune-mediated muscle disease. Vet Clin N Am, Sm Anim Pract 1994; 24(4):703–10.

594. Lifton SJ, King LG, Zerbe CA. Glucocorticoid-deficient hypoadrenocorticism in dogs—18 cases (1986–1995). JAVMA 1996; 209(12):2076–81.
595. Lightfoot RM, Cabral L, Gooch L, et al. Retinal pigment epithelial dystrophy in briard dogs. Res Vet Sci 1996; 60:17–23.
596. Lincoln JD. Cervical vertebral malformation/malarticulation syndrome in large dogs. Vet Clin N Am 1992; 22(4):923–35.
597. Lindley DM. Diseases of the eyelids. In: Morgan RV, ed. Handbook of small animal Practice. 3d ed. Philadelphia: WB Saunders, 1997:973–85.
598. Ling GV, Case LC, Nelson H, et al. Pharmacokinetics of allopurinol in Dalmatian dogs. J Vet Pharmacol and Therapeutics 1997; 20(2):134–8.
599. Ling GV, Franti CE, Ruby AL, et al. Urolithiasis in dogs I. Mineral prevalence and interrelations of mineral composition, age, and sex. Am J Vet Res 1998; 59(5): 624–9.
600. Ling GV, Franti CE, Ruby AL, Johnson DL. Urolithiasis in dogs II. Breed prevalence, and interrelations of breed, sex, age, and mineral composition. Am J Vet Res 1998; 59(5): 630–42.
601. Ling GV, Sorenson JL. Management and prevention of urate urolithiasis. In: Kirk's current veterinary therapy XII, Small animal practice. Philadelphia: WB Saunders, 1995: 985–9.
602. Lingaas F, Aarskaug T, Sletten M, et al. Genetic markers linked to neuronal ceroid lipofuscinosis in English setter dogs. Anim Genet 1998; 29(5): 371–6.
603. Lingvaas F, Sorensen A, Juneja RK, et al. Toward construction of a canine linkage map—establishment of 16 linkage groups. Mammalian Genome 1997; 8:218–21.
604. Lipsitz D. Hypomyelination in the Weimaraner and chow chow. Proc 16th ACVIM Forum, San Diego, 1998, 323–4.
605. Littman MP, Giger U. Familial protein-losing enteropathy (PLE) and/or protein-losing nephropathy (PLN) in soft-coated wheaten terriers (SCWT). J Vet Intern Med 1990; 4:133.
606. Liu PC, Chen YW, Shibuya H, et al. A length polymorphism in an intron of the canine polycystic kidney disease 1 Gene. Anim Genet 1998; 29(4): 322–3.
607. Liu S-K, Dorfman HD. A condition resembling human localized myositis ossificans in two dogs. J Sm Anim Pract 1976; 17:371–7.
608. Lobetti RG, Leisewitz AL, Spencer JA. *Pneumocystis carinii* in the miniature dachshund —case report and literature review. J Sm Anim Pract 1996; 37(6):280–5.
609. Lohmann B, Klesen S. Cataract and microphthalmia in a litter of Russian terriers. Praktische Tierarzt 1997; 78(11):981–3.
610. Lorenz MD, Cork LC, Griffin JW, et al. Hereditary spinal muscular atrophy in Brittany spaniels: clinical manifestations. JAVMA 1979; 175:833–9.
611. Lothrop CD Jr. Pathophysiology of canine growth hormone-responsive alopecia. Compend Contin Educ Pract Vet 1988; 10(12):1346–49.
612. Luescher AU. Compulsive behaviour in dogs. Vet Internat 1998; 10(2): 7–14.
613. Lulich JP, Osborne CA. Diseases of the urinary bladder. In: Morgan RV, ed. Handbook of small animal practice. 3d ed. Philadelphia: WB Saunders, 1997:531–43.
614. Lulich JP, Osborne CA, Parker ML, et al. Canine calcium oxalate urolithiasis. Detection, treatment, and prevention. In: Kirk RW, ed. Current veterinary therapy X, Small animal practice. Philadelphia: WB Saunders, 1989, 1182–8.
615. Lulich JP, Osborne CA, Polzin DJ. Diagnosis and long-term management of protein-losing glomerulonephropathy. Vet Clin N Am, Sm Anim Pract, 1996; 26(6):1401–16.
616. Lulich JP, Osborne CA, Smith CL. Canine calcium oxalate urolithiasis: risk factor management. In: Current veterinary therapy XI, Small animal practice. Philadelphia: WB Saunders, 1992:892–99.
617. Lulich JP, Osborne CA, Unger LK, et al. Prevalence of calcium oxalate uroliths in miniature schnauzers. Am J Vet Res 1991; 52:1579–82.
618. Lust G. An overview of the pathogenesis of canine hip dysplasia. JAVMA 1997; 210(10):1443–5.
619. Luttgen, PJ. Deafness in the dog and cat. Vet Clin N Am, Sm Anim Pract 1994; 24(5):981–9.
620. Lyon K. Personal communication, 1998.
621. Lyon K, Ackerman L. Dog owner's guide to proper dental care. Neptune City, NJ: TFH Publications, 1993. 33 p.

M

622. Machino H, Miki Y, Kawatsu T, et al. Successful dietary control of tyrosinemia II. J Am Acad Derm 1983; 9:533–9.
623. MacLachlan NJ, Breitschwerdt EB, Chambers JM, et al. Gastroenteritis of basenji dogs. Vet Path 1988; 25(1):36–41.
624. Maggio-Price L, Emerson CL, Hinds T, et al. Hereditary nonspherocytic hemolytic anemia in beagles. JAVMA 1988; 49(7):1020–25.
625. Magne ML. Selective IgA deficiency in German shepherd dogs. J Vet Allerg Clin Immunol 1996; 4(1):23–4.
626. Mahony OH, Knowles KE, Braund KG, et al. Laryngeal paralysis-polyneuropathy complex in young Rottweilers. J Vet Intern Med 1998; 12(5): 330–7.
627. Malik R, Church DB. Congenital mitral insufficiency in bull terriers. J Sm Anim Pract 1988; 29(8):549–57.
628. Mandara MT, DiMeo A. Lower motor neuron disease in the Griffon Briquet Vendeen dog. Vet Path 1998; 35(5):412–414,
629. Mandigers PJJ, Vannes JJ, Knol BW et al. Hereditary necrotizing myelopathy in Kooiker dogs. Res Vet Sci 1993; 54(1):118–23.
630. Mann GE, Stratton J. Dermoid sinus in the Rhodesian ridgeback. J Sm Anim Pract 1966; 7:631–42.
631. Manners HK, Hart CA, Getty B, et al. Characterization of intestinal morphologic, biochemical, and ultrastructural features in gluten-sensitive Irish setters during controlled oral gluten challenge exposure after weaning. Am J Vet Res 1998; 59(11): 1435–40.
632. Marcellin-Little DJ, DeYoung DJ, Ferris KK, et al. Incomplete ossification of the humeral condyle in spaniels. Vet Surg 1995; 23: 475–87.
633. March PA. Degenerative brain disease. Vet Clin N Am, Sm Anim Pract 1996; 26(4): 945–71.
634. March PA, Wurzelmann S, Walkley SU. Morphological alterations in neocortical and cerebellar GABAergic neurons in a canine model of juvenile Batten disease. Am J Med Genetics 1995; 57(2): 204–12.
635. Marks A, Vandenbroek AHM, Else RW. Congenital hypotrichosis in a French bulldog. J Sm Anim Pract 1992; 33:450–52.
636. Marks SL, Farman CA, Peaston A. Nodular dermatofibrosis and renal cystadenomas in a golden retriever. Vet Derm 1993; 4(3):133–7.
637. Marmor M, Willeberg P, Glickman LT, et al. Epizootiologic patterns of diabetes mellitus in dogs. Am J Vet Res 1982; 43:465–70.
638. Martin RA. Congenital portosystemic shunts in the dog and cat. Vet Clin N Am, Sm Anim Pract 1993; 23(3):609–623.
639. Marx J. Genetic diseases. A lst step toward gene therapy for hemophilia B. Science 1993; 262(5130):29–30.
640. Mason KV, Halliwell RE, McDougal BJ. Characterization of lichenoid-psoriasiform dermatosis of springer spaniels. JAVMA 1986; 189(8): 897–901.
641. Mason LT. The occurrence and pedigree analysis of a hereditary sensory neuropathy in the English Springer Spaniel. 15th Proceedings of AAVD/AACVD meeting 1999; Maui Hawaii, 23–24.
642. Mason NJ, Day MJ. Renal amyloidosis in related English foxhounds. J Sm Anim Pract 1996; 37(6):255–60.
643. Mathet JL, Bensignor E, Segault P. Canine demodicosis. A review. Recueil de Medecine Veterinaire 1996; 172(3–4): 149–65.
644. Mathews KA, Ayres SA, Tano CA, et al. Cyclosporine treatment of perianal fistulas in dogs. Can Vet J 1997; 38(1):39–41, 1997.
645. Matic SE. Congenital heart disease in the dog. J Sm Anim Pract 1988; 29(12):743–59.
646. Matthews KA, Sukhiani HR. Randomized controlled trial of cyclosporine for treatment of perianal fistulas in dogs. JAVMA 1997; 211(10):1249–53.
647. Mattson A. Pharyngeal disorders. Vet Clin N Am, Sm Anim Pract 1994; 24(5):825–54.

648. Matushek KJ, Rosin E. Perianal fistulas in dogs. Compend Contin Educ Pract Vet 1991; 13(4):621–7.
649. Mauldin EA, Scott DW, Miller WH Jr., Smith CA. Malassezia dermatitis in the dog: a retrospective histopathological and immunopathological study of 86 cases (1990–95). Vet Derm 1997; 8:191–202.
650. Mauser AE, Whitlark J, Whitney KM, et al. A deletion mutation causes hemophilia B in Lhasa apso dogs. Blood 1996; 88:3451–5.
651. McAloose D, Casal M, Patterson DF, Dambach DM. Polycystic kidney and liver disease in 2 related West Highland white terrier litters. Vet Path 1998; 35(1):77–81.
652. McCutcheon LJ, Cory CR, Nowack L, et al. Respiratory chain defect of myocardial mitochondria in idiopathic dilated cardiomyopathy of Doberman pinscher dogs. Can J Physiol Pharmacol 1992; 70:1529–33.
653. McDermott MF, Aksentijevich I, Galon J, et al. Germline mutations in the extracellular domains of the 55 kDa TNF Receptor, TNFR1, define a family of dominantly inherited autoinflammatory syndromes. Cell 1999; 97:133–144.
654. McEwan NA, Macartney L. Fanconi's syndrome in a Yorkshire terrier. J Sm Anim Pract 1987; 28(8):737–42.
655. McKeever PJ, Torres SMF, O'Brien TD. Spiculosis. J Am Anim Hosp Assoc 1992; 28(3):257–62.
656. McKerrell RE, Braund KG. Hereditary myopathy of Labrador retrievers. In: Kirk RW, ed. Current veterinary therapy X, Small animal practice. Philadelphia: WB Saunders, Philadelphia, 1989:820–2.
657. McKerrell RE, Braund KG. Hereditary myopathy in Labrador retrievers: clinical variations. J Sm Anim Pract 1987; 28(6):479–89.
658. McKiernan BC. Diseases of the nasal and nasopharyngeal cavities and paranasal sinuses. In: Morgan RV, ed. Handbook of small animal practice. 3d ed. Philadelphia: WB Saunders, 1997:138–47.
659. McLaughlin R Jr, Tomlinson J. Alternative surgical treatments for canine hip dysplasia. Vet Med 1996; 91(2):137–43.
660. McLaughlin R Jr, Tomlinson J. Radiographic diagnosis of canine hip dysplasia. Vet Med 1996; 91(1):36–47.
661. McLaughlin R Jr,Tomlinson, J. Treating canine hip dysplasia with triple pelvic osteotomy. Vet Med 1996; 91(2):126–36.
662. Mehta JR, Braund KG, McKerrel RE, Toivio-Kinnucan M. Analysis of muscle elements, water, and total lipids from healthy dogs and Labrador retrievers with hereditary muscular dystrophy. Am J Vet Res 1989; 50(5):640–4.
663. Mehta JR, Braund KG, McKerrel RE, Toivio-Kinnucan M. Isolectric focusing under dissociating conditions for analysis of muscle protein from clinically normal dogs and Labrador retrievers with hereditary muscular dystrophy. Am J Vet Res 1989; 50(5):633–9.
664. Melian C, Peterson ME. Diagnosis and treatment of naturally-occurring hypoadrenocorticism in 42 dogs. J Sm Anim Pract 1996; 37(6): 268–75.
665. Mellersh CS, Langston AA, Acland GM, et al. A linkage map of the canine genome. Genomics 1997; 46:326–36.
666. Mellersh CS, Ostrander EA. The canine genome. Molecular Genetics, Gene Transfer, and Therapy, 1997; 40:191–216.
667. Melniczek J, Dambach D, Prociuk U, et al. Sry-Negative XX sex reversal in Norwegian elkhounds. Canine Pract 1998; 23(1):50–1.
668. Menon KP, Tieu PT, Neufeld EF. Architecture of the canine IDUA gene and mutation underlying canine mucopolysaccharidosis I. Genomics 1992; 14:763–8.
669. Meric SM. Breed-specific meningitis in dogs. In: Current veterinary therapy XI, Small animal practice. Philadelphia: WB Saunders, 1992: 1007–9.
670. Meric SM, Child G, Higgins, RJ. Necrotizing vasculitis of the spinal pachyleptomeningeal arteries in three Bernese mountain dog littermates. J Am Anim Hosp Assoc 1986; 22(4):459–65.
671. Mertens PA, Dodman NH. Drug treatment for acral lick dermatitis. Kleintierpraxis 1996; 41(5):327–31.
672. Merton DA. Selective breeding in the dog and cat. Part I. Fundamentals of inheritance and planned breeding. Compend Contin Educ Pract Vet 1982; 4(3):251–7.
673. Merton DA. Selective breeding in the dog and cat. Part II. Known and suspected genetic diseases. Compend Contin Educ Pract Vet 1982; 4(4):332–56.
674. Meurs KM. Myocardial disease. In: Morgan RV, ed. Handbook of small animal practice. 3d ed. Philadelphia: WB Saunders, 1997:103–12.
675. Meurs KM, Brown WA. Update on boxer cardiomyopathy. Proc 16th ACVIM Forum, San Diego, 1998, 119–20.
676. Meurs KR. Insights into the hereditability of canine cardiomyopathy. Vet Clin N Am, Sm Anim Pract 1998; 28(6): 1449–57.
677. Meyer DJ, Harvey JW. Veterinary laboratory medicine: interpretation & diagnosis. Philadelphia: WB Saunders, 1998. 373 p.
678. Meyer HP, Rothuizen, J, Ubbink GJ, Vandeningh TS. GAM: Increasing incidence of hereditary intrahepatic portosystemic shunts in Irish wolfhounds in the Netherlands (1984–1992). Vet Rec 1995; 136:13–16.
679. Meyers KM, Wardrop KJ, Meinkoth J. Canine von Willebrand's disease: pathobiology, diagnosis, and short-term treatment. Compend Contin Educ Pract Vet 1992; 14(1):13–22.
680. Meyers VN, Jezyk PF, Aguirre GD, Patterson DF. Short-limbed dwarfism and ocular defects in the Samoyed dog. JAVMA 1983; 183(9):975–9.
681. Meyers-Wallen VN. Genetics of sexual differentiation and anomalies in dogs and cats. J Reprod and Fertil 1993; 47(Suppl):441–52.
682. Meyers-Wallen VN, Bowman L, Acland GM, et al. Sry-negative XX sex reversal in the German shorthaired pointer dog. J Hered 1995; 86(5):369–74.
683. Meyers-Wallen VN, Lee MM, Manganaro TF, et al. Mullerian-inhibiting substance is present in embryonic testes of dogs with persistent Mullerian duct syndrome. Biol of Reprod 1993; 48(6):1410–18.
684. Meyers-Wallen VN, Palmer VL, Acland GM, Hershfield B. Sry-negative XX sex reversal in the American cocker spaniel dog. Molecular reproduction and development, 1995 41(3):300–5.
685. Meyers-Wallen VN, Patterson DF. Disorders of sexual development in dogs and cats. In: Kirk RW, ed. Current veterinary therapy X, Small animal practice. Philadelphia: WB Saunders, 1989: 1261–9.
686. Mignot E, Bell RA, Rattazzi C, et al. An immunoglobulin switchlike sequence is linked with canine narcolepsy. Sleep 1994; 17(8):S68–S76.
687. Mignot E, Nishino S, Sharp LH, et al. Heterozygosity at the canarc–1 locus can confer susceptibility for narcolepsy—induction of cataplexy in heterozygous asymptomatic dogs after administration of a combination of drugs acting on monoaminergic and cholinergic systems. J Neuroscience 1993; 13:1057–64.
688. Miller LM, Lennon VA, Lambert EH, Reed SM, et al. Congenital myasthenia gravis in 13 smooth fox terriers. JAVMA 1983; 182(7):694–7.
689. Miller MA, Dunstan RW. Seasonal flank alopecia in boxers and Airedale terriers: 24 cases (1985–1992). JAVMA, 1993; 203(11):1567–72.
690. Miller MW. Cardiomyopathy, dilated—dogs. In: Tilley LP and Smith FWK Jr., eds. The five minute veterinary consult. Baltimore: Williams & Wilkins, 1997:418–19.
691. Miller MW, Bonagura JD. Congenital heart disease. In: Kirk RW, ed. Current veterinary therapy X, Small animal practice. Philadelphia: WB Saunders, 1989: 224–31.
692. Miller PE. Glaucoma. In: Current veterinary therapy XII, small animal practice. Philadelphia: WB Saunders, 1995:1265–72.
693. Miller PE, Stanz KM, Dubielzig RR, Murphy CJ. Mechanisms of acute intraocular pressure increases after phacoemulsification lens extraction in dogs. Am J Vet Res 1997; 58(10):1159–65.
694. Miller WH Jr. Alopecia associated with coat color dilution in two Yorkshire terriers, one saluki, and one mix-breed dog. J Am Anim Hosp Assoc 1991; 27(1):39–43.
695. Miller WH Jr. Colour dilution alopecia in Doberman pinschers with blue or fawn coat colours: a study on incidence and histopathology of this disorder. Vet Derm 1990; 1:113–22.

696. Miller WH Jr. Epidermal dysplastic disorders of dogs and cats. In: Kirk's current veterinary therapy XII, Small animal practice. Philadelphia: WB Saunders, 1995: 597–600.
697. Miller WH Jr, Scott DW. Follicular dysplasia of the Portuguese water dog. Vet Derm 1995; 6(2):67–74.
698. Miller WH Jr, Scott DW, Cayatte SM, et al. Clinical efficacy of increased dosages of milbemycin oxime for treatment of generalized demodicosis in adult dogs. JAVMA 1995; 207(12):1581–1584.
699. Miller WH Jr, Wellington JR, Scott DW. Dermatologic disorders of Chinese shar peis: 58 cases (1981–1989). JAVMA 1992; 200(7):986–90.
700. Miller WW, Albert RA. Canine entropion. Compend Contin Educ Pract Vet 1988; 10(4):431–8.
701. Millichamp NJ. Retinal dysplasia in the dog. Calif Vet 1985; 39:10–12, 49.
702. Millichamp NJ, Curtis R, Barnett KC. Progressive retinal atrophy in Tibetan terriers. JAVMA 1988; 192(6):769–76.
703. Mills JN, Labuc RH, Lawley MJ. Factor VII deficiency in an Alaskan malamute. Australian Vet J 1997; 75(5):320–22.
704. Milne KL, Hayes HM. Epidemiologic features of canine hypothyroidism. Cornell Vet 1981; 71:3–11.
705. Minor RR, Lein DH, Patterson DF et al. Defects in collagen fibrillogenesis causing hyperextensible, fragile skin in dogs. JAVMA 1983; 182(2):142–8.
706. Mischke R. Ramirez PAR, Deniz A, et al. Hemophilia A in the dog—symptoms, blood coagulation analysis and therapy. Berliner und Munchener Tierarztliche Wochenschrift 1996; 109(8):279–87. [Sib, GSD]
707. Miyamoto T, Wakizaka S, Matsuyama, et al. A control of a golden retriever with renal dysplasia. J Vet Med Sci 1997; 59(10):939–42.
708. Modiano JF, Helfand SC. Diseases of the thymus. In: Morgan RV, ed. Handbook of small animal medicine. 3d ed. Philadelphia: WB Saunders, 1997:805–7.
709. Moe L. Hereditary polyneuropathy of Alaskan malamutes. In: Kirk's current veterinary therapy XI, Small animal practice. Philadelphia: WB Saunders, 1992: 1038–39.
710. Moe L, Lium B. Computed tomography of hereditary multifocal renal cystadenocarcinomas in German shepherd dogs. Vet Radiol & Ultrasound 1997; 38(5):335–43.
711. Moe L, Lium B. Hereditary multifocal renal cystadenocarcinomas and nodular dermatofibrosis in 51 German shepherd dogs. J Sm Anim Pract 1997; 38(11):498–505.
712. Moise NS. Tricuspid valve dysplasia in the dog. In: Kirk's current veterinary therapy XII, Small animal practice. Philadelphia: WB Saunders, 1995:813–16.
713. Moise NS, Gilmour RF, Riccio ML, Flahive WF. Diagnosis of inherited ventricular tachycardia in German shepherd dogs. JAVMA 1997; 210(3): 403–410.
714. Moise NS, Gilmour RF Jr. Inherited sudden cardiac death in German shepherds. In: Current veterinary therapy XI, Small animal practice. Philadelphia: WB Saunders, 1992: 749–51.
715. Monahan PE, Samulski RJ, Tazelaar J et al. Direct intramuscular injection with recombinant aav vectors results in sustained expression in a dog model of hemophilia. Gene Therapy 1998; 5:40–9.
716. Monestierm J, Novick KE, Daram ET, et al. Autoantibodies to histone, DNA and nucleosome antigens in canine systemic lupus erythematosus. Clin Exp Immunol 1995; 99:37–41.
717. Monnet E, Orton EC, Gaynor JS, et al. Open resection for subvalvular aortic stenosis in dogs. JAVMA 1996; 209:1255–61.
718. Montgomery R. Canine hip dysplasia. Compend Contin Educ Pract Vet 1998; 20(7): 781–91.
719. Montgomery RD, Hathcock JT, Milton JL, et al. Osteochondrosis dissecans of the canine tarsal joint. Compend Contin Educ Pract Vet 1994; 16:835–44.
720. Montgomery RD, Milton, JL, Henderson RA, Hathcock JT. Osteochondritis dissecans of the canine stifle. Compend Contin Educ Pract Vet 1989; 11(10):1199–205.
721. Moon-Fanelli AA, Dodman NH. Description and development of compulsive tail chasing in terriers and response to clomipramine treatment. JAVMA 1998; 212(8):1252–7.
722. Moore CP. Disorders of the conjunctiva and third eyelid. In: Morgan RV, ed. Handbook of small animal practice. 3d ed. Philadelphia: WB Saunders, 1997:986–97.
723. Moore CP, Constantinescu GM. Surgery of the adnexa. Vet Clin N Am, Sm Anim Pract 1997; 27(5):1011–22.
724. Moore CP, Whitley RD. Visual disturbance in the dog. Part II. Diseases of the retina and optic papilla. In: Glaze MB, ed. Ophthalmology in small animal practice. Trenton, NJ: Veterinary Learning Systems, 1996:60–77.
725. Moore FM, Thornton GW. Telangiectasia of Pembroke Welsh corgi dogs. Vet Path 1983; 20:203–8.
726. Moore KW, Read, RA. Rupture of the cranial cruciate ligament in dogs—Part I. Compend Contin Educ Pract Vet 1996; 18(3):223–30.
727. Moore KW, Read RA. Rupture of the cranial cruciate ligament in dogs—Part I. Diagnosis and Management. Compend Contin Educ Pract Vet 1996; 18(4):381–9.
728. Moore MP. Approach to the patient with spinal disease. Vet Clin N Am 1992; 22(4):751–80.
729. Moore MP, Reed SM, Hegreberg GA, et al. Electromyographic evaluation of adult Labrador retrievers with type-II muscle fiber deficiency. Am J Vet Res 1987; 48(9):1332–6.
730. Moore PF, Rosin A. Malignant histiocytosis of Bernese mountain dogs. Vet Path 1986; 23(1):1–10.
731. Moore PF. Systemic histocytosis of Bernese mountain dogs. Vet Path 1984; 21:554–63.
732. Morgan RV. Vogt-Koyanagi-Harada syndrome in humans and dogs. Compend Contin Educ Pract Vet, 1989; 11(10):1211–8.
733. Morgan JP, Bahr A, Franti CE, Bailey CS. Lumbosacral transitional vertebrae as a predisposing cause of cauda-equina syndrome in German-shepherd dogs—161 cases (1987–1990). JAVMA 1993, 202(11):1877–82.
734. Morgan RV, Duddy JM, McClurg K. Prolapse of the gland of the 3d eyelid in dogs. A retrospective study of 89 cases (1980–1990). J Am Anim Hosp Assoc 1993; 29(1):56–60.
735. Moroff SD, Hurvitz AI, Peterson ME, et al. IgA deficiency in shar-pei dogs. Vet Immunology and Immunopathology 1986; 13:181–8.
736. Morrison WB, Frank DE, Roth JA, et al. Assessment of neutrophil function in dogs with primary ciliary dyskinesia. JAVMA 1987; 191(4):425–30.
737. Morrison WB, Wilsman NJ. Primary ciliary dyskinesia in the dog. J Vet Intern Med 1987; 1(2):67–74.
738. Morton LD, Sanecki RK, Gordon DE, et al. Juvenile renal disease in miniature schnauzer dogs. Vet Path 1990; 27:455–58.
739. Moser J, Meyers KM, Meinkoth JH, Brassard JA. Temporal variation and factors affecting measurement of canine von Willebrand factor. Am J Vet Res 1996; 57(9):1288–93.
740. Moser J, Meyers KM, Russon RH. Inheritance of von Willebrand factor deficiency in Doberman pinschers. JAVMA 1996; 209(6):1103–6.
741. Moser J, Meyers KM, Russon RH, Reeves JJ. Plasma von Willebrand factor changes during various reproductive cycle stages in mixed-breed dogs with normal von Willebrand factor and in Doberman pinschers with type I von Willebrand's disease. Am J Vet Res 1998; 59(1):111–8.
742. Muir P, Dubielzig RR, Johnson KA. Panosteitis. Compend Contin Educ Pract Vet 1996; 18(1):29–38.
743. Muir P, Dubielzig RR, Johnson KA, Shelton GD. Hypertrophic osteodystrophy and calvarial hyperostosis. Compend Contin Educ Pract Vet 1996; 18(2):143–51.
744. Muldoon MM, Birchard SJ, Ellison GW. Long-term results of surgical correction of persistent right aortic arch in dogs—25 cases (1980–1995). JAVMA 1997; 210(12):1761–65.
745. Muller GH. Skin diseases of the Chinese shar-pei. Vet Clin N Am 1990; 20(6):1655–70.
746. Muñana KR. Disorders of the brain. In: Morgan RV, ed. Handbook of small animal practice. 3d ed. Philadelphia: WB Saunders, 1997: 230–51.
747. Muñana KR. Encephalitis and meningitis. Vet Clin N Am, Sm Anim Prac 1996; 26(4): 857–74.
748. Munjar TA, Austin CC, Breur GJ. Comparison of risk factors for hypertrophic osteodystrophy, craniomandibular osteopathy

and canine distemper virus infection. Vet and Comparative Orthopaedics and Traumatology 1998; 11(1):42–8.
749. Murphy CJ. Disorders of the cornea and sclera. In: Kirk's current veterinary therapy XI, Small animal practice. Philadelphia: WB Saunders, 1992: 1101–11.
750. Murphy CJ, Belhorn RW, Thirkill C. Anti-retinal antibodies associated with Vogt-Koyanagi-Harada-like syndrome in a dog. J Am Anim Hosp Assoc 1991; 27(4):399–402.

N

751. Nachreiner RF, Refsal KR, Graham PA, et al. Prevalence of autoantibodies to thyroglobulin in dogs with nonthyroidal illness. Am J Vet Res 1998; 59(8): 951–5.
752. Nagata M, Iwasaki T, Masuda H, Shimizu H. Nonlethal junctional epidermolysis bullosa in a dog. Br J Derm 1997; 137(3):445–9.
753. Nagata M, Iwasaki TT, Masuda H, Shimizu H. Mitis junctional epidermolysis bullosa in a dog. In: Kwochka KW, Willemse T, and von Tscharner C, eds. Advances in veterinary dermatology, Vol 3. Oxford, England: Butterworth-Heinemann, 1998:528–9.
754. Nagata M, Shimizu H, Masunaga T, et al. Dystrophic form of inherited epidermolysis bullosa in a dog (Akita inu). Br J Derm 1995; 133:1000–3.
755. Nap RC, Hazewinkel HAW, Voorhout G, et al. The influence of the dietary protein content on growth in giant breed dogs. Vet and Comp Orthopaedics and Traumatology, 1993; 6:1–8.
756. Narfstrom K. Cataracts in the West Highland white terrier. J Sm Anim Pract 1981; 22:467–71.
757. Narfstrom K, Ekesten B. Electroretinographic evaluation of papillons with and without hereditary retinal degeneration. Am J Vet Res 1998; 59(2):221–6.
758. Narfstrom K, Wrigstad A, Ekesten B, Nilsson SEG. Hereditary retinal dystrophy in the briard dog. Clinical and hereditary characteristics. Vet & Comp Ophthal 1994; 4(2):85–96.
759. Narfstrom K, Wrigstad A, Nilsson SEG. The briard dog—a new animal model of congenital stationary night blindness. Br J Ophthal 1989; 73:750–6.
760. Nash AS, Kelly DF, Gaskell CJ. Progressive renal disease in soft-coated wheaten terriers: possible familial nephropathy. J Sm Anim Pract 1984; 25:479–87.
761. Nasisse MP. Canine ulcerative keratitis. In: Glaze MB, ed. Ophthalmology in small animal practice Trenton, NJ: Veterinary Learning Systems, 1996:45–59.
762. Neer TM, Dial SM, Pechman R, et al. Mucopolysaccharidosis VI in a miniature pinscher. J Vet Intern Med 1995; 9(6):429–33.
763. Neer TM, Kornegay JN. Leucoencephalomalacia and cerebral white matter vacuolization in two related Labrador retriever puppies. J Vet Intern Med 1995; 9:100–7.
764. Neff M, Broman KW, Mellersh CS, et al. A second-generation genetic linkage map of the domestic dog, Canis familiaris. Genetics 1999; 151(2):803–820.
765. Nell B, Kneissl S, Henninger W, Bago Z. Nodular dermatofibrosis and renal cystadenocarcinoma in a German shepherd crossbred dog. Wienner Tierarzliche Monatsschrift 1998; 85(4):123–9.
766. Nell B, Walde I, Stur I. Evidences of the iridocorneal angle in Siberian huskies with regard to the predisposition to glaucoma. Kleintierpraxis 1993; 38(6):353–6.
767. Nelson RW, Duesberg CA, Ford SL, et al. Effect of dietary insoluble fiber on control of glycemia in dogs with naturally acquired diabetes mellitus. JAVMA 1998; 21(3):380–6.
768. Nesbitt GH, Ackerman L. Canine & feline dermatology. Trenton, NJ: Veterinary Learning Systems, 1998. 498 p.
769. Nesbitt GH, Izzo J, Peterson L, et al. Canine hypothyroidism: a retrospective study of 108 cases. JAVMA 1980; 177:1117–20.
770. Ness MG. Treatment of fragmented coronoid process in young dogs by proximal ulnar osteotomy. J Sm Anim Pract 1998; 39(1):15–8.
771. Neumann W, Schulteneumann, AL. Use of cyclosprine-A (optimmune eye ointment) in dogs. Praktische Tierarzt 1997; 78(11):954–7.
772. Nicholas FW. Introduction to veterinary genetics. Oxford, England: Oxford University Press, 1996. 317 p.
773. Nicholas FW, Harper PAW. Inherited disorders: the comparative picture. Austral Vet J 1996; 73(2):64–6.
774. Nichols R, McDonald RK, Thompson L. Diseases of the pituitary gland. In: Morgan RV, ed. Handbook of small animal practice. 3d ed. Philadelphia: WB Saunders, 1997:440–6.
775. Nichols R, Peterson ME, Thompson, L. Diseases of the adrenal gland. In: Morgan RV, ed. Handbook of small animal practice. 3d ed. Philadelphia: WB Saunders, 1997:471–90.
776. Nickel RF, Ubbink G, Vandergaag I, Vansluijs FJ. Persistent Mullerian duct syndrome in the basset hound. Tijdschrift voor Diergeneeskunde 1992; 117:S31-S33.
777. Nishino S, Arrigoni J, Shelton J, et al. Effects of thyrotropin-releasing hormone and its analogs on daytime sleepiness and cataplexy in canine narcolepsy. J Neuroscience 1997; 17(16):6401–8.
778. Nonaka I. Animal models of muscular dystrophies. Lab Anim Sci 1998; 48(1):8–17.

O

779. Oakes MG, Lewis DD, Elkins, AD, et al. Evaluation of shelf arthroplasty as a treatment for hip dysplasia in dogs. JAVMA 1996; 208(11):1838–45.
780. Obrien PJ. Deficiencies of myocardial troponin-T and creatine kinase MB Isoenzyme in dogs with idiopathic dilated cardiomyopathy. Am J Vet Res 1997; 58(1):11–6.
781. Obrien PJ, Li G. Rapid, simple and sensitive microassay for skeletal muscle homogenates in the functional assessment of the Ca-release channel of sarcoplasmic reticulum—application to diagnosis of susceptibility to malignant hyperthermia. Molecular and Cellular Biochem 1997; 167(1–2):61–72.
782. O'Brien DP, Shibuya H, Zhou T, et al. X-linked cerebellar ataxia in English pointer dogs: phenotype and linkage data. Canine Pract 1998; 23(1):46.
783. O'Brien DP, Zachary JF. Clinical features of spongy degeneration of the central nervous system in two Labrador retriever littermates. JAVMA 1985; 186:1207–10.
784. O'Brien, JA. Laryngeal paralysis in dogs. In: Kirk RW, ed. Current veterinary therapy IX, Sm Anim Pract. Philadelphia: WB Saunders, 1986:789–92.
785. O'Brien JA, Hendricks J. Inherited laryngeal paralysis. Analysis in the Husky cross. Vet Quarterly 1986; 8:303.
786. O'Brien RT, Dueland RT, Adams WC, Meinen J. Dynamic ultrasonographic measurement of passive coxofemoral joint laxity in puppies. J Am Anim Hosp Assoc 1997; 33:275–81.
787. O'Brien TD, Osborne CA, Yano BL, et al. Clinicopathologic manifestations of progressive renal disease in Lhasa apso and shih tzu dogs. JAVMA 1982; 180:658–64.
788. Occhiodoro T, Anson DS. Isolation of the canine alpha-1-Fucosidase cDNA and definition of the fucosidosis mutation in English springer spaniels. Mammalian Genome 1996; 7(4): 271–4.
789. O'Grady MR, Holmberg DL, Miller CW, Cockshutt JR. Canine congenital aortic stenosis: a review of the literature and commentary. Can Vet J 1989; 30(10):811–5.
790. Ohlerth S, Busato A, Gaillard C, et al. Epidemiologic and genetic study of canine hip dysplasia in a colony of Labrador retrievers. Deutsche Tierarztliche Wochenschrift 1998; 105(10): 378–83.
791. Olby NJ, Chan KK, Targett MP, Houlton JEF. Suspected mitochondrial myopathy in a Jack Russell terrier. J Sm Anim Pract 1997; 38(5):213–6.
792. Olivry T, Fine J-D., Dunston S, et al. Canine epidermolysis bullosa acquisita: circulating autoantibodies target the aminoterminal non-collagenous (NC1) domain of collagen VII in anchoring fibrils. Vet Derm 1998; 9:19–31.
793. Olivry T, Fine J-D, Dunston S, et al. Canine epidermolysis bullosa acquisita: circulating autoantibodies target collagen VII epitopes. In: Kwochka KW, Willemse T, and von Tscharner C. Advances in veterinary dermatology, Vol 3. Oxford, England: Butterworth-Heinemann, 1998: 525–6.

794. Olivry T, Mason IS. Genodermatoses: inheritance and management. In: Kwochka KW, Willemse T, von Tscharner, eds. Advances in Vet Derm, Vol 3. Oxford, England: Butterworth-Heinemann, 1998: 365–8.
795. Olivry T, Poujadedelverdier A, Dunston SM, et al. Absent expression of collagen XVII (Bpag2, Bp180). Canine familial localized junctional epidermolysis bullosa. Vet Derm 1997; 8(3):203–12.
796. Olson PN, Seim HB, Park RD, et al. Female pseudohermaphroditism in three sibling greyhounds. JAVMA, 1989; 194(12): 1747–1749.
797. O'Neill CS. Hereditary skin disease in the dog and the cat. Compend Contin Educ Pract Vet 1981; 3(9):791–800.
798. Ori J, Yoshikai T, Yoshimura S, Takenaka S. Persistent hyperplastic primary vitreous (PHPV) in 2 Siberian husky dogs. J Vet Med Sci 1998; 60(2):263–5.
799. Ortega TM, Feldman ED, Nelson RW, et al. Systemic arterial blood pressure and urine protein/creatinine ratio in dogs with hyperadrenocorticism. JAVMA 1996; 209:1724–9.
800. Osborne CA, Unger LK, Lulich JP. Canine and feline nephroliths. In: Kirk's current veterinary therapy XII, Small animal practice. Philadelphia: WB Saunders, 1995:981–9.
801. Otto CM, Dodds WJ, Greene CE. Factor XII and partial prekallikrein deficiencies in a dog with recurrent gastrointestinal hemorrhage. JAVMA 1991; 198:129–31.

P

802. Padgett GA. Control of canine genetic diseases. New York: Howell Book House 1998,
803. Padgett GA, Madewel BR, Keller ET, et al. Inheritance of histiocytosis in Bernese mountain dogs. J Sm Anim Pract 1995; 36(3):93–8.
804. Padgett GA, Mostovsky UV. The mode of inheritance of craniomandibular osteopathy in West Highland white terrier dogs. Am J Med Genet 1986; 25:9–13.
805. Padgett GA, Mostosky UV, Probst CW, et al, The inheritance of osteochondritis dissecans and fragmented coronoid process of the elbow joint in Labrador retrievers. J Am Anim Hosp Assoc 1995; 31(4):327–30.
806. Padrid P. Diseases of the lower airway. In: Morgan RV, ed. Handbook of small animal practice, 3d ed. Philadelphia: WB Saunders: 164–72.
807. Pagé N. Hereditary nasal hyperkeratosis in labrador retrievers. 15th Proceedings of AAVD/ACVD meeting 1999, Maui Hawaii, 41–42.
808. Palmer AC, Blakemore WF. A progressive neuronopathy in the young Cairn terrier. J Sm Anim Pract 1989; 30(2): 101–106.
809. Palmer AC, Payne JE, Wallace ME. Hereditary quadriplegia and amblyopia in the Irish setter. J Sm Anim Pract 1973; 14:343–53
810. Palmer DN, Tyynela J, Vanmil HC, et al. Accumulation of sphingolipid activator protein A and protein D (Sapa and Sapd) in granular osmiophilic depositis in miniature schnauzer dogs with ceroid lipofuscinosis. J Inherited Metabol Dis 1997; 20(1):74–84.
811. Panciera D. Thyroid-function testing: Is the future here? Vet Med 1997; 92(1):50–7.
812. Panciera DL. Clinical manifestations of canine hypothyroidism. Vet Med 1997; 92(1):44–52.
813. Panciera DL. Treatment of hypothyroidism—consequences and complications. Canine Pract 1997; 22(1):57–8.
814. Panciera DL, Vail DM. Diseases of the pituitary gland. In: Morgan RV, ed. Handbook of small animal practice. 3d ed. Philadelphia: WB Saunders, 1997: 440–6.
815. Paradis M, Page N. Topical (pour-on) ivermectin in the treatment of chronic generalized demodicosis in dogs. Vet Derm 1998; 9(1):55–9.
816. Parent JM. Epilepsy. In: Tilley LP, Smith FWK, eds. The 5 minute veterinary consult. Baltimore: Williams & Wilkins, 1997: 558–9.
817. Parker AJ. "Little white shakers" syndrome: generalized, sporadic, acquired, idiopathic tremors of adult dogs. In: Kirk's current veterinary therapy XII, Small animal practice. Philadelphia: WB Saunders, 995: 1126–7.
818. Parker WM, Foster RA. Cutaneous vasculitis in five Jack Russell terriers. Vet Derm 1996; 7:109–15.
819. Parker PHH, Ballew M, Greene HL. Nutritional management of glycogen storage disease. Ann Rev Nutr 1993; 13: 83–109.
820. Paterson S. Sterile idiopathic pedal panniculitis in the German shepherd dog—Clinical presentation and response to treatment of 4 cases. J Sm Anim Pract; 36(11):498–501, 1995.
821. Patterson DF, Haskins ME, Jezyk PF, et al. Research on genetic diseases: Reciprocal benefits to animals and man. JAVMA 1988; 193(9):1131–44.
822. Patterson DF, Pexieder T, Schnarr WR, et al. A single major gene defect underlying cardiac conotruncal malformations interferes with myocardial growth during embryonic development. Studies in the CTD line of keeshond dogs. Am J Hum Genet 1993; 52:388–397.
823. Patterson WR, Estry DW, Schwartz KA, et al. Absent platelet aggregation with normal fibrinogen binding in basset hound hereditary thrombopathy. Thrombosis and Haemostasis 1989; 62:1011–15.
824. Paulsen ME, Lavach JD, Snyder SP, et al. Nodular granulomatous episclerokeratitis in dogs: 19 cases (1973–1985). JAVMA 1987; 190(12):1581–7.
825. Peelman LJ, Vanzeveren A, Coopman F, Bouquet Y. Genetic disease of the dog (*Canis familiaris*) and their molecular, genetic and biochemical characterization. Vlaams Diergeneeskundig Tijdschrift 1996; 65(5):242–52.
826. Peiffer RL Jr. Glaucoma. In: Morgan RV, ed. Handbook of small animal practice. 3d ed. Philadelphia: WB Saunders, 1997: 1030–5.
827. Peiffer RL Jr. Inherited ocular diseases in the dog and cat. In: Glaze MB, ed. Ophthalmology in small animal practice. Trenton, NJ: Veterinary Learning Systems, 1996: 142–54.
828. Pemberton PW. Lobley RW, Holmes R, et al. Gluten-sensitive enteropathy in Irish setter dogs. Characterization of jejunal microvillar membrane proteins by 2-dimensional electrophoresis. Res Vet Sci 1997; 62(2):191–3.
829. Perry W. Generalised nodular dermatofibrosis and renal cystadenoma in a series of 10 closely related German shepherd dogs. Australian Vet Practitioner 1995; 25:90–3.
830. Peterson ME, Kintzer PP. Medical treatment of pituitary dependent hyperadrenocorticism—mitotane. Vet Clin N Am, Sm Anim Pract 1997; 27(2):255–74.
831. Peterson ME, Kintzer PP, Kass PH. Pretreatment clinical and laboratory findings in dogs with hypoadrenocorticism—225 cases (1979–1993). JAVMA 1996; 208(1): 85–91.
832. Peterson ME, Melian C, Nichols R. Measurement of serum total thyroxine, triiodothyronine, free thyroxine, and thyrotropin concentrations for diagnosis of hypothyroidism in dogs. JAVMA 1997; 211(11):1396–1402.
833. Peterson-Jones, SM. A review of research to elucidate the causes of the generalized progressive retinal atrophies. Vet J 1998; 155(1):5–18.
834. Philips JM, Felton TM. Hereditary umbilical hernia in dogs. J Hered 1934; 30: 433–5.
835. Pickett JP. Glaucoma. In: Tilley LP and Smith FWK, eds. The 5 minute veterinary consult. Baltimore: Williams & Wilkins, 1997, 630–1.
836. Picut CA, Lewis RM. Juvenile renal disease in the Doberman pinscher: ultrastructural changes of the glomerular basement membrane. J Comp Path 1987; 97: 587–95.
837. Pion PD, Sanderson SL, Kittelson MD. The effectiveness of taurine and levocarnitine in dogs with heart disease. Vet Clin N Am, Sm Anim Pract 1998; 28(6): 1495–514.
838. Pioro EP, Mitsumoto H. Animal models of ALS. Clin Neurosci 1995; 3(6): 375–85.
839. Podberscek AL, Serpell JA. Aggressive behavior in English cocker spaniels and the personality of their owners. Vet Rec 1997; 141(3):73–6.
840. Podberscek AL, Serpell JA. Environmental influences on the expression of aggressive behavior in English cocker spaniels. Appl Anim Behav Sci 1997; 52(3–4):215–27.

841. Podell M. Seizures in dogs. Vet Clin N Am, Sm Anim Pract 1996; 26(4):779–809.
842. Podell M. Seizures and sleep disorders. In: Morgan RV, Handbook of small animal practice. 3d ed., Philadelphia: WB Saunders, 1997:220–9.
843. Podell M, Hadjiconstantinou M. Cerebrospinal fluid gamma-aminobutyric acid and glutamate values in dogs with epilepsy. Am J Vet Res 1997; 58(5):451–6.
844. Polvi A, Garden OA, Houlston RS, et al. Genetic susceptibility to gluten-sensitive enteropathy in Irish setter dogs is not linked to the major histocompatibility complex. Tissue Antigens 1998; 52(6):543–549.
845. Poncelet L, Heimann M, Coignoul F, Balligand M. Globoid cell leukodystrophy in seven West Highland white terrier pups. Annales de Medecine Veterinaire 1994; 138: 513–9.
846. Popovitch CA, Smith GK, Gregor TP, et al. Comparison of susceptibility for hip dysplasia between rottweilers and German shepherd dogs. JAVMA 1995; 206:648–50.
847. Post K, Dignean MA, Clark EG. Hair follicle dysplasia in a Siberian husky. J Am Anim Hosp Assoc 1988; 24(6):659–62.
848. Potter KA, Tucker RD, Carpenter JL. Oral eosinophilic granuloma of Siberian huskies. J Am Anim Hosp Assoc 1980; 16(4):595–600.
849. Power HT, Ihrke PJ, Stannard AA, Backus KQ. Use of etretinate for treatment of primary keratinization disorders (idiopathic seborrhea) in cocker spaniels, West Highland white terriers, and basset hounds. JAVMA 1992; 201(3):419–29.
850. Priat C, Hitte C, Vignaux F, et al. A whole-genome radiation hybrid map of the dog genome. Genomics 1998; 54:361–378.
851. Prieur DJ, Wilkerson MJ, Lewis DC, et al. Iduronate–2 sulfatase deficiency in a dog: canine hunter syndrome. Am J Hum Genet 1995; 57:A182.
852. Probst CW. Fragmented medial coronoid process and osteochondritis dissecans of the elbow. Companion Anim Pract 1988; 2(5):27–33.]
853. Prockop DJ, Kivirikko KI. Heritable diseases of collagen. N Engl J Med 1984; 311:376–86.
854. Puerto DA, Smith GK, Gregor TP, et al. Relationships between results of the Ortolani method of hip joint palpation and distraction index, Norberg angle, and hip score in dogs. JAVMA 1999; 214(4):487–501.
855. Pugh CR, Miller WW. Retinal and skeletal dysplasia in the Labrador retriever. Vet Med 1995; 90(6):593–6.
856. Pullen RP, Somberg RL, Felsburg PJ, Henthorn PS. X-linked severe combined immunodeficiency in a family of Cardigan Welsh corgis. J Am Anim Hosp Assoc 1997; 33(6):494–9.

R

857. Rand JS, Best SJ, Matthews KA. Portosystemic vascular shunts in a family of American cocker spaniels. J Am Anim Hosp Assoc 1988; 24(3):265–72.
858. Randolph JF, Center SA, Kallfelz FA, et al. Familial nonspherocytic hemolytic anemia in poodles. Am J Vet Res 1986; 47:687–95.
859. Randolph JF, Center SA, McEntee M, Goldberg EH. H-Y antigen-positive XX true bilateral hermaphroditism in a German shorthaired pointer. J Am Anim Hosp Assoc 1988; 24(4):417–20.
860. Randolph JF, Toomey J, Center SA, et al. Use of the urine cortisol-to-creatinine ratio for monitoring dogs with pituitary-dependent hyperadrenocorticism during induction treatment with mitotane (o,p'DDD). Am J Vet Res 1998; 59(3):258–61.
861. Rapp E, Kolbl S. Ultrastructural study of unidentified inclusions in the cornea and iriocorneal angle of dogs with pannus. Am J Vet Res 1995; 56(6):779–85.
862. Ray J, Haskins ME, Ray K. Molecular diagnostic tests for ascertainment of genotype at the Mucopolysaccharidosis type VII locus in dogs. Amer J Vet Res 1998; 59(9): 1092–5.
863. Ray K, Baldwin VJ, Acland GM, Aguirre GD. Molecular diagnostic tests for ascertainment of genotype at the rod cone dysplasia 1 (rcd1) locus in Irish setters. Current Eye Research 1995; 14:243–7.
864. Raymond SL, Jones, DW, Brooks MB, Dodds WJ. Clinical and laboratory features of a severe form of von Willebrand disease in Shetland sheepdogs. JAVMA 1990; 197:1342–6.
865. Read RA. Cyclosporine and its treatment of ophthalmic diseases in animals. Austral Vet Practitioner 1996; 26(2):86–9.
866. Rendon MI, Cruz PD Jr, Sontheimer RD, Bergstresser PR. Acanthosis nigricans: a cutaneous marker of tissue resistance to insulin. J Am Acad Derm 1989; 21:461–9.
867. Renooij W, Schmitz MGJ, Vangaal PJ, Slappendel, RJ. Gastric mucosal phospholipids in dogs with familial stomatocytosis-hypertrophic gastritis. European J Clin Invest 1996; 26(12):1156–9.
868. Rest JR, Forrester D, Hopkins JN. Familial vasculopathy of German shepherd dogs. Vet Rec 1996; 138(6):144.
869. Reusch C, Hoerauf A, Lechner J, et al. A new familial glomerulonephropathy in Bernese mountain dogs. Vet Rec 1994; 134:411–5.
870. Reuser AJJ. Molecular biology, therapeutic trials and animal models of lysosomal storage diseases—type II glycogenosis as an example. Annales de Biologie Clinique 1993; 51:218–9.
871. Richardson DC. The role of nutrition in canine hip dysplasia. Vet Clin N Am, Sm Anim Pract 1992; 22(3):525–40.
872. Richardson DC, Zentek J. Nutrition and osteochondrosis. Vet Clin N Am, Sm Anim Pract 1998; 28(1):115–35.
873. Richtsmeier JT, Sack GH, Grausz HM, Cork LC. Cleft palate with autosomal recessive transmission in Brittany spaniels. Cleft Palate—Craniofacial J 1994; 31:364–71.
874. Rishniw M, Wilerson MJ, Delahunta A. Myelodysplasia in an Alaskan malamute dog with adult-onset of clinical signs. Prog in Vet Neurol 1994; 5(1):35–8.
875. Ristic Z, Medleau L, Paradis M, Whiteweithers NE. Ivermectin for treatment of generalized demodicosis in dogs. JAVMA 1995; 207(10):1308–10.
876. Rivas AL, Tintle L, Argentieri D, et al. A primary immunodeficiency syndrome in shar-pei dogs. Clin Immunology and Immunopathology 1995; 74(3):243–51.
877. Rivres B, Walter PA, McKeever PJ. Treatment of canine acral lick dermatitis with radiation therapy—17 cases (1979–1991). J Am Anim Hosp Assoc 1993; 29(6):541–4.
878. Robbins GR. Unilateral renal agenesis in the beagle. Vet Rec 1965; 77: 1345–7.
879. Roberts SM. Pannus. In: Current veterinary therapy XII, Small animal practice. Philadelphia: WB Saunders, 1995: 1245–8.
880. Robertson BF, Roberts SM. Lateral canthus entropion in the dog. 1. Comparative anatomic studies. Veterinary & Comparative Ophthal 1995; 5(3):151–6.
881. Robertson BF, Roberts SM. Lateral canthus entropion in the dog. 2. Surgical correction. Results and follow-up from 21 cases (1991–1994). Veterinary & Comparative Ophthal 1995; 5(3):162–9.
882. Robinson R. Chinese crested dog. J Hered 1985; 76:217–8.
883. Robinson R. Genetic aspects of umbilical hernia incidence in cats and dogs. Vet Rec 1977; 100: 9–13.
884. Robinson R. Genetics for dog breeders. 2d ed. Oxford, England: Pergamon Press, 1990 280 p.
885. Robinson R. Legg-Calve-Perthes disease in dogs—genetic aetiology. J Sm Anim Pract 1992; 33:275–6.
886. Robinson WF, Huxtable CR, Gooding JP. Familial nephropathy in cocker spaniels, Aust Vet, 1985; 62:109–12.
887. Rodriguez F, Herraez P, Delosmonteros AE, et al. Collagen dysplasia in a litter of Garafiano shepherd dogs. Zentralblatt für Veterinarmedizin—Reihe A 1996; 43:509–12.
888. Roels S, Schoofs S, Ducatelle R. Juvenile nephropathy in a Weimaraner dog. J Sm Anim Pract 1997; 38(3):115–8.
889. Rolfe DS, Twedt DC. Copper-associated hepatopathies in dogs. Vet Clin N Am, Sm Anim Pract 1995; 25:399–417.
890. Romagnoli SE. Canine cryptorchidism. Vet Clin N Am, Sm Anim Pract 1991; 21(3):533–44.
891. Roperto F, Cerundolo R. Restucci B, et al. Colour dilution alopecia (CDA) in ten Yorkshire terriers. Vet Derm 1995; 6:171–8.
892. Roperto F, Papparella S, Crovace A. Legg-Calvé-Perthes disease in dogs: histological and ultrastructural investigations. J Am Anim Hosp Assoc 1992; 28(2):156–62.

893. Rosin A, Moore P, Dubielzig R. Malignant histiocytosis in Bernese mountain dogs. JAVMA 1986; 188(9J):1041–5.
894. Ross DL. Orthodontics for the dog. Bite evaluation, basic concepts, and equipment. Vet Clin N Am, Sm Anim Pract 1986; 16(5):955–6.
895. Rosser EJ. German shepherd pyoderma. Compend Contin Educ Pract Vet 1998; 20(7): 831–40.
896. Rosser EJ Jr. German shepherd dog pyoderma: a prospective study of 12 dogs. J Am Anim Hosp Assoc 1997; 33:355–63.
897. Rosser EJ Jr, Dunstan RW, Breen PT, Johnson GR. Sebaceous adenitis with hyperkeratosis in the standard poodle: a discussion of 10 cases. J Am Anim Hosp Assoc 1987; 23(3):341–5.
898. Rosychuk RAW. Cutaneous manifestations of endocrine disease in dogs. Compend Contin Educ Pract Vet 1998; 20(3):287–98.
899. Rothstein E, Scott DW, Miller WH Jr., Baglad MS. A retrospective study of dysplastic hair follicles and abnormal melanization in dogs with follicular dysplasia syndromes or endocrine skin disease. Vet Derm 1998; 9: 235–41.
900. Roudebush P, Maslin WR, Cooper RC. Canine tumoral calcinosis. Compend Contin Educ Pract Vet 1988; 10(10):1162–5.
901. Roush JK. Nonselection and nonresponse bias in clinical research. JAVMA 1998; 213(9): 1270–3.
902. Rovesti GL, Fluckiger R, Margini A, Marcellin-Little DJ. Fragmented coronoid process and incomplete ossification of the humeral condyle in a rottweiler. Vet Surg 1998; 27(4):354–7.
903. Rubin LF. Inherited eye diseases in purebred dogs. Baltimore: Williams & Wilkins, 1989, 363 p.
904. Rubin LF, Bournme TKR, Lord LH. Hemeralopia in dogs: heredity or hemeralopia in Alaskan malamutes. Am J Vet Res 1967;28:355–9.
905. Ruhli MB, Spiess BM. Goniodysgenesis in the Bouvier des Flandres dog. Schweizer Archiv fur Tierheilkunde 1996; 138:307–11.
906. Rybnicek J, Affolter VK, Moore PF. Sebaceous adenitis: an immunohistological examination. In: Kwochka KW, Willemse T, and von Tscharner C, eds. Advances in veterinary dermatology, Vol 3 . Oxford, England: Butterworth-Heinemann, 1998:539–40.
907. Ryder EJ, Holmes NG, Suter N, et al. Seven new linkage groups assigned to the DogMap reference families. Animal Genetics 1999; 30(1): 63–65.

S

908. Sacre BJ, Cummings JF, Delahunta A. Neuroaxonal dystrophy in a Jack Russell terrier pup resembling human infantile neuroaxonal dystrophy. Cornell Vet 1993; 83(2):133–42.
909. Salisbury M-A. Keratoconjunctivitivis sicca. In: Kirk's current veterinary therapy XII, Small animal practice. Philadelphia: WB Saunders, 1995:1231–9.
910. Saunders GK, Wood PA, Myers RK, et al. GM1 gangliosidosis in Portuguese water dogs: pathologic and biochemical findings. Vet Path 1988; 25(4):265–9.
911. Savill J, Azzarelli B, Siakotos AN. Early detection of canine ceroid lipofuscinosis (CCL): an ultrastructural study. Am J Med Genet 1995; 57:250–3.
912. Scarlett, JM: Epidemiology of thyroid diseases of dogs and cats. Vet Clin N Am, Sm Anim Pract, 1994; 24(3):477–86.
913. Schaer M. Acute pancreatitis in dogs. Compend Contin Educ Pract Vet 1991; 13(12):1769–80.
914. Schaer M, Harvey JW, Calderwood Mays MB, et al. Pyruvate kinase deficiency causing hemolytic anemia with secondary hemochromatosis in a cairn terrier dog. J Am Anim Hosp Assoc 1992; 28: 233–8.
915. Schaible RH. Genetic predisposition to purine urolithis in dalmatian dogs. Vet Clin N Am, Sm Anim Pract 1986; 16(1):127–31.
916. Schaible RH, Ziech J, Glickman NW, et al. Predisposition to gastric dilatation-volvulus in relation to genetics of thoracic conformation in Irish setters. J Am Anim Hosp Assoc 1997; 33(5):379–83.
917. Schatzberg S, Keene B, Atkins, C et al. A polymerase chain reaction (PCR) screening strategy for the canine dystrophin promoter. Canine Pract 1998; 23(1):44–5.
918. Schellenberg D, Yi Q, Glickman NW, Glickman LT. Influence of thoracic conformation and genetics on the risk of gastric dilatation-volvulus in Irish setters. J Am Anim Hosp Assoc 1998; 34(1):64–73.
919. Schmeitzel LP. Canine dermatomyositis: an immune-mediated disease with a link to canine lupus erythematosus. Compend Contin Educ Pract Vet 1992; 14:867–71.
920. Schmeitzel LP. Sex hormone-related and growth hormone-related alopecias. Vet Clin N Am, Sm Anim Pract 1990; 20(6): 1579–1601.
921. Schmeitzel LP, Lothrop CD Jr, Rosenkranz WS. Congenital adrenal hyperplasia-like syndrome. In: Kirk's current veterinary therapy XII, Small animal practice. Philadelphia: WB Saunders, 1995:600–4.
922. Schmutz SM, Moker JS, Clark EG, Shewfelt R. Black hair follicular dysplasia, an autosomal recessive condition in dogs. Can Vet J 1998; 39(10): 644–6.
923. Schnapper A, Waibl H. Morphometric studies on thoracolumbar intervertebral discs in the dachshund. Kleintierpraxis 1998; 43(10): 731–6.
924. Schrader SC. Differential diagnosis of nontraumatic causes of lameness in young growing dogs. In: Kirk's current veterinary therapy XII, Small animal practice. Philadelphia: WB Saunders, 1995:1171–80.
925. Schunk KL. Seizure disorders. In: Morgan RV, ed. Handbook of small animal medicine, 2d ed. New York: Churchill Livingstone, 1992:243–50.
926. Schwarz PD. Patellar luxation. In: Tilley L, Smith, F., eds. The 5 minute veterinary consult. Baltimore: Williams & Wilkins, 1997:912–3.
927. Scott DW. Cutaneous eosinophilic granuloma with collagen degeneration in the dog. J Am Anim Hosp Assoc 1983; 19(4):529–32.
928. Scott DW. Granulomatous sebaceous adenitis in dogs. J Am Anim Hosp Assoc 1986; 22(5):631–4.
929. Scott DW. Vitamin A-responsive dermatosis in the cocker spaniel. J Am Anim Hosp Assoc 1986; 22(1):125–9.
930. Scott DW. Vitiligo in the rottweiler. Canine Pract 1990; 15(3):22–5.
931. Scott DW, Anderson WI. Panniculitis in dogs and cats: a retrospective analysis of 78 cases. J Am Anim Hosp Assoc 1988; 24(5):551–9.
932. Scott DW, Buerger RG. Idiopathic calcinosis circumscripta in the dog: a retrospective analysis of 130 cases. J Am Anim Hosp Assoc 1988; 24(6):651–8.
933. Scott DW, Miller WH Jr. Primary seborrhea in English springer-spaniels—a retrospective study of 14 cases. J Sm Anim Pract 1996; 37:4:173–8.
934. Scott DW, Randolph JF. Vitiligo in two old English sheepdog littermates and in a dachshund with juvenile-onset diabetes mellitus. Compan Anim Pract 1989; 19(3):18–22.
935. Scott DW, Rousselle S, Mille WHH Jr. Symmetrical lupoid onychodystrophy in dogs: a retrospective analysis of 18 cases (1989–1993). J Am Anim Hosp Assoc. 1995; 31(3):194–201.
936. Scott DW, Walton DK. Clinical evaluation of oral vitamin E for the treatment of primary canine acanthosis nigricans. J Am Anim Hosp Assoc 1985; 21(3):345–50.
937. Scott DW, Walton DK. Hyposomatotropism in the mature dog: a discussion of 22 cases. J Am Anim Hosp Assoc 1986; 22(4):467–73.
938. Scott DW, Walton DK, Slater MR, et al. Immune-mediated dermatoses in domestic animals: ten years after—Part 1. Compend Contin Educ Pract Vet 1987; 9(4):424–35.
939. Scott DW, Walton DK, Slater MR. Immune-mediated dermatoses in domestic animals: ten years after—Part 2. Compend Contin Educ Pract Vet 1987; 9(5):539–49.
940. Scott-Moncrieff JC, Hawkins EC, Cook JR Jr. Canine muscle disorders. Compend Contin Educ Pract Vet 1990; 12(1):31–9.
941. Scott-Moncrieff JCR, Snyder PW, Glickman LT, et al. Systemic necrotizing vasculitis in nine young beagles. JAVMA 1992; 201(10):1553–8.
942. Seim HB III. Wobbler syndrome in the Doberman pinshcer. In: Kirk RW, ed. Current veterinary therapy X, Small animal practice. Philadelphia: WB Saunders, 1989:858–62.

943. Selcer EA, Helman RG, Selcer RR. Dermoid sinus in a shih tzu and a boxer. J Am Anim Hosp Assoc 1984; 20(4):634–6.
944. Selden JR: The intersex dog: classification, clinical presentation, and etiology. Compend Contin Educ Pract Vet 1979; 1(6):435–41.
945. Selmanowitz VJ, Kramer KM, Orentreich N. Canine hereditary black hair follicular dysplasia. J Hered 1972; 63: 43–4.
946. Selmanowitz VJ, Kramer KM, Orentreich N. Congenital ectodermal defect in miniature poodles. J Hered 1970; 61: 196–9.
947. Shaker E, Hurvitz AI, Peterson ME. Hypoadrenocorticism in a family of standard poodles. JAVMA 1988; 192:1091–2.
948. Shakir SA, Sundarara A. Canine acanthosis nigricans. A report of 3 cases. Indian Vet J 1996; 73(8):826–8.
949. Shanley KJ. The seborrheic disease complex. Vet Clin N Am, Sm Anim Pract 1990; 20(6):1557–77.
950. Shanley KJ, Miller WH Jr. Panniculitis in the dog: a report of 5 cases. J Am Anim Hosp Assoc 1985; 21(4):545–50.
951. Sharp NJH, Cofone M, Robertson ID et al. Computed tomography in the evaluation of caudal cervical spondylomyelopathy of the Doberman pinscher. Vet Radiol & Ultrasound 1995; 36(2):100–8.
952. Sharp NJH, Kornegay N, Lane SB. The muscular dystrophies. Seminars in Vet Med and Surg (Small Animal) 1989; 4(2):133–40.
953. Shastry BS, Reddy VN. Studies on congenital hereditary cataract and micophthalmia of the miniature schnauzer dog. Biochem and Biophys Res Comm 1994; 203:1663–7.
954. Shell LG, Jortner BS, Leib MS. Familial motor neuron disease in rottweiler dogs: neuropathologic studies. Vet Path 1987; 24(2):135–9.
955. Shell LG, Jortner BS, Leib MS. Spinal muscular atrophy in two rottweiler littermates. JAVMA 1987; 190(7):878–80.
956. Shell LG, Potthoff A, Carithers R, et al. Neuronal-visceral GM1 gangliosidosis in Portuguese water dogs. J Vet Intern Med 1989; 3(1):1–7.
957. Shires PK, Shultz KS. The musculoskeletal system. In: Hoskins JD, ed. Veterinary pediatrics. Philadelphia: WB Saunders, 1995:427–50.
958. Shores A, Redding RW, Braund KG, Simpson ST. Myotonia congenita in a chow chow pup. JAVMA 1986; 188(5):532–3.
959. Shull RM, Lu XC, Mcentee MF, et al. Myoblast gene therapy in canine mucopolysaccharidosis I—abrogation by an immune response to alpha-l-iduronidase. Human Gene Therapy 1996; 7:1595–603.
960. Sjöström L. Ununited anconeal process in the dog. Vet Clin N Am, Sm Anim Pract 1998; 28(1):75–86.
961. Simpson KW. Current concepts of the pathogenesis and pathophysiology of acute pancreatitis in the dog and cat. Compend Contin Educ Pract Vet 1993; 15(2):217–53.
962. Simpson ST. Hydrocephalus. In: Kirk RW, ed. Current veterinary therapy X, Small animal practice. Philadelphia; WB Saunders, 1989, 842–7.
963. Simpson ST. Intervertebral disc disease. Vet Clin N Am, Sm Anim Pract 1992:22(4):889–97.
964. Singer HS, Cork LC. Canine GM2 gangliosidosis—morphological and biochemical analysis. Vet Path, 1989; 26:114–20.
965. Sisson DD, Thomas WP. Myocardial diseases. In: Ettinger SJ, Feldman EC, eds. Textbook of veterinary internal medicine. 4th ed. Philadelphia: WB Saunders, 1995: 995–1032.
966. Skelly BJ, Sargan DR, Herrtge ME, Winchester BG. The molecular basis of canine fucosidosis. J Med Genet 1996; 33:284–8.
967. Skelly CM, McAllister H, Donnelly WJC. Avulsion of the tibial tuberosity in a litter of greyhound puppies. J Sm Anim Pract 1997; 38(10):445–9.
968. Slappendel RJ. Von Willebrand's disease in Dutch Kooiker dogs. Veterinary Quarterly 1995; 17(Suppl. 1):S21-S22.
969. Slater MR, Scarlett, JM, Donoghue S, et al. Diet and exercise as potential risk factors for osteochondritis dissecans in dogs. Am J Vet Res, 1992; 53(11):2119–24.
970. Slaughter J, Padgett G, Blanchard G, et al. Canine essential hypertension. Probably mode of inheritance. J Hypertens 1986; 4:S170-S171.
971. Smallwood LJ, Barsanti JA. Hypoadrenocorticism in a family of Leonbergers. J Am Anim Hosp Assoc 1995; 31(4):301–5.
972. Smeak DD. Abdominal hernias. In: Textbook of small animal surgery, 2d ed. D Slatter, ed., Philadelphia, WB Saunders Co. 1993; 433–54.
973. Smedile LE, Houston DM, Taylor SM, et al. Idiopathic, asymptomatic thrombocytopenia in Cavalier King Charles spaniels—11 cases (1983–1993). J Am Anim Hosp Assoc 1997; 33(5):411–5.
974. Smith BF, Henthorn PS, Rajpurohit Y, et al. A cDNA-encoding canine muscle type phosphofructokinase. Gene 1996; 168(2):275–6.
975. Smith BF, Stedman H, Rajpurohit Y, et al. Molecular baasis of canine muscle type phosphofructokinase deficiency. J Biol Chem 1996; 271:20070–4.
976. Smith CA. Veterinarians probe greyhound idiosyncracies. JAVMA 1995; 206(11):1689–93.
977. Smith FWK Jr, Buoen LC, Weber AF, et al. X-chromosomal monosomy (77,XO) in a Doberman pinscher with gonadal dysgenesis. J Vet Intern Med 1989; 3(2):90–5.
978. Smith GK. Advances in diagnosing canine hip dysplasia. JAVMA 1997; 210(10):1451–7.
979. Smith GK, Biery DN, Gregor TP. New concepts of coxofemoral joint stability and the development of a clinical stress-radiographic method for quantitating hip joint laxity in the dog. JAVMA 1990, 196:59–70.
980. Smith GK, Hill CM, Gregor TP, Olson K. Reliability of the hip distraction index in two-month-old German shepherd dogs. JAVMA 1998; 212:1560–3.
981. Smith GK, Popovitch CA, Gregor TP, Shofer FS. Evaluation of risk factors for degenerative joint disease associated with hip dysplasia in dogs. JAVMA 1995; 206(5):642–7.
982. Smith MO, Wenger DA, Hill SL, Matthes J. Fucosidosis in a family of American-bred English springer spaniels. JAVMA 1996; 209(12):2088–90.
983. Smith PJ, Brooks DE, Lazarus JA, et al. Ocular hypertension following cataract surgery in dogs—139 cases (1992–1993). JAVMA 196; 209(1):105–11.
984. Smith RIE, Sutton RH, Joly RD, Smith KR. A retinal degeneration associated with ceroid lipofuscinosis in adult miniature schnauzers. Vet & Compar Ophthal 1996; 6(3):187–91.
985. Smucker ML, Kaul S, Woodfield JA, et al. Naturally occurring cardiomyopathy in the Doberman pinscher—a possible large animal model of human cardiomyopathy. J Am Coll Cardiol 1990; 16:200–6.
986. Snaps FR, Balligand, MH, Saunders JH, et al. Comparison of radography, magnetic resonance imaging, and surgical findings in dogs with elbow dysplasia. Am J Vet Res 1997; 58(12):1367–70.
987. Snyder PS. Canine hypertensive disease. Compend Contin Educ Pract Vet 1991; 13(12):1785–92.
988. Snyder PW, Kazacos EA, Felsburg PJ. Histologic characterization of the thymus in canine X-linked severe combined immunodeficiency. Clin Immunology and Immunopathology 1993; 67(1):55–67.
989. Snyder PW, Kazacos EA, Scott-Montcrieff JC, et al. Pathological features of naturally occurring juvenile polyarteritis in beagle dogs. Vet Path, 1995; 32(4):337–45.
990. Somberg RL, Pullen RP, Casal ML, et al. A single nucleotide insertion in the canine interleukin–2 receptor y chain results in X-linked severe combined immunodeficiency disease. Vet Immunol and Immunopathol 1995; 47:203–13.
991. Somberg RL, Tipold A, Hartnett BJ, et al. Postnatal development of T-cells in dogs with X-linked severe combined immunodeficiency. J Immunol 1996; 156(4):1431–5.
992. Sorenson JL, Ling GV. Diagnosis, prevention, and treatment of urate urolithiasis in Dalmatians. JAVMA 1993; 203(6):863–9.
993. Sorenson JL, Ling GV. Metabolic and genetic aspects of urate urolithiasis in Dalmatians. JAVMA 1993; 203(6):857–62.
994. Sorensen SH, Proud FJ, Rutgers HC. A blood test for intestinal permeability and function—a new tool for the diagnosis of chronic intestinal disease in dogs. Clinica Chimica Acta 1997; 264(1):103–15.
995. Speciale J, Dayrell-Hart B. Signalment: an aid for recognition of uncommon and diagnostically challenging neurologic diseases in dogs. Compend Contin Educ Pract Vet 1996; 18(10):1099–109.

996. Speeti M, Eriksson J, Saari S, Westermarck E. Lesion of subclinical Doberman hepatitis. Vet path 1998; 35(5): 361–369.
997. Spiess BM. Inherited ocular diseases in the Entlebucher mountain dog. Schweizer Archiv fur Tierheilkunde 1994; 136(3):105–10.
998. Spiess BM. Tonography in the dog—methodology and normal values. Wiener Tierarztliche Monatsschrift 1995; 82(8):245–50.
999. Srenk P, Jaggy A, Gaillard C, et al. Genetic aspect of idiopathic epilepsy in the golden retriever. Tierarztliche Praxis 1994; 22:574–8.
1000. Staaden RV. Cardiomyopathy of English cocker spaniels. JAVMA 1981; 178:1289–92.
1001. Stades FC, Boeve MH, Verbruggen AMJ. Diseases of the vitreous and hyaloid system in the dog. Pratique Medicale et Chirurgicale de L'Animal de Compagnie 1997; 32 (Suppl 4):193–202.
1002. Stades FC, Wyman M, Boev, MH, Neumann W. Ophthalmology for the veterinary practitioner. Hanover Germany, Schlütersche 1998,
1003. Stalis IH, Chadwick B, Dayrell-Hart B, et al. Necrotizing meniogoencephalitis of Maltese dogs. Vet Path 1995; 32:230–5.
1004. Steinberg SA, Klein E, Killens RL, Unde TW. Inherited deafness among nervous pointer dogs. Hered 1994; 85(1):56–9.
1005. Stepien RL. Dysrhythmias. In: Morgan RV, ed. Handbook of small animal practice, 3d ed. Philadelphia: WB Saunders, Philadelphia, 1997:63–84.
1006. Stigen O. Calcification of intervertebral discs in the dachshund—a radiographic study of 115 dogs at 1 and 5 years of age. Acta Veterinaria Scandinavica 1996, 37(3):229–37.
1007. Stogdale L, Botha WS, Saunders GN. Congenital hypotrichosis in a dog. J Am Anim Hosp Assoc 1982; 18(1): 184–7.
1008. Stokol T, Parry BW. The effect of modified-live virus vaccination on von Willebrand factor antigen concentrations and platelet counts in dogs. Vet Clin Path 1997; 26(3):135–7.
1009. Stoltzfus LJ, Sosapineda B, Moskowitz SM, et al. Cloning and characterizaion of cDNA encoding canine alpha-L-Iduronidase–messenger RNA deficiency in mucopolysaccharidosis I dog. J Biol Chem 1992; 267:6570–5.
1010. Stone EM, Fingert JH, Alward WLM, et al. Identification of a gene that causes primary open-angle glaucoma. Sci 1997; 275(5300): 668–70.
1011. Strain GM. Aetiology, prevalence and diagnosis of deafness in dogs and cats. Brit Vet J 1996; 152(1):17–35.
1012. Strain GM. Congenital deafness in dogs and cats. Compend Contin Educ Pract Vet 1991; 13(2):245–50.
1013. Subden RE, Fletch SM, Smart MA, et al. Genetics of the Alaskan malamute chondrodysplasia syndrome. J Hered 1972; 63:149–52.
1014. Sudo RT, Nelson TE. Changes in ryanodine-induced contractures by stimulus frequency in malignant hyperthermia susceptible and malignant hyperthermia nonsusceptible dog skeletal muscle. J Pharmacol & Experimental Therapeutics 1997; 282:1331–6.
1015. Sueki H, Shanley K, Goldschmidt MH, et al. Dominantly inherited epidermal acantholysis in dogs, simulating human benign familial chronic pemphigus (Hailey-Hailey disease). Br J Derm 1997; 136:190–6.
1016. Sukhiani HR, Parent JM, Atilola MAO, Holmberg DL. Intervertebral disk disease in dogs with signs of back pain alone: 25 cases (1986–1993). JAVMA 1996; 209(7):1275–9.
1017. Swenson L, Audell L, Hedhammar A. Prevalence and inheritance of and selection for elbow arthrosis in Bernese mountain dogs and rottweilers in Sweden and benefit-cost analysis of a screening and control program. JAVMA 1997; 210(2):215–9.
1018. Swenson L, Audell L, Hedhammar A. Prevalence and inheritance of and selection for hip dysplasia in 7 breeds of dogs in Sweden and benefit-cost analysis of a screening and control program. JAVMA 1997; 210(2):207–11.
1019. Swenson L, Häggström J, Kvart C, Juneja RK. Relationship between parental cardiac status in Cavalier King Charles spaniels and prevalence and severity of chronic valvular disease in offspring. JAVMA 1996; 208(12):2009–12.
1020. Swift S. The problem of inherited diseases. 2. Subaortic stenosis in boxers. J Sm Anim Pract 1996; 37(7):351–2.
1021. Switonski M, Reimann N, Bosma AA, et al. Report on the progress of standardization of the G-banded canine (*Canis familiaris*) karyotype. Chromosome Res 1996; 4: 306–9.

T

1022. Takahashi JL, Farrow CS, Presnell KR. Primary lymphedema in a dog: case report. J Am Anim Hosp Assoc 1984; 20(5):849–54.
1023. Tammen I, Klippert H, Kuczka A, et al. An improved DNA test for bovine leukocyte adhesion deficiency. Res in Vet Sci 1996; 60(3):218–21.
1024. Taylor RM, Farrow BRH, Healy PJ. Canine fucosidosis: clinical findings. J Sm Anim Pract 1987; 28(4):291–300.
1025. Tennant B. The problem of inherited diseases. 3. Hemophilia in the German shepherd. J Sm Anim Pract 1996; 37(8):405–6.
1026. Thacker EL, Refsal KR, Bull RW. Prevalence of autoantibodies to thyroglobulin, thyroxine, or triiodothyronine and relationship to autoantibodies and serum concentrations of triodothyroinines in dogs. Am J Vet Res 1995; 53:449–53.
1027. Thomas JS. Von Willebrand's disease in the dog and cat. Vet Clin N Am, Sm Anim Pract 1996; 26(5):1089–110.
1028. Thomas WB. Disorders of the spinal cord. In: Morgan RV, ed. Handbook of small animal practice. 3d ed. Philadelphia: WB Saunders, 1997:252–71.
1029. Thomas WP. Therapy of congenital pulmonic stenosis. In: Kirk's current veterinary therapy XII, Small animal practice. Philadelphia: WB Saunders, 1995:817–21.
1030. Thornburg LP. A study of canine hepatobiliary diseases (Pt 4): Copper and liver disease. Compan Anim Pract 1988; 2(7):3–6.
1031. Thornburg LP. Histomorphological and immunohistochemical studies of chronic active hepatitis in Doberman pinschers. Vet Path 1998; 35(5): 380–385.
1032. Thornburg LP, Dolan M, Raisbeck M. Copper toxicosis in dogs. (Pt 3): Diagnosis and conclusion. Canine Pract 1986; 13(1):10–14.
1033. Thornburg LP, Shaw D, Dolan M, et al. Hereditary copper toxicosis in West Highland white terriers. Vet Path 1986; 23:148–54.
1034. Tidholm A, Haggstrom J, Jönsson L. Prevalence of attenuated wavy fibers in myocardium of dogs with dilated cardiomyopathy. JAVMA 1998; 212(11):1732–4.
1035. Tidholm A, Jönsson L. Dilated cardiomyopathy in the Newfoundland: a study of 37 cases (1983–1994). J Am Anim Hosp Assoc 1996; 32(6):465–70.
1036. Tidholm A, Joönsson L. A retrospective study of canine dilated cardiomyopathy (189 cases). J Am Anim Hosp Assoc 1997, 33:544–50.
1037. Tidholm AEM. Canine dilated cardiomyopathy—a study of 189 cases in 38 breeds. Vet Quarterly 1996; 18:S34-S35.
1038. Tinlin S, Webster S, Giles AR. The development of homologous (canine anticanine) antibodies in dogs with hemophilia A (factor VIII deficiency)—a 10-year longitudinal study. Thrombosis and Haemostasis 1993; 69(1):21–4.
1039. Tipold A, Fatzer R, Jaggy A, et al. Necrotizing encephalitis in Yorkshire terriers. J Sm Anim Pract 1993; 34:623–8.
1040. Tipold A, Pfister H, Jungi TW. IgA deficiency in the dog. Praktische Tierarzt 1996; 77(3):181–3.
1041. Tisdall PLC, Hunt GB, Bellenger CR, Malik R. Congenital portosystemic shunts in Maltese and Australian cattle dogs. Australian Vet J 1994; 71:174–8.
1042. Todhunter RJ, Lust G. Polysulfated glycosaminoglycan in the treatment of osteoarthritis. JAVMA 1994; 204(8):1245–51.
1043. Toenniessen JG, Morin DE. Degenerative myelopathy—a comparative review. Compend on Contin Educ for Pract Vet 1995; 17(2):271–9.
1044. Tomlinson J, McLaughlin R Jr. Canine hip dysplasia: developmental factors, clinical signs, and initial examination steps. Vet Med 1996; 91(1):26–33.
1045. Tomlinson J, McLaughlin R Jr. Medically managing canine hip dysplasia. Vet Med 1996; 91(1):48–53.
1046. Tomlinson J, McLaughlin R Jr. Total hip replacement: the best treatment for dysplastic dogs with osteoarthrosis. Vet Med 1996; 91(2):118–24.

1047. Toombs JP. Cervical intervertebral disk disease in dogs. Compend Contin Educ Pract Vet 1992; 14(11):1477–87.
1048. Toth J, Dioszegi Z, Fenyves B. New form of osteochondrosis—apophyseolysis of tuber calcanei in young rottweiler and Doberman dogs (Severs disease). Magyar Allatorvosok Lapja 1997; 119(7):399–402.
1049. Trepanier LA, van Schoick A, Schwark WS, Carrillo J. Therapeutic serum drug concentrations in epileptic dogs treated with potassium bromide alone or in combination with other anticonvulsants: 122 cases (1992–1996). JAVMA 1998; 213(10): 1449–53.
1050. Trowaldwigh G, Hakansson L, Johannisson A, et al. Leucocyte adhesion protein deficiency in Irish setter dogs. Vet Immunology and Immunopathology 1992; 32:261–80.
1051. Trowaldwigh G, Hohannisson A, Hakansson L. Canine neutrophil adhesion proteins and Fc-Receptors in healthy dogs and dogs with adhesion protein deficiency, as studied by flow cytometry. Vet Immunology and Immunopathology 1993; 38(3–4):297–310.
1052. Tsai GC, Cork LC, Slusher BS, et al. Abnormal acidic amino acids and N-acetylaspartylglutamate in hereditary canine motorneuron disease. Brain Res 1993; 629(2):305–9.
1053. Turecek PL, Gritsch H, PichlerL, et al. In vivo characterization of recombinant von Willebrand factor in dogs with von Willebrand disease. Blood 1997; 90(9):3555–67.

U

1054. Ubbink GJ, Vandebroek J, Hazewinkel HAW, Rothuizen J. Cluster analysis of the genetic heterogeneity and disease distributions in purebred dog populations. Vet Rec 1998; 142(9):209–213.
1055. Ubbink GJ, Vanderbroek J, Hazewinkel HAW, Rothuizen J. Risk estimates for dichotomous genetic disease traits based on a cohort study of relatedness in purebred dog populations. Vet Rec 1998; 142(13):328–31.
1056. Uchida Y, Moonfanelli AA, Dodman N, et al. Serum concentrations of zinc and copper in bull terriers with lethal acrodermatitis and tail-chasing behavior. Am J Vet Res 1997; 55(8):808–10.

V

1057. Vaden S. PLE/PLN in soft-coated wheaten terriers. Canine Pract 1998; 23(1):12–3.
1058. Vajner L. Lymphocytic thyroiditis in beagle dogs in a breeding colony—findings of serum autoantibodies. Veterinarni Medicina 1997; 42(11):333–8.
1059. Valentine BA, Kornegay JN, Cooper BJ. Clinical electromyographic studies of canine X-linked muscular dystrophy. Am J Vet Res 1989; 50(12):2145–7.
1060. Valentine BA, Winand NJ, Pradhan D, et al. Canine X-linked muscular dystrophy as an animal model of Duchenne muscular dystrophy—a review. Am J Med Genet, 1992; 42: 352–56.
1061. Vanderwoerdt A, Stades FC, Vanderlindesipman JS, Boeve MH. Multiple ocular anomalies in 2 related litters of soft coated wheaten terrires. Vet & Compar Ophthalmol 1995; 5(2):78–82.
1062. Vandevelde M. Degenerative diseases of the spinal cord. Vet Clin N Am 1980; 10(1):147–54.
1063. Van Ee RT, Gibson K, Robets ED. Osteochondritis dissecans of the lateral ridge of the talus in a dog. JAVMA 1988; 193(10):1284–6.
1064. Van Ee RT, Palminteri A. Tail amputation for treatment of perianal fistulas in dogs. J Am Anim Hosp Assoc 1987; 23(1):95–100.
1065. Van Gundy T. Canine Wobbler syndrome (Pt I) Pathophysiology and diagnosis. Compend Contin Educ Pract Vet 1989; 11(2):144–57.
1066. Van Gundy T. Vascular ring anomalies. Compend Contin Educ Pract Vet 1989; 11(1):36–48.
1067. Van Gundy TE. Disc-associated Wobbler syndrome in the Doberman pinscher. Vet Clin N Am, Sm Anim Pract 1988; 18(3):667–96.
1068. Vanham LML, Desmidt M, Tshamala M, et al. Canine X-linked muscular dystrophy in Belgian Groenendaeler shepherds. J Am Anim Hosp Assoc 1993; 29:570–4.
1069. Van Liew CH, Greco DS, Salman MD. Comparison of results of adrenocortiocotropic hormone stimulation and low-dose dexamethasone suppression tests with necropsy findings in dogs: 81 cases (1985–1995).
1070. Van Nes JJ. Electrophysiological evidence of sensory nerve dysfunction in 10 dogs with acral lick dermatitis. J Am Anim Hosp Assoc 1986; 22(2):157–60.
1071. Van Wijk PA, Rijnberk A, Croughs RJM, et al. Molecular screening for somatic mutations in corticotropic adenomas of dogs with pituitary-dependent hyperadrenocorticism. J Endocrinol Invest 1997; 20:1–7.
1072. Vanzuilen CD, Nickel RF, Reijngoud DJ. Xanthinuria (xanthine oxidase deficiency) in two Cavalier King Charles spaniels. Vet Quarterly 1996; 18(1):S24-S25.
1073. Vanzuilen CD, Nickel RF, Vandijk TH, Reijngoud DJ. Xanthinuria in a family of Cavalier King Charles spaniels. Vet Quarterly 1997; 19(4):172–4.
1074. Vasseur, PB Foley P, Stevenson S, Heitter D. Mode of inheritance of Perthes disease in Manchester terriers. Clin Orthopaedics and Related Res 1989; 12:281–92.
1075. Venker-van Haagen AJ, Bouw J, Hartman W. Hereditary transmission of laryngeal paralysis in Bouviers. J Am Anim Hosp Assoc 1981; 17:75–80.
1076. Venter IJ, Vanderlugt JJ, Vanrensburg IBJ, Petrick SW. Multiple congenital eye anomalies in bloodhound puppies. Vet & Compar Ophthalmol 1996; 6(1):9–13.
1077. Verbruggen AJ, Boroffka SAEB, Boeve MH, Staaades FC. Persistent hyperplastic tunica vasculosa lentis and persistent hyaloid artery in a 2-year-old basset hound. Vet Quarterly 1997; 19(1):S66-S67.
1078. Verlander MW, Gorman NT, Dodds WJ. Factor IX deficiency (hemophilia B) in a litter of Labrador retrievers. JAVMA 1984; 185:83–4.
1079. Veske A, Nilsson SE, Narfstrom K, Gal A. Retinal dystrophy of Swedish Briard/Briard-beagle dogs is due to a 4-bp deletion in RPE65. Genomics 1999; 57(1): 57–61.
1080. Victoria T, Rafi MA, Wenger DA. Cloning of the canine Galc cDNA and identification of the mutation causing globoid cell leukodystrophy in West Highland white and Cairn terriers. Genomics 1996; 33(3):457–62.
1081. Vignaux F, Priat C, Jouquand S, et al. Toward a dog radiation hybrid map. J Hered 1999; 90: 62–67.
1082. Vilafranca M, Ferrer L. Juvenile nephropathy in Alaskan malamute littermates. Vet Path 1994; 31:375–7.
1083. Vilafranca M, Wohlsein P, Borras D, et al. Muscle fiber expression of transforming growth factor beta–1 and latent transforming growth factor-beta binding protein in canine masticatory muscle myositis. J Compar Path 1995; 12(3):299–306.
1084. Villagomez DAF, Alonso RA. A distinct Mendelian autosomal recessive syndrome involving the association of anotia, palate agenesis, bifid tongue, and polydactyly in the dog. Can Vet J 1998; 39(10): 642–3.
1085. Visonneau S, Cesano A, Tran T, et al. Successful treatment of canine malignant hisitiocytosis with the human major histocompatability complex nonrestricted cytotoxic T-cell line tall–104. Clin Cancer Res 1997; 3(10):1789–97.
1086. Vite CH, Cozzi F, Rich M, et al. Myotonic myopathy in a miniature schnauzer—Case report and data suggesting abnormal chloride conductance across the muscle membrane. J Vet Intern Med 1998; 12(5): 394–7.
1087. Vogt JC, Krahwinkel DJ, Brigh, RM, et al. Gradual occlusion of extrahepatic portosystemic shunts in dogs and cats using the ameroid constrictor. Vet Surg 1996; 25(6):495–502.
1088. Vonbomhard D, Kraft W. Idiopathic mucinosis cutis of Chinese shar-pei dogs—epidemiology, clinical features, histopathologic findings and treatment. Tierarztliche Praxis Ausgabe Kleintiere Heimtiere 1998; 26(3):189–96.
1089. Vroom MW, Theaker MJ, Rest JR, White SD: Lupoid dermatosis in 5 German short-haired pointers. Vet Derm 1995; 6(2):93–8.

W

1090. Wada M, Minamisono T, Ehrhart L, et al. Familial hyperlipoproteinemia in beagles. Lefe Sciences 1977; 20:999–1008.
1091. Wagner SO, Podell M, Fenner WR. Generalized tremors in dogs: 24 cases (1984–1995). JAVMA 1997; 211(6):731–5.
1092. Waldman L. Seasonal flank alopecia in affenpinschers. J Sm Anim Pract 1995; 36:271–3.
1093. Walvoort HC, van Nes JJ, Stokhof AA, Wolvekamp WTC. Canine glycogen storage disease type II: a clinical study of four affected Lapland dogs. J Am Anim Hosp Assoc 1984; 20(2):279–86.
1094. Waring GGO, MacMillan A, Reveles P. Inheritance of crystalline corneal dystrophy in Siberian huskies. J Am Anim Hosp Assoc 1986; 22(5):655–8.
1095. Waters DJ, Roy RG, Stone EA. A retrospective study of inguinal hernia in 35 dogs. Vet Surg 1993; 22: 44–8.
1096. Watson ADJ, Adams WM, Thomas CB. Craniomandibular osteopathy in dogs. Compend Contin Educ Pract Vet 1995; 17(7):911–8.
1097. Watson P, Simpson KW, Bedford PGC. Hypercholesterolemia in briards in the United Kingdom. Res Vet Sci 1993; 54(1):80–5.
1098. Watson PJ, Herrtage ME. Medical management of congenital portosystemic shunts in 27 dogs—a retrospective study. J Sm Anim Pract 1998; 39(2):62–8.
1099. Weber UT, Carrel T, Lang J, Lombard GW. Palliative treatment of Tetralogy of Fallot in a dog using a PTFE (polytetrafluorethylene) vascular graft. Schweizer Archiv fur Tierheilkunde 1995; 137:480–4.
1100. Weichselbaum RC, Feeney DA, Jessen CR, et al. Evaluation of the morphologic characteristics and prevalence of canine urocystoliths from a regional urolith center. Amer J Vet Res 1998; 59(4); 379–87.
1101. Weinstein MJ, Mongil CM, Rhodes WH, Smith GK. Orthopedic conditions of the rottweiler (Pt II). Compend Contin Educ Pract Vet 1995; 17(7):925–33.
1102. Weinstein MJ, Mongil CM, Smith GK. Orthopedic conditions of the rottweiler (Pt. I). Compend Con Educ Pract Vet 1995; 17(6):813–21.
1103. Weir JAM, Yager JA, Caswell JL et al. Familial cutaneous vasculopathy of German shepherds—clinical, genetic and preliminary pathological and immunological studies. Can Vet J 1994; 35(12):763–9.
1104. Weissenbock H, Obermaier G, Dahme E. Alexander's disease in a Bernese mountain dog. Acta Neuropathologica 1996; 91:200–4.
1105. Wellman ML, Davenport DJ, Morton D, Jacobs RM. Malignant histiocytosis in four dogs. JAVMA 1985; 187(9): 919–21.
1106. Westermarck E. The hereditary nature of canine pancreatic degenerative atrophy in the German shepherd dog. Acta Vet Scand 1980; 21:389–94.
1107. Westermarck E, Pamilo P, Wiberg M. Pancreatic degenerative atrophy in the collie breed—a hereditary disease. J Vet Med (Series A—Animal physiology, pathology and clinical veterinary medicine). Zentralblatt fur Veterinarmedizin Reihe A 1989; 36:549–54.
1108. Wheeler CA. Disorders of the posterior segment. In Morgan RV, ed. Handbook of ssmall animal practice. 3d ed. Philadelphia: WB Saunders, 1997:1047–64.
1109. White RN, Burton CA, Mcevoy FJ. Surgical treatment of intrahepatic portosystemic shunts in 45 dogs. Vet Rec 1998; 142(14):358–65.
1110. White SD. Naltrexone for treatment of acral lick dermatitis in dogs. JAVMA 1990; 196(7):1073–6.
1111. White SD, Batch S. Leukotrichia in a litter of Labrador retrievers. J Am Anim Hosp Assoc 1990; 26(3):320–1.
1112. White SD, Gross TL. Hereditary lupoid dermatosis of the German shorthaired pointer. In: Kirk's current veterinary therapy XII, Small animal practice. Philadelphia: WB Saunders, 1995:606–607.
1113. White SD, Rosychuk RAW, Schultheiss P, Scott KV. Nodular dermatofibrosis and cystic renal disease in three mixed-breed dogs and a boxer dog. Vet Derm 1998; 9:119–26.
1114. White SD, Rosychuk RAW, Scott KV, et al. Acquired aurotrichia ("gilding syndrome") of miniature schnauzers. Vet Derm 1992; 3(1):37–42.
1115. White SD, Rosychuk RAW, Scott KV, et al. Sebaceous adenitis in dogs and results of treatment with isotretinoin and etretinate: 30 cases (1990–1994). JAVMA 1995; 207(2):197–200.
1116. White SD, Rosychuk RAW, Stewart LJ, et al. Juvenile cellulitis in dogs: 15 cases (1979–1988). JAVMA 1989; 195(11):1609–11.
1117. White SD, Shelton GD, Sisson A, et al. Dermatomyositis in an adult Pembroke Welsh corgi. J Am Anim Hosp Assoc 1992; 28(5):398–401.
1118. Whitehair JG, Vasseur PB, Willits NH. Epidemiology of cranial cruciate ligament rupture in dogs. JAVMA 1993; 203(7):1016–9.
1119. Whitley RD, McLaughlin SA. Update on eye disorders of purebred dogs. Vet Med 1995; 90(6):574–92.
1120. Whitley RD, McLaughlin SA, Whitley EM, Gilger BC. Cataract removal in dogs—the surgical techniques. Vet Med 1993; 88(9):859–66.
1121. Whitney KM, Goodman SA, Bailey EM, Lothrop CD. The molecular basis of canine pyruvate kinase deficiency. Experim Hematol 1994; 22(9):866–74.
1122. Whitney KM, Lothrop CD. Genetic test for pyruvate kinase deficiency of basenjis. JAVMA 1995; 207(7):918–21.
1123. Wiberg ME, Lautala H-M, Westermarck E. Response to long-term enzyme replacement treatment in dogs with exocrine pancreatic insufficiency. JAVMA 1998; 213(1):86–90.
1124. Wilcock BP, Yager JA. Focal cutaneous vasculitis and alopeciaa at sites of rabies vaccinations in dogs. JAVMA 1986; 188(10): 1174–7.
1125. Wilkes MK, Palmer, AC. Congenital deafness and vestibular deficit in the Doberman. J Sm Anim Pract 1992; 33:218–24.
1126. Willard MD, Simpson RB, Delles EK, et al. Effects of dietary supplementation of fructo-oligosaccharides on small intestinal bacterial overgrowth in dogs. Am J Vet Res 1994; 55(5):654–9.
1127. Willard MD, Simpson RB, Fossum TW, et al. Characterization of naturally developing small intestinal bacterial overgrowth in 16 German shepherd dogs. Am J Vet Res 1994; 204(8):1201–6.
1128. Williams DA. Diseases of the small intestine. In: Morgan RV, ed. Handbook of small animal practice. 3d ed. Philadelphia: WB Saunders, 1997: 353–70.
1129. Williams DA, Scott-Moncrieff C, Bruner J, et al. Validation of an immunoassay for canine thyroid-stimulating hormone and changes in serum concentration following induction of hypothyroidism in dogs. JAVMA 1996; 209(10):1730–2.
1130. Williams DL, Boydell IP, Long RD. Current concepts in the management of canine cataract. A survey of techniques used by surgeons in Britain, Europe and the USA and review of recent literature. Vet Rec 1996; 138:347–53.
1131. Williams ML, Elias PM. Ichthyosis. Genetic heterogeneity, genodermatoses, and genetic counseling. Arch Derm 1986; 122:529–31.
1132. Willis AM, Martin CL, Stiles J, Kirschner SE. Brow suspension for treatment of ptosis and entropion in dogs with redundant facial skin folds. JAVMA 1999; 214(5): 660–662.
1133. Willis MB. A review of the progress in canine hip dysplasia control in Britain. JAVMA 1997; 210:1480–2.
1134. Willis MB. Practical genetics for dog breeders. New York: Howell Book House: 1992. 239 p.
1135. Wilsson E, Sundgren PE. The use of a behavior test for selection of dogs for service and breeding. 2. Heritability for tested parameters and effect of selection based on service dog characteristics. Appl Anim Behav Sci 1997; 54(2–3):235–41.
1136. Winand N, Pradham D, Cooper B, et al. Molecular characterization of severe Duchenne-type muscular dystrophy in a family of rottweiler dogs. Proc. of Molecular mechanisms of neuromuscular disease, Muscular Dystrophy Association, Tucson, AZ, 1994.
1137. Wisselink MA. Vitiligo-poliosis in the male rottweiler. Tijdschrift voor Diergeneeskunde 1993; 118:659–70.

1138. Wood JLN, Lakhani HK. Deafness in Dalmatians—does sex matter? Prev Vet Med 1998; 36(1):39–50.
1139. Wood JLN, Lakhani HK. Prevalence and prevention of deafness in the Dalmatian—assessing the effect of parental hearing status and gender using ordinary logistic and generalized random litter effect models. Vet J 1997; 154(2):121–33.
1140. Woodard JC. Canine hypertrophic osteodystrophy. A study of the spontaneous disease in littermates. Vet Path 1982; 19:337–40.
1141. Woods JP, Bartels KE, Stair EL, et al. Laser-induced shock-wave lithotripsy of canine urocystoliths and nephroliths. Lasers in Surg 1997; 2970:227–31.
1142. Woods P, Sharp N, Schatzberg S. Muscular dystrophy in Pembroke corgis and other dogs. Proc. 16th ACVIM Forum, San Diego, 1998, 301–3.
1143. Wosar MA, Lewis DD, Neuwirth L, et al. Radiographic evaluation of elbow joints before and after surgery in dogs with possible fragmented medial coronoid process. JAVMA 1999; 214(1): 52–8.
1144. Wright JC. Canine aggression toward people. Vet Clin N Am, Sm Anim Pract 1991; 21(2): 299–314.
1145. Wrigstad A, Narfstrom K, Nilsson SEG. Slowly progressive changes of the retina and retinal pigment epithelium in briard dogs with hereditary retinal dystrophy. A morphological study. Documenta Ophthalmologica 1994; 87(4):337–54.
1146. Wrigstad A, Nilsson SEG, Dubielzig R, Narfstrom, K. Neuronal ceroid lipofuscinosis in the Polish Owczarek Nizinny (PON) dog—a retinal study. Documenta Ophthalmologica 1995; 91:33–47.

Y

1147. Yakely WL. A study of inheritability of cataracts in the American cocker spaniel. JAVMA 1978; 172:814–20.
1148. Yasuba M, Okimoto K, Iida M, Itakura C. Cerebellar cortical degeneration in beagle dogs. Vet Path 1988; 25(4):315–7.
1149. Yuzbasiyan-Gurkan V, Halloran-Blanton S, Cao Y, et al. Linkage of a microsatellite marker to the canine copper toxicosis gene in the Bedlington terrier. Am J Vet Res 1997; 58(1):23–7.

Z

1150. Zaal MD, Vandeningh TSGAM, Goedegebuure SA, Vannes JJ. Progressive neuronopathy in 2 Cairn terrier littermates. Vet Quarterly 1997; 19(1):34–6.
1151. Zentek J, Buhl K, Wolf S, et al. Unusual high frequency of liver cirrhosis with copper storage in German shepherds. Praktische Tierarzt 1999; 80(3): 170–175.

Index

Note: f. after a page number indicates a figure; t. indicates a table.

About the Author

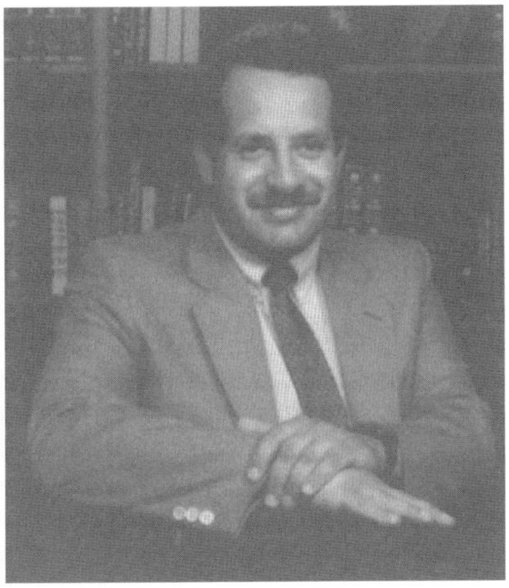

Dr. Lowell Ackerman is a graduate of the Ontario Veterinary College and a Diplomate of the American College of Veterinary Dermatology. A practicing veterinarian, frequent author and lecturer, and national radio personality, Dr. Ackerman has taken a special interest in the fields of genetics, dermatology, nutrition, and behavior. He is currently the genetics counselor and Director of Clinical Resources for Mesa Veterinary Hospital, a general specialty, emergency, and teaching hospital in Mesa, Arizona with 19 affiliated veterinarians. Dr. Ackerman has authored or co-authored 66 books and over 150 book chapters and articles on pet health care issues. His book credits include *Healthy Dog!*, *Dermatology for the Small Animal Practitioner*, *Owner's Guide to Dog Health*, and *Behavior Problems of the Dog and Cat*. Dr. Ackerman is a member of the National Society of Genetic Counselors and President of the American Veterinary Society of Genetic Counseling.